Phlebotomy Simplified

Second Edition

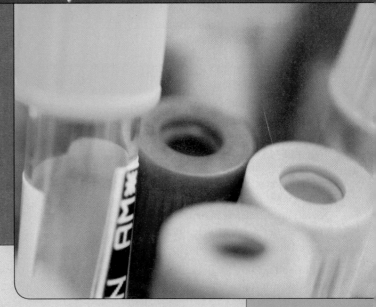

Diana Garza, EdD, MT(ASCP)[CM]

Medical Writer/Editor
Health Care Consultant
Houston, Texas

Kathleen Becan-McBride, EdD, MT(ASCP)[CM]

Director, Workforce and Resource Development
Medical School Professor, Department of Family & Community Medicine
The University of Texas Health Science Center at Houston
Texas Medical Center, Houston, Texas

PEARSON

Boston   Columbus   Indianapolis   New York   San Francisco   Upper Saddle River
Amsterdam   Cape Town   Dubai   London   Madrid   Milan   Munich   Paris   Montreal   Toronto
Delhi   Mexico City   Sao Paulo   Sydney   Hong Kong   Seoul   Singapore   Taipei   Tokyo

Publisher: Julie Levin Alexander
Publisher's Assistant: Regina Bruno
Editor-in-Chief: Mark Cohen
Executive Editor: John Goucher
Associate Editor: Melissa Kerian
Editorial Assistant: Erica Viviani
Development Editor: Cathy Wein
Director of Marketing: David Gesell
Executive Marketing Manager: Katrin Beacom
Marketing Specialist: Michael Sirinides
Senior Managing Editor: Patrick Walsh
Project Manager: Patricia Gutierrez
Senior Operations Supervisor: Ilene Sanford
Operations Specialist: Lisa McDowell
Photographer: Rocky Kneten Photography
Design Director: Andrea Nix

Art Director: Maria Guglielmo
Text Designer: Dina Curro
Cover Designer: Wanda Espana
Cover Art: © Simon Jarratt/AGE Fotostock
Chapter Opening Image: Jupiter Images PictureArts
    Corporation/Brand X Royalty Free
Video camera, Vector icon: Courtesy of
    Z-art/Shutterstock.com
Media Editor: Amy Peltier
Lead Media Project Manager: Lorena Cerisano
Full-Service Project Management: Patty Donovan
Composition: Laserwords
Printer/Binder: R.R. Donelley/Willard
Cover Printer: Lehigh-Phoenix/Hagerstown
Text Font: 10/12 ITC Garamond

Credits and acknowledgments for content borrowed from other sources and reproduced, with permission, in this textbook appear on appropriate page within text.

Notice:The authors and the publisher of this volume have taken care that the information and technical recommendations contained herein are based on research and expert consultation, and are accurate and compatible with the standards generally accepted at the time of publication. Nevertheless, as new information becomes available, changes in clinical and technical practices become necessary.The reader is advised to carefully consult manufacturers' instructions and information material for all supplies and equipment before use, and to consult with a health care professional as necessary.This advice is especially important when using new supplies or equipment for clinical purposes.The authors and publisher disclaim all responsibility for any liability, loss, injury, or damage incurred as a consequence, directly or indirectly, of the use and application of any of the contents of this volume.

Library of Congress Cataloging-in-Publication Data
Garza, Diana.
  Phlebotomy simplified / Diana Garza, Kathleen Becan-McBride. — 2nd ed.
    p. ; cm.
  Includes bibliographical references and index.
  ISBN-13: 978-0-13-278432-0
  ISBN-10: 0-13-278432-7
  I. Becan-McBride, Kathleen   II. Title.
  [DNLM: 1. Phlebotomy—methods. QY 25]
  616.07'561—dc23
                                            2012000405

10 9 8 7 6

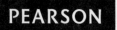

ISBN-10: 0-13-278432-7
ISBN-13: 978-0-13-278432-0

"To my husband, Peter McLaughlin, my daughters, Lauren and Kaitlin, my son Kevin, and my parents for their affection and continuous support."

—Diana Garza

"To my husband, Mark, my sons, Patrick and Jonathan, and daughters-in-law, Danielle and Ade, and grandchildren, Finnaveir and Madeleine, my parents, my sister, and my parents-in-law for their support and devotion."

—Kathleen Becan-McBride

Brief Contents

Contents

CHAPTER 9   Capillary Blood Specimens   215

CHAPTER 10   Pediatric and Geriatric Procedures   233

Procedures

Preface

Phlebotomy Simplified, 2nd edition is designed for beginning health care students and practitioners who are responsible for blood and specimen collections (medical assistants, nurses, phlebotomists, medical laboratory technicians and technologists, respiratory therapists, and others). The primary goal of the book is to link novice health care workers to the most updated standards of phlebotomy practice that are basic, yet essential for safe and effective blood collection. It is tailored to entry-level phlebotomists, for example, the medical terminology section provides practice with terms that entry-level phlebotomists need to know to begin their first job. *Phlebotomy Simplified, 2nd edition* provides introductory competencies, including communication, clinical, technical, and safety skills, that all health care workers will use for the entry-level practice of phlebotomy. It has been updated using guidelines from the latest Clinical and Laboratory Standards Institute (CLSI) and the National Accrediting Agency for Clinical Laboratory Sciences (NAACLS). We view this textbook as a fundamental and essential guide to basic standards of practice in the field.

The style format and length of the second edition is similar to the popular first edition. It is an easy, step-by-step, practice-oriented approach to blood collection procedures that can be implemented in a variety of settings, including hospitals, ambulatory clinics, home health care, and pediatric clinics. This edition has many new images, figures, and charts, including anatomical figures, and photos of new technology, equipment, and supplies.

The *Table of Contents*, organized in 11 chapters, follows the order in which a phlebotomist is educated and how he or she approaches the patient.

Chapter 1   Phlebotomy Practice and Quality Assessment Basics
Chapter 2   Ethical, Legal, and Regulatory Issues
Chapter 3   Basic Medical Terminology, the Human Body, and the Cardiovascular System
Chapter 4   Safety and Infection Control
Chapter 5   Documentation, Specimen Handling, and Transportation
Chapter 6   Blood Collection Equipment
Chapter 7   Preexamination/Preanalytical Complications
Chapter 8   Venipuncture Procedures
Chapter 9   Capillary Blood Specimens
Chapter 10   Pediatric and Geriatric Procedures
Chapter 11   Special Collections
Appendices
Glossary

At the end of each chapter are study questions, problem-solving cases, competency assessments, and a new section entitled Advocating Patient Safety. This new section in each chapter focuses on preventable errors, a major focus for health care professionals. This section covers a short commentary or case analysis with discussion questions that specifically relates to the patient's safety.

The Appendices provide practical procedures (e.g., Finding a Job, Using Military Time, etc.) and important updated terms, phrases, and symbols for beginning workers. For example, new phrases in English/Spanish are included for a more comprehensive and safe approach to patient and specimen identification. In addition, the Glossary provides definitions that relate to phlebotomy practice and includes all key terms from the text.

All in all, we have made this textbook as practical, educational, and useful as possible for those who are striving to begin a career in phlebotomy.

Key Features of the Second Edition

- Anatomical artwork depicting relationship of blood vessels to nerves in the arm.
- Expanded section about vein selection and basic hemostasis.
- Incorporation of new CLSI standards.
- Updates and new images of the latest phlebotomy equipment and supplies.
- Expanded sections on venipuncture complications and methods to avoid them.
- New section at the end of each chapter about "Advocating Patient Safety"
- Expanded section on "Finding a Job"
- Updated sections on equipment, supplies, and barcode technology.
- Colorful photographs that show procedural steps and equipment.
- Flowcharts provide additional easy-to-follow procedures.
- Case studies to encourage problem solving.
- Updated medical terminology section and glossary terms that are pertinent to phlebotomists.
- Sections on age-related competencies and communication.
- Self-assessment exercises.
- Clinical alert symbols throughout the text indicate that extra caution is needed.
- Step-by-step procedural information is presented using an on-the-job perspective.
- Key terms, objectives, cases, and study questions are provided for each chapter.
- A color chart of types of blood collection tubes relates appropriate color coding with additives.
- Appendices contain essential elements for Spanish phrases, symbols and units of measurement, military time, and NAACLS Competencies.
- Vital to instructors and students, NAACLS Competencies are linked to the level of coverage and specific content in the text and our more advanced text entitled *Phlebotomy Handbook, 8th edition.*

Companion Website

A companion website was developed to integrate knowledge in a multisensory manner. It can be accessed by clicking on **www.myhealthprofessionskit.com.** It is organized to correlate with the textbook chapters and is a valuable tool for students and instructors. Features of this exciting new ancillary include interactive games and more.

Video Program

The series contains 38 segments demonstrating a wide array of blood specimen collection procedures and patient interactions. The video is based on current Clinical and Laboratory Standards Institute (CLSI) guidelines and standards, and emphasizes safety, infection control, effective communication, quality assessment, and avoiding errors. The video series is ideal for independent self-study or review for those aiming to enhance their understanding and performance. It is also an ideal classroom teaching tool for instructors who wish to supplement their teaching with dynamic footage of experts in action. The series helps fulfill National Association for Accreditation of Clinical Laboratory Sciences (NAACLS) competencies for accredited programs in Phlebotomy.

Additional Resources for Educators

The 2nd edition has companion resources that are cross-referenced to the text. The *Instructor's Resource Manual* contains a wealth of material to help faculty plan and manage their course. It includes a detailed lecture outline, teaching tips, and more for each chapter. A complete test bank as well as PowerPoint lectures that contain discussion points with embedded color images from the book, as well as animations and videos is included.

An Accompanying Guide for Examination Review

Available for separate purchase is Pearson's *SUCCESS! in Phlebotomy:* 7th edition. This is an aid to students and health care workers preparing for a certification examination. It has over 850 exam-type questions and an accompanying website with a simulated board examination and referenced explanatory answers. Students can practice taking the simulated examination in print or via computer.

Acknowledgments

We are grateful to many generous people, product suppliers, manufacturing companies, professional organizations, and health care organizations for assistance in preparing this text. We are particularly indebted to BD Vacutainer Systems, the University of Texas Health Science Center at Houston, and many colleagues at health care institutions in the Texas Medical Center in Houston.

We greatly appreciate our working relationships with our editors and copy editors who have encouraged us and improved this second edition. Special thanks go to Cathy Wein and Melissa Kerian.

We are eternally thankful to our families who have encouraged and supported our work throughout the years. They hold a special place in our hearts.

Diana Garza
Kathleen Becan-McBride

Drs. Diana Garza and Kathleen Becan-McBride have a passion for phlebotomy practice and the people who work in this field. They have been collaborators for over 28 years on numerous educational programs, textbooks, and curricular materials; they have participated as presenters at national and international meetings, and as advisors for educational programs in phlebotomy and clinical laboratory sciences. Their vast work experience has covered all areas in the clinical laboratory beginning with their experience in the microbiology (Garza) and clinical chemistry (Becan-McBride) laboratories, moving into management and education as their careers evolved. Drs. Garza and Becan-McBride were involved in numerous courses for laboratory technologists/scientists, nurses, and physicians to teach phlebotomy techniques. As young faculty members, they began to develop curriculum materials for their own use, and in 1984 collaborated in publishing one of the first comprehensive textbooks focused entirely on phlebotomy practices. Their successful coauthoring partnership has endured for almost 3 decades. Both became tenured professors at their respective institutions and over the years they received numerous grants for phlebotomy education as well as other health care initiatives. Their experience spans from academic medical centers, to smaller clinical laboratories, to industry, to international collaborations and consultations; they have also served on certification and accreditation committees, both for clinical/medical laboratory scientists and for phlebotomists; and they have had editorial responsibilities for several journals and continuing education publications, both in print and electronic versions.

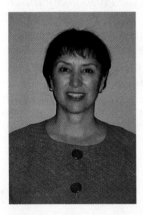

Diana Garza received her Bachelor of Science degree in Biology from Vanderbilt University in Nashville, TN followed by an additional year to complete her Medical Technology requirements at Vanderbilt University Medical Center. Her interest in laboratory sciences and in teaching led her to earn a Masters in Science Education at the Peabody School of Vanderbilt University. She worked at Vanderbilt Medical Center in the Microbiology department while she was a graduate student. A move back to her home state of Texas led her to a collaborative graduate program with Baylor College of Medicine and the University of Houston, and resulted in her Doctorate of Education in Allied Health Education and Administration, all while she worked in the Microbiology Section at the University of Texas M.D. Anderson Cancer Center (MDACC). Her laboratory and teaching experience continued at the University of Texas Health Science Center at Houston and for many years at MDACC, where she later became the Administrative Director of the Division of Laboratory Medicine. In 1990, she joined the faculty of Texas Woman's University-Houston Center, where she taught Internet-based quality improvement courses, interdisciplinary management courses, and became editor of several journals and continuing education publications. She was extensively involved in curriculum review processes, and program and university accreditation. She has taught extensively; been a reviewer/inspector in many regulatory processes; participated in accreditation procedures; and authored, edited, and published numerous manuscripts in the field of phlebotomy, health care, and quality management. She currently sits on numerous advisory boards, selectively consults with health care organizations and companies, and continues her medical writing/editing career.

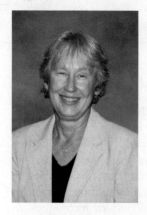

Kathleen Becan-McBride is Director of Workforce and Resource Development at The University of Texas Health Science Center at Houston (UTHSCH) and tenured Medical School Professor in the Department of Family and Community Medicine at UTHSCH. She has a B.S. in Biology from the University of Houston, M.Ed. in Allied Health Education and Administration from the University of Houston and a Doctorate in Higher Education Administration from the University of Houston. She went through the St. Luke's Episcopal Hospital Medical Technology Internship Program to receive her Board Certification as a Medical Laboratory Scientist. Prior to her professional career at UTHSCH, she taught at Houston Community College in the MLT Program and at UTMB-Galveston in the Medical Technology and Physician Assistant Programs.

She has published 23 books and more than 50 articles and has been on numerous national and international health care advisory boards and several editorial boards for health care journals. Dr. Becan-McBride has had research projects related to the medical laboratory sciences and also community (i.e, UV/TB Prevention Research Project in Homeless Shelters in Houston). She is on educational advisory boards for medical laboratory science educational programs and statewide community outreach programs. She has had invitational medical laboratory science presentations nationally and internationally to countries including Singapore, China, Russia, France, South America and most recently, New Zealand. Also, she was the invited "Guest of Honor" and speaker at the Philippine Association of Medical Technologists (PAMET)—USA 20th Anniversary Convention. She and Dr. Garza received the American Medical Writers' Association (AMWA) Book award for the *Phlebotomy Handbook* in October, 2006. For the ASCP Board of Certification, she was the elected Chair of the Board of Governors from 2008–2010. Dr. Becan-McBride has been educating students in the health professions since 1973. She has taught medical students, medical laboratory technician students, physician assistant students, medical laboratory science students among others in several areas related to medical laboratory sciences including infection control, biological safety, chemical safety, radiation safety, diagnostic microbiology, clinical chemistry, and several other medical and safety areas.

Reviewers

Evelyn Paxton, MS, MT(ASCP)
Rose State College
Midwest City, Oklahoma

Timothy Sandor, BS, CLS (NCA), MT(ASCP)
Lake Superior College
Duluth, Minnesota

Julie H. Simmons, MPH, MT(ASCP) SBB
Wake Forest University Baptist Medical Center
Winston-Salem, North Carolina

Anh Strow, MPH, MT(ASCP), CLS (NCA)
Illinois Central College
Peoria, Illinois

Susan B. Thomasson, MEd, MT(ASCP) SH, LMBT
Carolinas College of Health Sciences
Charlotte, North Carolina

Chapter 1

Phlebotomy Practice and Quality Assessment Basics

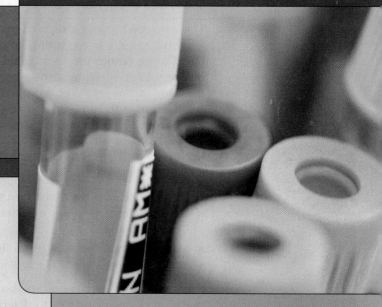

KEY TERMS

active listening

ambulatory care

American Society for Clinical Laboratory Science (ASCLS)

American Society for Clinical Pathology (ASCP)

blood sample

blood specimen

competency statement

continuous quality improvement (CQI)

culture

expiration date

iatrogenic anemia

National Phlebotomy Association (NPA)

personal protective equipment (PPE)

phlebotomist

point-of-care

preexamination (preanalytical) phase

quality

quality control

skin puncture

standard operating procedure (SOP)

venipuncture

zone of comfort

CHAPTER OBJECTIVES

Upon completion of Chapter 1, the learner should be able to do the following:

1. Define *phlebotomy* and describe phlebotomy services.
2. List professional competencies for phlebotomists.
3. List skills for effective communication.
4. Describe the essential steps for a job search.
5. Describe basic principles of quality and list examples of quality assessments for phlebotomy.

Phlebotomy Practice and Definition

The term *phlebotomy* is derived from the Greek words *phlebo,* which relates to veins, and *tomy,* which relates to cutting. In ancient times, phlebotomy was practiced to withdraw blood using various means including knives, crude lancets, leeches, blood cups or bowls, pumps, and glass syringes. In some cultures, phlebotomy was thought to cleanse or purify the body and/or get rid of unwanted spirits. However, today the current definition can be summarized as the incision of a vein for the purpose of collecting a **blood sample** (a portion of blood removed that is small enough so as not to cause harm) for laboratory testing or other therapeutic purposes (e.g., blood donations). Modern phlebotomy equipment and practices have improved significantly. For purposes of this text, phlebotomy practices that are covered relate to the two most common techniques:

- **Venipuncture**—withdrawing a venous (from a vein, not an artery) blood sample using a needle attached to an evacuated tube system or other collection devices (covered in Chapters 6 and 8);
- **Skin puncture**—puncturing a finger with a specially designed safety lancet to withdraw a smaller amount of capillary blood (covered in Chapters 6 and 9).

Patients' **blood specimens** are discrete portions of blood taken for laboratory analysis of one or more characteristics to determine the character of the whole body.[1] Laboratory test results are used for three important reasons:

- Diagnostic and screening tests—to figure out what is wrong with the patient or to screen for abnormalities;
- Therapeutic assessments—to develop the correct treatment or choose the right drug for the patient's medical condition;
- Monitoring health status—to make sure that the therapy or treatment is working.

The **phlebotomist,** or blood collector, is the individual who performs phlebotomy. Phlebotomists can also assist in the collection and transportation of specimens other than venous blood (e.g., arterial blood, urine, tissues, and sputum) and may also perform clinical, technical, or clerical functions. However, the primary function of the phlebotomist is to assist the health care team in the accurate, safe, and reliable collection and transportation of high-quality specimens for clinical laboratory analyses. This means that each and every patient's specimen should be correctly identified, collected, and transported to the laboratory. The reliability and accuracy of *all* patient test results depend on the **preexamination (preanalytical) phase** of specimen collection—that is, the part of the process that occurs *before* the actual testing and analysis are performed. The preanalytical process is the fundamental and crucial domain of every phlebotomist (Figure 1-1 ■).

Members of the Health Care Team and Phlebotomy Duties

Phlebotomists' duties vary in scope depending on the setting (Box 1-1 ■). They may have duties related to all phases of laboratory analysis or may be assigned to duties in only one area of a hospital. Technology has also enabled laboratory testing to be performed closer to the **point-of-care** (e.g., at the patients' bedside, at ancillary or mobile sites, or even in the home). Point of care testing (POCT) includes low risk laboratory tests or clinical procedures such as glucose screening, hematocrit, fecal occult blood tests (FOBT), urine dip sticks, throat swabs, etc. In some cases, health professionals—such as nurses, medical assistants,

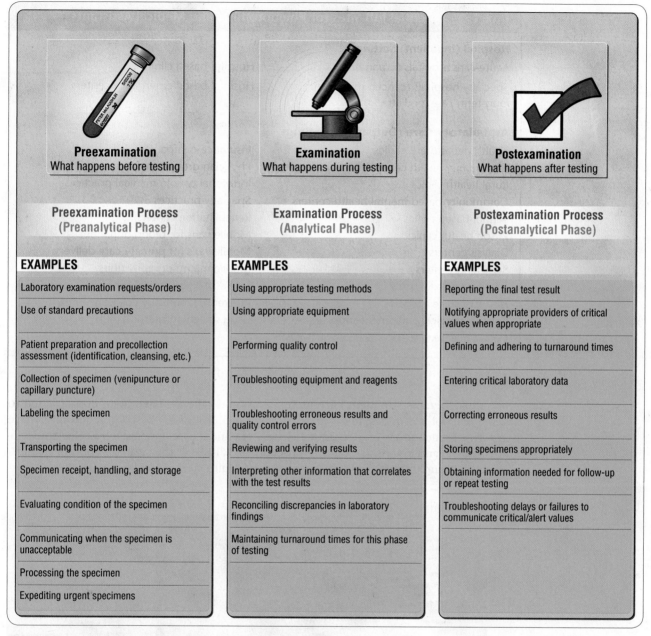

Preexamination
What happens before testing

Preexamination Process
(Preanalytical Phase)

EXAMPLES

Laboratory examination requests/orders

Use of standard precautions

Patient preparation and precollection assessment (identification, cleansing, etc.)

Collection of specimen (venipuncture or capillary puncture)

Labeling the specimen

Transporting the specimen

Specimen receipt, handling, and storage

Evaluating condition of the specimen

Communicating when the specimen is unacceptable

Processing the specimen

Expediting urgent specimens

Examination
What happens during testing

Examination Process
(Analytical Phase)

EXAMPLES

Using appropriate testing methods

Using appropriate equipment

Performing quality control

Troubleshooting equipment and reagents

Troubleshooting erroneous results and quality control errors

Reviewing and verifying results

Interpreting other information that correlates with the test results

Reconciling discrepancies in laboratory findings

Maintaining turnaround times for this phase of testing

Postexamination
What happens after testing

Postexamination Process
(Postanalytical Phase)

EXAMPLES

Reporting the final test result

Notifying appropriate providers of critical values when appropriate

Defining and adhering to turnaround times

Entering critical laboratory data

Correcting erroneous results

Storing specimens appropriately

Obtaining information needed for follow-up or repeat testing

Troubleshooting delays or failures to communicate critical/alert values

FIGURE ■ 1-1 The Clinical Laboratory's Workflow Pathway

The Clinical and Laboratory Standards Institute (CLSI) describes the basic workflow of a clinical laboratory as beginning with a request for a laboratory test and ending with laboratory examination results and their interpretation by a health care provider. The workflow concept is depicted here in general terms but in reality involves many steps and actions; only a few examples are listed under each heading. The importance of these processes cannot be overstated because any failure to perform them correctly or completely can result in harm to patients, medical errors, waste of resources, and repeated work. All steps in each of these domains must be done according to standards of practice and must be traceable to the individual who performs the tasks. Standards of practice are procedural guidelines set by governmental, accreditation, certification agencies; professional organizations; and/or manufacturing and equipment requirements.

Box 1-1 Potential Job Sites for Phlebotomists and Medical Assistants

Hospital (Inpatient) Settings

Acute-care hospitals (urban or rural)

Specialty hospitals (cancer, psychiatric, long-term care, pediatric)

Hospital-based clinics

Hospital-based emergency centers

Ambulatory Care (Outpatient) Settings

Health department clinics

Community health centers (CHCs)

Rural health clinics

Community-based mental health centers

School-based clinics

Prison health clinics

Dialysis centers

Screening centers

Home health agencies

Home hospice agencies

Durable medical equipment suppliers

Health maintenance organizations (HMOs)

Insurance companies

Physician group practices

Individual or solo medical practices

Specialty practices

Rehabilitation centers

Mobile vans for blood donations

Mobile vans for primary care delivery

Mobile mammography units

Free-standing surgical centers

Reference laboratory collection sites

Drug screening sites

---

respiratory therapists, patient care technicians, and others—have been cross-trained to assume phlebotomy duties; in other cases, traditional laboratory-based phlebotomists have been cross-trained to assume expanded clerical or patient-care duties, such as electrocardiograms (EKGs) and low-risk laboratory procedures. Whatever the case, phlebotomists must work closely and professionally with a variety of health care professionals (Figure 1-2 ■).

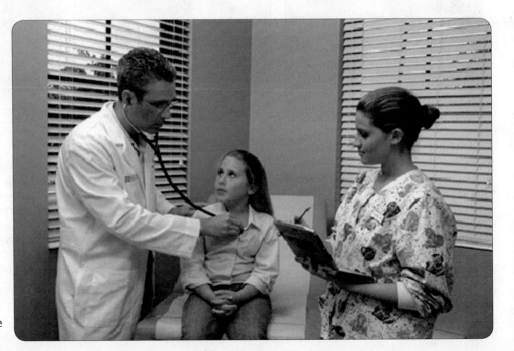

FIGURE ■ 1-2
Phlebotomists Work with All Members of the Health Care Team

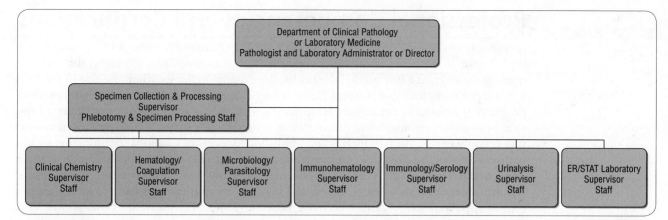

FIGURE ■ 1-3 Example of a Hypothetical Organizational Chart for a Hospital-Based Laboratory

The clinical or medical laboratory is closely linked to all phlebotomists because it is the final stop for blood specimens that are collected and analyzed. There are many types and sizes of laboratories, however Figure 1-3 ■ provides one example of a clinical laboratory and Box 1-2 ■ describes laboratory personnel with whom a phlebotomist would likely work.

Box 1-2   Clinical Laboratory Personnel

- **Pathologists**—physicians (medical doctors, MDs) who have extensive training in pathology (the study and diagnosis of disease).
- **Administrative/Management staff**—individuals who may have a graduate degree in health care administration or business.
- **Technical supervisors**—medical laboratory scientists with additional experience and education in a laboratory specialty area, such as hematology, microbiology, or clinical chemistry.
- **Medical Laboratory Scientists (MLS)**—certified professionals with a bachelor's degree in a biological science. Educational requirements include one or more years of study in a MLS program. Licensing is required in some states. Roles and responsibilities include performing chemical, microscopic, microbiologic, or immunologic tests pertaining to patient care; recording and reporting test results; participating in research and development of new test methods; performing preventive maintenance, troubleshooting, and quality control of instruments and reagents; maintaining safety in the clinical laboratory; and teaching residents and fellows in pathology and laboratory sciences.
- **Medical Laboratory Technicians (MLT)**—individuals who have a two-year certificate or associate degree. The MLT may perform designated tests and procedures, prepare specimens for testing and transport, prepare reagents, perform quality control measures, and assist the MLS in numerous preanalytic and postanalytic processes, as well as performing limited analytical processes.
- **Phlebotomists or Phlebotomy Technicians**—individuals with a high school diploma and specialized phlebotomy educational and clinical training; most phlebotomists take a certification examination. More information is presented in the following section.
- **Medical Assistants (MA)**—individuals who have completed a medical assisting certificate, often in conjunction with an associates degree. The MA in a laboratory setting may perform phlebotomy procedures, specified low-risk laboratory tests, basic patient assessments (blood pressure, etc.), specimen processing and handling, and clerical duties.
- **Certified Specialists**—individuals who complete required experiences and a certification examination in a specified area of the laboratory, such as blood banking, hemapheresis, microbiology, clinical chemistry, hematology, laboratory safety, or laboratory management.
- **Other laboratory personnel**—doctoral-level scientists who specialize in specific areas such as immunology or microbiology, laboratory information systems (LIS) operators and programmers, clerical staff, quality management staff, infection control officers, and biomedical equipment specialists.

Professional Competencies and Certifications

A high-school diploma or its equivalent is most often required to enter a phlebotomy training program in hospitals, community colleges, or technical schools. Typically, the length of training varies from a few weeks to months, depending on the location, the size of the facility, and the complexity of patients being served. Prior to acceptance and/or employment, programs will request a criminal background check, a drug screen, and/or evidence of specific immunizations, including the Hepatitis B vaccination series. Employers often require phlebotomy certification, which is accomplished by passing a national certification examination. Certification provides career advantages through job opportunities, career advancement, and portability (i.e., it is recognized from state to state). Some states (e.g., California) require phlebotomists to be licensed and may accept applications from students trained only at approved schools and who have passed approved certification examinations. Thus it is important to double-check the requirements in different areas of the country prior to entering an educational program.

Professional organizations that recognize phlebotomists are listed in Table 1-1 ■. Many of these organizations have developed **competency statements** to describe the entry-level skills, tasks, and roles performed by designated health care workers. In addition, some offer continuing educational opportunities via conferences, webinars, or online course work. Professional organizations may provide guidelines for health care organizations to set **standard operating procedures (SOP)** covering the practices, conduct, behaviors, and actions that are acceptable in the field. The organizations listed in Table 1-1 have an interest in promoting and improving the practice of phlebotomy.

Table 1-1 Professional Organizations for Phlebotomists

The organizations listed here have an interest in promoting and improving the practice of phlebotomy. They differ slightly in their membership requirements, fees, member benefits, continuing education (CE) courses, availability of certification examinations specifically for phlebotomists, and their profit motives (some are nonprofit and others are for-profit or proprietary; i.e., private ownership). The eligibility requirements and documentation for each certification also differ among these groups. Before applying for one or more of the certification examinations, double-check to see which ones are more reputable, secure, and accepted in the local community or state. Sometimes health care organizations have preferences for specific certifications and will adjust salaries accordingly. Likewise, local community colleges and universities can also provide recommendations about which certification examination to take. Because some states have credentialing or continuing education requirements for phlebotomists, it is important to know which organizations are approved by the state health departments to provide the examination or CE programs. In addition to those organizations listed below, numerous private companies market phlebotomy-related products and sometimes offer continuing education programs as well.

Nonprofit Organizations

The American Society for Clinical Laboratory Science (ASCLS)

6701 Democracy Boulevard, Suite 300
Bethesda, MD 20817
(301) 657-2768
(301) 657-2909 (fax)
www.ascls.org

ASCLS has recognized clinical laboratory personnel for more than 50 years. Several types of memberships are available, depending on the education and experience of the individual. Phlebotomists may join ASCLS as associate members in the Phlebotomy Section.

American Society for Clinical Pathology (ASCP)

33 W. Monroe Street, Suite 1600
Chicago, IL 60603
(312) 541-4999; (800) 267-2727
(312) 541-4998 (fax)
www.ascp.org

ASCP offers many levels of certification, through the Board of Certification (BOC), including a Phlebotomy Technician Examination, PBT, Donor Phlebotomy Technician (DPT), and an international certification examination for PBT (ASCP[i]). It also provides educational programs, teleconferences, webinars, workshops, phlebotomy scholarships, and online CE for phlebotomists. The certification exam covers the entry-level skills of a phlebotomist and uses taxonomy levels that assess recall (recognize facts), interpretive skills (use knowledge to interpret numeric data), and problem-solving skills (use applications of specific information to solve problems). Over 13,000 phlebotomists have been certified by ASCP since 1989.

American Society of Phlebotomy Technicians (ASPT)

P.O. Box 1831
Hickory, NC 28603
(828) 294-0078
(828) 327-2969 (fax)
www.aspt.org

ASPT offers a CPT (ASPT) certification examination. It also offers certification examinations for point-of-care technician, EKG technician, drug collection specialist, paramedical insurance examiner, and patient care technician.

National Accrediting Agency for Clinical Laboratory Sciences (NAACLS)

5600 N. River Road, Suite 720
Rosemont, IL 60018-5119
 (773) 714-8880
(773) 714-8886 (fax)
www.naacls.org

NAACLS accredits educational programs in clinical laboratory sciences including phlebotomy. No certification examinations are provided.

National Phlebotomy Association (NPA)

1901 Brightseat Road
Landover, MD 20785
(301) 386-4200
(301) 386-4203 (fax)
www.nationalphlebotomy.org

NPA was established in 1978 to recognize the phlebotomist as a distinctive and identifiable part of the health care team. NPA has established professional standards, a code of ethics, educational opportunities, and an annual certification examination resulting in a CPT (NPA). NPA has trained and certified approximately 15,000 phlebotomists in all 50 states and abroad and has accredited 75 teaching programs. Accredited programs must include the following topic areas: Historical Perspective, Medical Terminology, Anatomy and Physiology, Communication, Phlebotomy Practical, Cardio-Pulmonary Resuscitation (CPR), Stress Management, Phlebotomy Techniques, Human Relations, Legal Aspects, Infection Control, and Drug Awareness.

Commercial Organizations

American Certification Agency (ACA)

P.O. Box 58
Osceola, IN 46561
(574) 277-4538
(574) 277-4624 (fax)

Contact: Shirley Evans, Testing Specialist or Carole Mullins, Director

E-mail: info@acacert.com.
www.acacert.com

The ACA provides certification examinations for phlebotomy technicians and instructors.

continued

Table 1-1 Professional Organizations for Phlebotomists (*cont.*)

American Medical Technologists (AMT)

10700 West Higgins Road, Suite 150
Rosemont, IL 60018
(847) 823-5169 or (800) 275-1268
(847) 823-0458 (fax)
www.amt1.com

AMT offers several certification examinations including Phlebotomy Technician, Medical Laboratory Technician, Medical Laboratory Assistant, Medical Assistant, Medical Administrative Specialist, Allied Health Instructor, and Clinical Laboratory Consultant.

National Center for Competency Testing (NCCT/MMCI)

7007 College Blvd, Suite 705
Overland Park, KS 66211
(800) 875-4404
(913) 498-1243 (fax)
www.ncctinc.com

The NCCT provides certification and CE for phlebotomy technicians and instructors.

National Healthcareer Association (NHA)

National Headquarters
7 Ridgedale Avenue, Suite 203
Cedar Knolls, NJ 07927
(973) 605-1881 or (800) 499-9092
(973) 644-4797 (fax)
www.nha2000.com

Established in 1989, NHA was formed to create a network for health care professionals. NHA provides a certification examination for phlebotomists, CPT.

Table 1-2 ■ is an example of one organization's list of competencies for entry-level phlebotomy technicians. At minimum, these are the types of competencies that an employer might assess for the phlebotomist's performance evaluation. Competency statements describe the entry-level skills and tasks performed by phlebotomy technicians and measured on the certification examination. With regard to anatomy and physiology, specimen collection, specimen processing and handling, and laboratory operations related to phlebotomy, and in accordance with established procedures, the Phlebotomy Technician, PBT (ASCP), at career entry, should be able to accomplish the tasks listed in Table 1-2. Also refer to the appendices for a more detailed list of competencies from the National Accrediting Agency for Clinical Laboratory Sciences (NAACLS).

In addition to the competencies just discussed, Box 1-3 ■ encompasses duties and professional attributes, ability, and performance measures that employers might use for a phlebotomist's performance evaluation. Performance measures are observed through the phlebotomist's behavior, approach to the job, knowledge, and skills. There are many ways for supervisors to assess competency; direct observation, video recording, skills tests, reviewing worksheets or log books, reviewing quality control records, and using simulations or written examinations are some. Performance evaluations are important to both the employee and the employer, because they provide feedback, identify problems early, promote consistent evaluation, encourage employees to stay updated and to improve their skills, and provide a record of competency.

Table 1-2	American Society for Clinical Pathology (ASCP) Board of Certification Competency Statements for the Phlebotomy Technician

In regard to Circulatory System, Specimen Collection, Specimen Processing and Handling, Point-of-Care Testing, Non-Blood Specimens, and Laboratory Operations related to Phlebotomy, and in accordance with established procedures, the Phlebotomy Technician at career entry:

Applies Knowledge of

- principles of basic and special procedures
- basic anatomy and physiology
- preanalytic (preexamination) variables
- standard operating procedures (SOPs)
- medical terminology
- regulatory requirements
- fundamental biological characteristics
- patient and personal safety
- infection control

Selects Appropriate

- course of action
- equipment/methods/reagents/samples
- quality control procedures
- site for blood collection

Prepares Patients, Samples, and Equipment

Evaluates

- specimen and patient situation
- quality control procedures
- appropriate actions and methods
- sources of preanalytic (preexamination) variables
- common procedural/technical problems
- corrective action

Source: American Society for Clinical Pathology Board of Certification, www.ascp.org, 2011, with permission.

PROFESSIONAL CHARACTER TRAITS

Within the health professions, organizations such as the ASCP and NPA have developed standards of ethical conduct and behavior for members, and members are expected to adhere to those standards of performance. The major points are as follows:

- Do no harm to anyone intentionally.
- Perform according to sound technical ability and good judgment.
- Respect patients' rights (which include patients' confidentiality, privacy, the right to know about their treatment, and the right to refuse treatment).
- Have regard for the dignity of all human beings.

Box 1-3	Typical Clinical, Technical, and Clerical Duties and Attributes of Phlebotomists

What are the clinical duties of phlebotomists?

- Communicate professionally with patients and coworkers
- Identify the patient correctly
- Assess the patient before blood collection
- Prepare the patient accordingly
- Perform the puncture
- Withdraw blood into the correct containers/tubes
- Assess the degree of bleeding and pain
- Assess the patient after the phlebotomy procedure

What kind of technical duties do phlebotomists have to perform?

- Manipulate small objects, tubes, and needles
- Select and use appropriate equipment
- Perform quality control functions
- Transport the specimens correctly
- Prepare/process the sample(s) for testing/analysis
- Assist in laboratory testing procedures, washing glassware, and cleaning equipment

What clerical duties are expected of phlebotomists?

- Print/collate/distribute laboratory requisitions and reports
- Work on secure computers, facsimile machines, printers, and telephones
- Answer all queries as appropriate
- Demonstrate courtesy in all patient encounters
- Always respect privacy and confidentiality (on and off the job)

What kinds of policies must a phlebotomist adhere to?

- Safety in the laboratory and in patients' rooms
- Infection control, gowning/gloving, and hand hygiene
- Fire prevention and control
- Dress codes
- Attendance, sick leave, and vacation

What kind of communication skills do phlebotomists need?

- Verbal
- Nonverbal
- Listening skills
- Telephone etiquette
- Written communication
- Use of medical terminology appropriate for patients and coworkers
- Management of angry or difficult patients

How is the quality and productivity of a phlebotomist's work measured?

- Quality can be measured by waiting times, lack of complications or mistakes, contamination rates, etc.
- Productivity is often measured by the time and attention given to patients and to detailed procedures, and by the throughput of work based on how much work is completed during specified amounts of time.

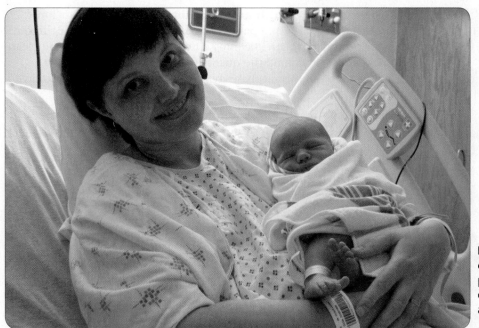

FIGURE ■ 1-4 When communicating, whether the patient is young or old, a parent or spouse, compassion is always appreciated.

Source: emin kuliyev/Shutterstock.com

Important character attributes for this career path include:

■ **Sincerity and compassion**—Phlebotomists must possess an intense desire to serve people and a sincere interest in learning about blood and specimen collection practices (Figure 1-4 ■).

■ **Emotional stability and maturity**—Health care workers must be able to cope daily with seeing others in pain, handling blood and body fluids, facing injury and trauma, seeing disease sites, and the possibility of observing death. Responses to harsh situations must be prompt, professional, and reassuring to the patients, their families, and the health care team.

■ **Accountability for doing things right**—Personal integrity, veracity (telling the truth), and "doing what is right when no one is looking" (e.g., washing hands between patient collections, observing precautions to gown and scrub in isolation, reporting one's own mistakes, and collecting timed tests at the proper time) reflect a health care worker's personal responsibility for his or her actions.

■ **Dedication to high standards of performance and precision**—Health care workers must continually upgrade and maintain the quality of their skills. They must seek knowledge about new techniques and safety procedures, new supplies and equipment, and computer technology through continuing education. They should be willing to ask for assistance when dealing with a difficult patient or procedure and have the desire to follow rigid standards of performance. They should only collect the specimens ordered and only those that they have been trained to collect.

■ **Respect for patients' dignity, privacy, confidentiality, and the right to know**—Phlebotomists have an obligation to respect all patients' rights, regardless of their personal opinions and biases. All patients must be treated with dignity and respect regardless of race, culture, religion, gender, age, or disabling conditions. Phlebotomists should have a full understanding of patients' rights to privacy, to confidentiality, and to knowing what procedures are being performed.

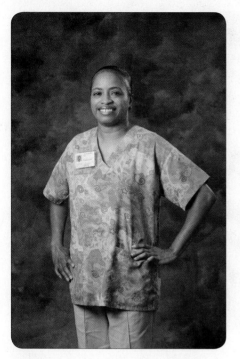

FIGURE ■ 1-5 Cleanliness and good health, along with a professional dress code, provide a positive image.

- **Propensity for health and cleanliness**—Phlebotomists must protect themselves and patients by accepting that sterile techniques, good personal hygiene, keeping a healthy mind and body, and cleanliness affect safety and the quality of health care (Figure 1-5 ■). This is more important than saving time or cutting corners to save money.

- **Pride, satisfaction, and self-fulfillment in the job**—Phlebotomists should attain professional satisfaction from continually improving their professional skills and knowledge, from knowing that others are dependent on the quality of their work, and from knowing that their skills contribute to the betterment of patients. The most successful, highly regarded phlebotomists are those who are most gratified with their work.

- **Working with team members**—Phlebotomists must be flexible enough to work with a diverse health care team in a wide range of settings. Health care teams can improve skills (more talent, expertise, and technical competence), communication (more ideas, mutual respect, crossing departmental lines), participation (increased job satisfaction, combined efforts valued above individual efforts), and effectiveness (solutions are more likely to be implemented because the team has shared ownership of decisions).

- **Take pleasure in communicating with patients**—The quality and ease of collecting blood specimens depends on both the technical skills of the health care worker and successful interactions with the patient (Figure 1-6 ■). Phlebotomists should learn about transcultural communication strategies, communication barriers, and gender- or age-related issues that affect communication.

The decision to become a phlebotomist requires a special person with multiple talents and internal drive. It can be a stressful job and individuals choosing this career path must be able to balance the challenges. The choice of this career path should not be taken lightly. (Test your career readiness level with the assessment in Box 1-4 ■). Box 1-5 ■ provides some tips for relieving stress and staying physically and emotionally healthy.

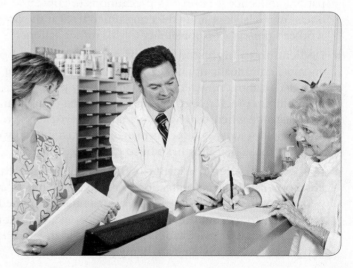

FIGURE ■ 1-6 Professional and courteous communication with patients is an essential job function.
Source: Lisa F. Young/Fotolia

Box 1-4   Phlebotomy Career Self-Assessment

If you are considering a career in phlebotomy, ask yourself the following questions. If there are doubts in your mind about your answers, think about whether you are willing to change or learn new skills.

1. Do I pay close attention to details?
2. Do I like to work with small objects such as needles and test tubes?
3. Do I follow procedures exactly?
4. Does it bother me if I am closely watched or supervised?
5. Do I mind seeing blood, sick patients, body tissues, or fluids or smelling unpleasant odors?
6. What is my reaction to inflicting the pain of a needlestick on someone?
7. Am I willing to admit my own mistakes? Will I be truthful even if the consequences are negative?
8. Do I like working with a team? Do I get along well with other people?
9. Am I willing to stand for long periods of time, walk extensively, reach, stoop, lift, or carry equipment?
10. Am I willing to work on holidays and weekends occasionally?

Box 1-5   Ten Tips for Relieving Stress

1. Find time to do your own thing. If you need privacy, structure some quiet time for yourself to meditate, pray, etc. If you need an outlet, structure time for a hobby or a diversion outside of work to remove yourself from the stress, even if it is a brief period of time each day or week.
2. Look for humor in daily situations or associate with gentle people who can help you laugh or lighten up.
3. Think of new ways to get exercise so that it does not get boring. Try adding a new exercise to your routine every few weeks. Try a new dance class or exercise form. If you cannot schedule an entire class, try short exercise sessions (10 minutes at three different times of the day is better than none at all).
4. Eat nutritious, low-fat foods and consider taking vitamins if your diet is not providing all the necessary nutrients. Think of your plate with at least 50% vegetables, 25% protein, and 25% carbohydrates.
5. Take more control over the sources of your stress. For example, if cooking meals after a hard day's work is stressful, cook multiple meals on your day off and freeze the rest so that they are easier to prepare during the busy workweek. If getting kids dressed and fed each morning is causing you to be late for work, lay out their clothes and breakfast foods the night before.
6. Read interesting books, listen to new music, or watch interesting movies.
7. Keep a life journal or a dream journal. If you forget to write in it, just skip a few days and pick it up again when you feel like it.
8. Go occasionally to a performance such as a concert, play, or dance program. Try to see an art exhibit or an art gallery open house.
9. Avoid harmful habits such as smoking, drinking excessively, or unnecessary drug use.
10. Do not be afraid to seek professional assistance when needed.

Professional Appearance and Personal Health

APPEARANCE, GROOMING, AND PHYSICAL FITNESS

Posture

Phlebotomists usually perform their work while standing. There are occasions, however, particularly with ambulatory patients, when it is more effective to sit adjacent to the patient for the blood collection procedure. Erect posture conveys a sense of confidence and pride in job performance. Slouching conveys a sense of laziness and apathy. Good posture minimizes back and neck strain, promotes better breathing, and eases the patient's mind about the confidence of the phlebotomist.

Grooming and Personal Hygiene

Physical appearance communicates a strong impression about an individual. Neatly combed hair; clean fingernails; a clean, pressed uniform; protective lab coat and gloves; and an overall tidy appearance communicate a commitment to cleanliness and infection control, and they instill confidence in a person. A daily bath or shower, followed by the use of deodorant, brushing teeth, using mouthwash, and appropriate dressing are also recommended. Hygiene is particularly important in today's health care environment, where patients and employees are deeply concerned about the spread of infectious diseases. Employers of health care workers are legally required to provide **personal protective equipment (PPE)** or barrier protection for workers handling biohazardous, infectious substances. This includes gowns, gloves, masks, laboratory coats or aprons, and face shields. Because of latex sensitivities and allergies, employers must provide an array of sizes and styles of gloves and gowns to protect their employees. Table 1-3 ■ describes a dress code policy.

NUTRITION, REST, AND EXERCISE

The role of a health care worker requires physical stamina because the pace is often hectic, and overtime work is common. Good health improves the health care worker's appearance, attitude, job performance, and ability to cope with stress. Appropriate eating habits, rest during lunch and break periods, and off-duty exercising are essential to an individual's well-being and stress reduction. Practicing a healthy lifestyle while on and off duty will facilitate a return to work with a refreshed and more productive attitude.

Communication Strategies for Phlebotomists

Face-to-face communication is the most effective form of communication and is part of a phlebotomist's job every day. Verbal interactions can be depicted as a communication loop that starts when the verbal message leaves the sender and is heard by the receiver (Figure 1-8 ■). The receiver completes the loop by providing feedback to the sender. Feedback can be in the form of a verbal acknowledgment or a nod of the head. Without feedback, the sender has no way of knowing whether the message was accurately heard or understood or if the message was somehow blocked by extraneous factors that can "filter out" meaning from a message. Filters (such as hallway noise, someone else talking, a telephone ringing, etc.) can be damaging to effective communication because these distractions do not allow the loop to be completed; thus, there is a risk that patients will not understand care instructions. Phlebotomists must be sure that the message they send is the same message received by the patient.

Table 1-3	Sample of a Dress Code Policy

Purpose: Presenting a professional and positive image to all patients, customers, and members of the community is a goal of this health care organization. Professional dress, good grooming, and personal cleanliness are important aspects of the overall effectiveness and morale of all employees. To establish a standard appearance, the following guidelines will be enforced. Employees who appear inappropriately dressed or groomed will be sent home. Please note that these are *minimum* guidelines and that individual departments are likely to have more rigid requirements because of safety, infection control, or patient preferences. Consult your supervisor regarding any questions you may have regarding these guidelines.

Identification   Name badges will be visibly worn at all times. Stickers, pins, or other types of tokens will not cover the employee or department name.

Daily hygiene   Having clean teeth, hair, clothes, and body are basic daily requirements. Clean, wrinkle-free clothes, scrubs, or uniforms that are in good condition should be worn.

Hair   Hair should be clean, neat, and trimmed. Moderate styles are recommended. Well-groomed, closely trimmed beards, sideburns, and mustaches are allowed. Shoulder-length hair should be pulled back and secured.

Nails   Because hands and nails are colonized with microorganisms that can easily be transmitted from one person to the next, nails should be clean, neatly manicured, and not more than 1/4 inch past the fingertip. Nail polish or gels and artificial nails are not recommended and are not allowed in many facilities in which employees have direct patient contact (Figure 1-7 ■).

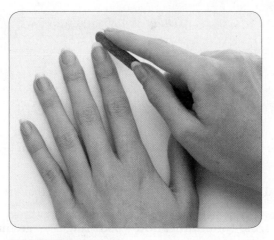

FIGURE ■ 1-7
Source: Dave King, Dorling Kindersley

Fragrances/scents   Perfumes and fragrances can be offensive and/or nauseating to patients who are ill. It is recommended that the use of fragrances be minimized or eliminated.

Make-up   Make-up should be conservative and lightly applied. Extreme or excessive make-up is not allowed.

Clothing   Denim clothing is not usually allowed, except on special occasions announced by the hospital administration. Tight-fitting clothing or clothes that are revealing or distracting are not permitted. Shirts should be buttoned up to the second button. Shirttails should be tucked in, and T-shirts with logos or athletic prints will not be allowed. Proper undergarments should be worn at all times. Skirts and dresses should not be shorter than 3 inches above the knee. Shorts are not permitted. Pants/slacks should be worn with a belt if they have belt loops. Tight-fitting leggings are not permitted. It is recommended that male employees who are not involved in patient care wear ties.

Shoes   Shoes should be comfortable, safe in the work environment, clean, and polished. Consideration should be made to minimizing noise when walking. Socks and/or proper hose or tights should be worn. Sandals, flip-flops, and cloth shoes are not permitted.

Jewelry   Excessive jewelry is not allowed. Because safety is a major concern, chains must be worn inside the collar, and long dangling earrings are not acceptable. Other types of exposed jewelry (facial piercings) may also pose hazards and/or may become irritated with the use of personal protective equipment; therefore, they are not recommended.

Tattoos   In general terms, tattoos are not perceived as part of a highly professional image. Therefore, tattoos should be covered by clothing so as not to pose a distraction in patient care encounters. In some departments/facilities, discreet, non-offensive tattoos may be permitted to show, but it varies based on individual department protocols. Infected tattoos may pose a significant health risk to the employee and to patients.

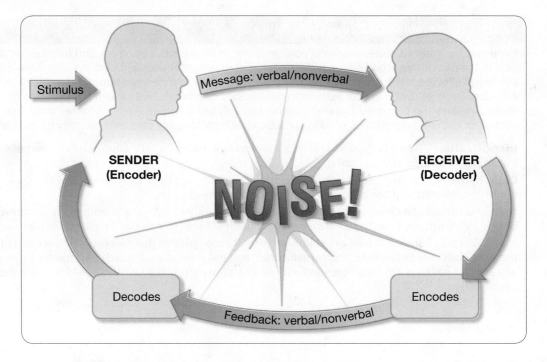

FIGURE ■ 1-8
Communication Loop

THE BASICS OF COMMUNICATION

The communication loop is complete when the sender receives feedback from the receiver about the intent of the message. Communication can be broken down into its three more detailed components:

> **Verbal communication**—The actual words that are spoken, the pace and tone of voice
>
> **Nonverbal communication**—Body language, gestures
>
> **Active listening**—Using verbal and nonverbal information to assess the situation

In patient care situations the most effective communication involves the following elements.

- Showing empathy (for waking up a patient, disturbing him or her, interrupting a meal) (Figure 1-9 ■)
- Showing respect (for privacy and confidentiality, for his or her condition, for family members)
- Building trust (maintain confidentiality, explain procedures clearly, tell the truth)
- Establishing a professional bond (use common courtesy, show interest)
- Listening actively (face the patient, maintain a nonjudgmental posture, lean toward the patient, establish eye contact, do not interrupt, relax and listen intently)
- Providing specific feedback (about the patient's behavior, about a procedure, about what the patient said)

VERBAL COMMUNICATION

Verbal communication involves conveying the right message in a professional tone of voice using language that is appropriate for the situation.

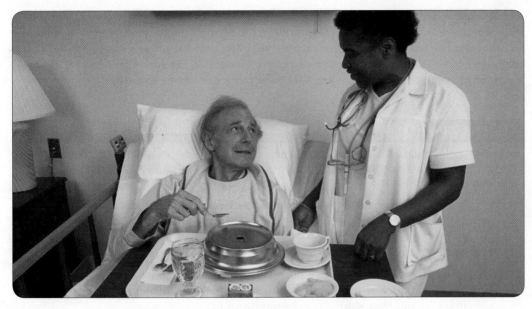

FIGURE ■ 1-9 Show Empathy for Patients

Note that the health care worker has a compassionate, caring look on her face. She is smiling and making eye contact with the patient in a pleasant and professional communication exchange.

Language

Phlebotomists should use simple, everyday vocabulary, particularly with children. Complex medical jargon should be avoided. Patients must *not* be told, "This won't hurt." Most blood collection procedures are, indeed, slightly painful; therefore, it is important that the patient be forewarned and prepared (e.g., "This might hurt a little, but it will be over soon.").

Sensory Impairments

Hearing or sight impairments (deafness or blindness) can have an impact on effective communication. However, many technological advances have enabled individuals with impairments a means to live independently and perform tasks of daily living. To assess whether a patient has understood, a question such as, "Is there a step you would like me to repeat before we begin?" or "Do you want me to explain the procedure again?" yields better clues that the patient has understood than saying, "Do you understand?" If it is obvious that the patient did not hear, the phlebotomist should use preprinted instructions or write down instructions for the patient. If the patient is deaf and requires communication in sign language, all efforts must be made to find an interpreter who can perform the sign language as needed. It is also recommended that writing tools be kept nearby.

For patients who are sight-impaired, it is most important to communicate the phlebotomist's identity and what he/she is going to do to the patient. Let the patient know who is in the room if there are others. Speak directly to the patient, not a companion if there is one, and do not be afraid to verbally offer your hand for a handshake as a way to introduce yourself.

Languages Other than English

The diversity of languages spoken in this country is extensive. In large city hospitals it is common to see signage in multiple languages and/or universal signs and pictorial graphics that are easy to understand. Patients who do not speak English can often understand some basics from nonverbal cues, but the phlebotomist must know how to locate an interpreter or use translation services when possible. In the absence of a translator, written instructions in other languages may facilitate the process. Printed cards in different languages can be used to transmit information about the phlebotomy procedures.

Because of the proximity of the United States to Central and South America, it is beneficial for some phlebotomists to develop skills in the Spanish language; however, it is recommended that the health care worker practice the phrases with someone who can speak the language before attempting to communicate with a patient, because mispronounced words may lead to confusion. Refer to Appendix 5 for basic phrases in Spanish.

Clinical Alert !

In some states, children are not permitted to serve as translators for their parents when health care issues are discussed. Phlebotomists should check with their supervisors about the applicable laws in their state.

Environmental Noise

A busy, noisy environment in a clinic or hospital room distracts both the sender and receiver, often resulting in an unclear message. Box 1-6 ∎ offers tips for dealing with some common situations that may interfere with clear communication.

Age

The vocabulary of a toddler is different from a teenager and also different from that of an adult or an elderly person. Phlebotomists should be sensitive to word usage for each age. Remember that it might take longer to explain a procedure to a young child who is more fearful about the pain than an adult. Whatever the case, be truthful about the pain and the procedure and use terms that are right for the situation.

Pace, Tone, and Volume of Voice

The tone (intonation or pitch) of one's voice and the inflection used can change a positive sentence into a negative-sounding statement. Volume is the "loudness" of the voice and ranges from a whisper to a shout. The pace, tone, and volume of voice should match the words that are spoken. Sarcasm is usually communicated just by changing one's tone of voice. Health care workers can avoid sending mixed messages to patients by practicing

Box 1-6   Communicating in a Noisy Environment

A busy hallway, visitors, a television, cellular phones, iPods, iPads, and/or headphones can prevent the patient from hearing accurately. In cases where the distractions may occur, the phlebotomist should take steps to reduce the sound level so that the patient can hear necessary instructions. Practice using the examples below:

To visitors: "Excuse me, please. It is important for me to explain this procedure to Mr. Jones. Would you mind if we have a few quiet moments together? Thank you for your cooperation."

For the television or movie video: "Mr. Jones, I am sorry to disrupt your movie or show, but would you mind if we lower the volume for a few minutes or pause it so we can go over the procedure for collecting your blood sample? Thank you; this should only take a few minutes."

For headphones: "Mr. Jones, it is important that we discuss this procedure before beginning. Would you mind taking off your headphones for a few minutes? I will be brief. Thank you for your cooperation."

Box 1-7	Improving Tone of Voice and Facial Expression

The following exercise is fun and useful for improving verbal and nonverbal communication skills. Practice it in front of a mirror or with a coworker.

Step 1. Using a nice tone of voice (i.e., a calm, compassionate, clear, professional tone), with a smile on your face, practice saying the following phrases:
  ■ "Please . . ."
  ■ "Good morning, Mr. Jones. Have you had your breakfast yet?"
  ■ "May I please check your identification wristband?"
  ■ "Thank you for your cooperation."

Step 2. Now, using a degrading and hurried voice (i.e., quick, sarcastic, whiny, angry tone), with a frustrated, disdainful look on your face, repeat the phrases listed in step 1.

Step 3. List the specific features you liked about the first method and those features you disliked about the second method. Try to contrast details of facial features (wrinkled eyebrows or smiling face), how the voice lowers or raises at the end of the statements, and how you feel when speaking in the two manners.

Step 4. Keep a mental impression (or actually take a picture) of the way you look and sound during the first step. Remember: A simple smile can often force a positive change in one's voice.

a calm, soothing, and confident tone of voice (as opposed to a fast, high-pitched, nervous voice). Box 1-7 ■ is a practice exercise for health care professionals to use in observing their own facial expressions and voice modifications.

Emergency Situations

Emergency, or "STAT," blood collections are common in emergency rooms and in complicated medical cases. Verbal communication must be fast, but professional, and accurate. The STAT phlebotomy procedures also require extra speed and accuracy without jeopardizing the "personal touch." Patients in emergency rooms may not have identification information with them and/or may be unconscious. All facilities, however, should have documented procedures for the identification process with which phlebotomists should be familiar. Individual patients should be considered in terms of their privacy, dignity, and individual needs, and never by nicknames such as "Mr. L down the hall" or "the broken leg in 3C." Each is entitled to professional, respectful care in all circumstances.

Bedside Manner

The climate established by a phlebotomist upon entering a patient's room affects the entire patient encounter. The feeling of confidence that comes from the knowledge that the blood collection tray is clean and well stocked is the first step in a good bedside manner. Entering the room with a feeling of optimism or positive energy stimulates cooperation. A calm professional tone of voice should begin the introduction. A pleasant facial expression, neat appearance, and professional manner set the stage for a positive interaction with the patient. The first 30 seconds after the phlebotomist enters the patient's room determine how that patient perceives the quality of patient care offered by that hospital. Most patients admit that the procedure they dread most is being "stuck" for blood collection, so phlebotomists should make every effort to communicate in an encouraging manner.

THE PATIENT ENCOUNTER

When encountering the patient for the first time, there are some basic procedures to follow:

■ Knock gently (do not pound) on the patient's hospital room door.

■ Introduce yourself and state that you are from the hospital unit or laboratory staff, whichever is the case (Box 1-8 ■).

■ Inform the patient that his or her specimen must be collected for a test ordered by the physician. (A statement indicating that this is routine hospital protocol often reassures the patient. A lengthy discussion of why a certain test was ordered is inappropriate. These questions should be referred to the patient's physician.)

■ The most important step in the initial patient encounter is patient identification and it will be covered in greater detail later in the text. However, the communication process should be a smooth transition from the phlebotomist's introduction to the actual identification procedure.

■ During all steps, remain calm, compassionate, and professional and limit conversations to essential information. If there are problems or discrepancies, the phlebotomist should calmly indicate to the patient that it may take a few more moments to double check the information.

■ Let the patient know how the procedure is going (e.g., provide feedback such as "this is going well," or "it is almost over").

■ Do not be distracted from the phlebotomy procedure by excessive talk of unrelated issues.

■ Before leaving the room, thank the patient for cooperating.

COMMUNICATION FOR PATIENT IDENTIFICATION

Clear communication practices for patient identification are essential. If the patient is hospitalized, identification should be accomplished by a match between the test requisition or labels and a unique identification number on the armband and by verbal confirmation from the patient. If a hospitalized patient does not have an armband (some long term care facilities do not require an armband), a positive confirmation must be made by a unit nurse or other authorized individual who knows the patient. This process should be well documented by the phlebotomist. Special identification procedures should also be well documented for ambulatory patients, especially in cases of home-bound patients, mobile vans, and other off-site locations. Armbands are not commonly used in ambulatory settings; however, some form of identification card usually is. It may include some demographic data and other identifying information, such as the patient's unique identification number, date of birth (DOB), a picture, address, or a combination of these. Identity must be confirmed by the patient and the phlebotomist prior to blood collection (Figure 1-10 ■).

Some health care facilities insist that the phlebotomist ask for the patient's complete address, whereas others require the mention of the patient's hometown, birth date, identification number, or street name to reinforce and confirm identity. Some prefer that patients spell out an unusual last name. This portion of the specimen collection procedure ensures that the remainder of the diagnostic testing protocol provides information on the correct person. Detailed identification procedures are covered in Chapter 8.

Box 1-8	**The Right Way to Communicate to Acquire Information**

The following scenario is a typical, but simplified one that might occur at the opening greeting between a phlebotomist and a hospitalized patient. Imagine both the verbal and nonverbal factors involved for the patient and the phlebotomist. The *wrong responses* are noted in italics and are sometimes the easiest way to respond so it is important to train oneself to avoid these phrases. This can be used as a discussion tool about how the phlebotomist can have either a positive or negative impact.

Phlebotomist: Good morning. My name is Sally, I am from the Laboratory, and I am here to collect a blood sample for your laboratory tests. (Pause for the patient to see you and give him/her an opportunity to speak. If the lights are off, turn on a low level light first so the patient can adjust.) I will need to check your identification. Could you please state your name and spell it?

Wrong response/action: Turn on the overhead lights and say "Hi, how are you doing . . . are you Mrs. Betty Smith?"

Patient (softly): My name is Betty Smith.

Phlebotomist: Could you please repeat that and spell it for me please?

Wrong response: Huh? What did you say? Could you speak up?

Patient: My name is Betty Smith, B-E-T-T-Y S-M-I-T-H.

Phlebotomist: Thank you, Mrs. Smith. I think I have it now but I also need to check the identification number on your armband. I will be taking a blood sample from your arm so that the laboratory can perform tests that your doctor ordered. Have you had breakfast yet?

Wrong response: Okay, got it . . . let's get on with it. I have a huge list of patients to draw this morning.

Patient: No breakfast yet; I just woke up.

Phlebotomist: Mrs. Smith, have you ever fainted during a blood collection procedure?

Wrong response: Ever fainted before?

Patient: No, I haven't fainted before but I don't like being stuck.

Phlebotomist: I can understand your feelings; most people feel that way. Have you ever had any problems during blood collections or are you allergic to any products such as latex?

Wrong response: Got any allergies?

Patient: I'm not allergic to anything.

Phlebotomist: Mrs. Smith, I need to look at your arms. Would you prefer your right side or left side?

Wrong response: Hold out this arm so I can check it out.

Patient: Nobody ever gets blood on the left side so we'd better try the right side.

Phlebotomist: Thanks for that info; we can check the right side. Please hold out your arm so that I can feel for your veins.

Wrong response: Oh, don't worry about a thing. I'm pretty good at drawing blood from tough veins. I can squeeze blood out of a turnip!

Patient: Okay, but will it hurt?

Phlebotomist: It will hurt a little, but I'll do my best to have it done quickly. Do you have any other questions?

Wrong response: No, it doesn't hurt.

Patient: Not really, just get it over with so I can go back to sleep.

Phlebotomist: Thanks for your cooperation, Mrs. Smith.

Wrong response: Well, I'm just doing what I was told.

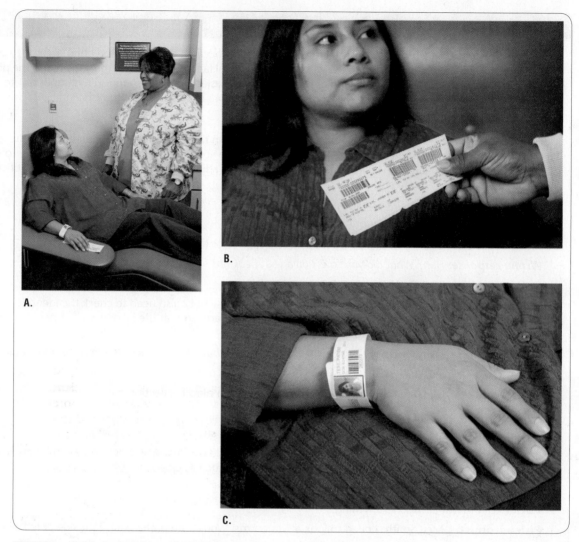

FIGURE ■ 1-10 Patient Identification Basics

Patient identification involves at least 3 steps: A. Ask the patient to verbally confirm and/or spell his or her name (often times facilities require the birthdate and/or address as well). B. Compare the information stated with the laboratory test requisitions/labels. C. Confirm the information from steps A and B with another source of reliable, verifiable identification (such as an armband).

COMMUNICATION IN A CLINIC OR IN THE HOME

Phlebotomists who collect specimens in a clinic or home setting must take extra steps to assure the phlebotomy procedure is successful. These steps include the following:

■ The phlebotomist must introduce him- or herself and clearly explain the purpose of the interaction.

■ The patient should be directed to sit in a chair with sides and arms or recline during the procedure. This may involve walking to a private area, blood collection booth, or special recliner.

- If the phlebotomy procedure is taking place in an unfamiliar setting, such as the patient's home, the phlebotomist must take extra time beforehand to find the nearest bathroom (for handwashing or blood spillage) and the nearest bed, in case there are complications during the phlebotomy procedure (fainting).

- In a patient's home, the phlebotomist should bring a mobile phone or computer to clarify laboratory orders or inquire about patient information.

- Information about the procedure should be fully explained (especially if it is a first-time blood collection for the patient or if it has been a long time since the last blood collection).

- Identifying the patient should be done meticulously and cautiously, using various methods to identify the patient positively (e.g., driver's license or identification card, confirmation of birthday and home address, or other identifiers, if available).

- The puncture site must be appropriately cared for, and it should be clear that bleeding from the puncture site has stopped and that the patient is physically fit to leave the area after the phlebotomy procedure. If the patient is homebound, the phlebotomist must be sure that the patient is no longer bleeding, that the puncture site has been appropriately bandaged, and that the patient is able to stay by him- or herself.

ROLE OF FAMILY, VISITORS, AND SIGNIFICANT OTHERS

Family members and friends of adult patients are often present when phlebotomists need to acquire specimens. It is important to realize that their presence can make the patient more secure and comfortable. Sometimes, however, families and visitors are much more difficult to deal with than the patients. They may make requests that are beyond the phlebotomist's scope of acceptable or authorized responsibilities, and it is better then to inform the appropriate health care team member of the family member's request. If several visitors are in the hospital room with the patient, they may be asked to step into the hall while the blood specimen is being drawn. If the health care worker believes that assistance is required (to give emotional support, etc.) and the patient agrees, a family member may be asked to stay during the procedure. Children should be accompanied by a parent or guardian. This can make the family members feel helpful and provide reassurance to patients.

Physicians, priests, and chaplains have the right to visit privately with patients. Unless the blood specimen is required at a specific time, i.e., "timed specimens" for monitoring drug levels, the health care worker should respect that privacy and return to the patient after completing the other draws in the unit or area. If the procedure is needed at a specified time or is a STAT request, the health care worker can apologize for the interruption, explain the nature of the request, and ask permission to collect the specimen.

Families and visitors of patients, except for parents/guardians of pediatric patients, should not be permitted in the clinical laboratory or provided with patient information, except by prior arrangement and permission of the patient. The patient's privacy and safety and the confidentiality of patient records must be considered.

NONVERBAL COMMUNICATION

Some theories suggest that communication consists of 10 to 20 percent verbal and 80 to 90 percent nonverbal messages. Nonverbal cues, or body language, can be positive—and facilitate understanding—or negative—and hinder effective communication (Table 1-4 ■ and Figure 1-11 ■).

Table 1-4	Nonverbal Communication/Body Language	
Positive Body Language	**Effects**	
Face-to-face positioning	Aids communication	
Relaxed hands, arms, shoulders	Alleviates tension or stress	
Erect posture	Promotes better breathing and appearance of professionalism	
Eye contact, eye level (avoid looking down on someone)		
Smiling		
Appropriate zone of comfort		
Negative Body Language	**Effects**	
Slouching, shrugged shoulders	Unprofessional posture	
Rolling eyes, wandering eyes	Gives the appearance of boredom	
Staring blankly or at ceiling	Causes discomfort, uneasiness	
Rubbing eyes, excessive blinking	Is distracting from effective communication	
Squirming, tapping foot or pencil, etc.		
Deep sighing, groaning		
Crossing arms, clenching fists		
Wrinkling forehead		
Thumbing through books or papers		
Stretching, yawning		
Peering over eyeglasses		
Pointing finger at someone		

Clinical Alert !

The patient should always be asked, "Could you please state your name and spell it?" not "Are you Ms. Smith?" The first question is a more reliable and direct way of confirming identity. The second question is inappropriate and less reliable because a patient who is heavily medicated may agree with anything that he or she is asked.

POSITIVE BODY LANGUAGE

Smiling

A simple, compassionate smile can open lines of communication by making each patient feel that he or she is the most important person at that moment. In addition, most people look better with smiles on their faces than they do with frowns. It takes fewer muscle movements to smile than it does to frown.

Eye Contact and Eye Level

Eye contact promotes a sense of trust and honesty between the patient and phlebotomist. There is an expression: "The eyes are the windows of the soul."

Eye level is also a consideration. Because bedridden patients must always "look up" to those in the room, it can create a feeling of intimidation, of being "looked down on," or of weakness. Most of the time, phlebotomists do not have the extra time to spend finding a chair to sit in so that they are at eye level; however, if a health care worker must explain a

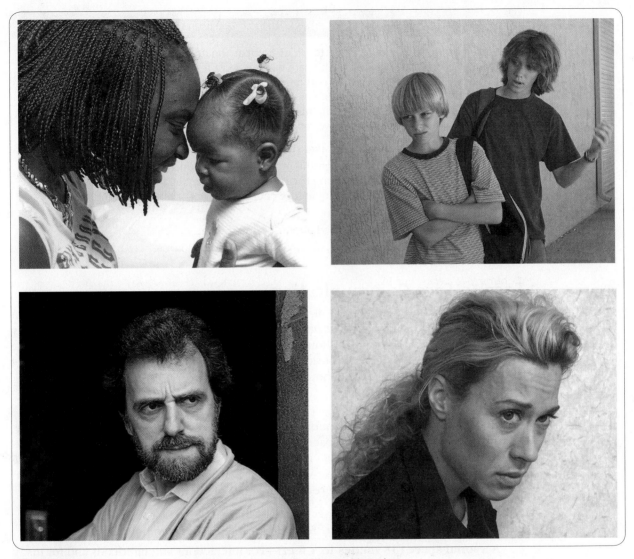

FIGURE ■ 1-11 Nonverbal Communication Can Be Positive or Negative
Note the effects of each look, eye expression, and body language.

lengthy procedure or if it is noted that the patient is particularly nervous about the procedure, the explanation should be done while seated at eye level with the patient (Box 1-9 ■).

A word of caution about eye contact is needed when dealing with patients of certain cultures. Generally speaking, Americans view eye contact as a positive aspect of human nature, and avoidance of eye contact might mean that someone is not being truthful. However, some Asian and Native American cultures believe that prolonged eye contact is rude and an invasion of privacy. Muslim women may avoid eye contact because of modesty.[2] Patients may not appreciate direct eye contact with a health care provider because it may make them feel self-conscious; it may be unacceptable in their culture or may not be acceptable with the opposite sex. The phlebotomist should take cues from the patient. If the patient does not look at the health care worker when he or she is speaking, perhaps he or she would feel more comfortable with more space between them or less direct eye contact. The phlebotomist can take the interaction at a slower pace to monitor the patient's comfort level. The more secure and comfortable the patient feels, the easier the procedure will be for the phlebotomist.

| Box 1-9 | Practice Exercise for Developing Sensitivity to Bedridden Patients |

Health care workers should strive to be as compassionate as possible. Bedridden patients often feel intimidated because health care workers must repeatedly "look down" on them to provide care. Sometimes these patients are frightened or depressed because of their condition or prognosis. This exercise will help you imagine yourself in the patient's condition and can make you a more compassionate member of the health care team. Practice the exercise with a coworker whom you do not know very well.

1. Lie on a bed while your coworker stands directly over you, looking down.
2. Have the coworker go through the motions of a venipuncture procedure, including the greeting and identification process. Try to imagine the anticipation of the needle-stick. Have the coworker maintain eye contact with you while conversing.
3. Repeat step 2, without eye contact.
4. List what you liked and disliked about this procedure.

Face-to-Face Communication

Phlebotomists should face patients directly. Otherwise, the patient may feel neglected, that he or she is being avoided, or that information is being withheld. If a patient turns away from a phlebotomist, however, it should be taken as a cue that the patient is uncomfortable for some reason. The phlebotomist should do everything possible to make the patient feel more comfortable during the phlebotomy procedure.

Zone of Comfort

Most individuals begin to feel uncomfortable when strangers get too close to them physically. A **zone of comfort** is the area of space around a patient that is private territory, so to speak, where they feel comfortable with an interaction. If that zone is crossed, feelings of uneasiness may occur.

For most Western cultures, there are four zones of interpersonal space:

Intimate space (direct contact up to 18 inches)—For close relationships and health care workers who bathe, feed, dress, and perform venipunctures

Personal space (18 inches to 4 feet)—For interactions among friends and for many patient encounters

Social space (4 feet to 12 feet)—For most interactions of everyday life

Public space (more than 12 feet)—For lectures, speeches, and so on

When a stranger gets too close, it can cause the patient to feel nervous, fearful, or anxious. Health care workers must be understanding and approach nervous patients slowly and gently, to avoid causing feelings of being threatened. This is particularly true with children, many of whom have a wide zone of comfort—that is, they do not like anyone to approach them except close relatives or friends. It is helpful to slowly approach the patient while crossing the zone of comfort, not to be too hasty, and to talk to patients during the process.

CULTURAL SENSITIVITY

Culture is a system of values, beliefs, and practices that stem from an individual's concept of reality (Box 1-10 ■). Culture influences decisions and behaviors in many aspects of life. Learning about various ethnic groups and cultures is important for health care professionals to understand the reasons for patients' behaviors during times of health and illness.

Box 1-10   What Is Culture?

Culture is an important aspect of our global society. Culture varies among groups of individuals, but it usually encompasses the following traits:

Values—The accepted principles of a group: individualism versus socialism, importance of education and financial security, competition versus cooperation, sanctity of life, and so on.

Beliefs—Doctrine or faith of a person or group: spiritual orientation, family bonds, and so on.

Traditions and practices—Customs and behaviors associated with groups: holidays, foods, music, dance, health care practices, and so on.

Specific traits that vary among cultures have been addressed previously (e.g., eye contact and zone of comfort). However, with the changing demographics of the U.S. population, it is vital for all health care workers to become more sensitive and compassionate about accepting cultural practices that vary from our own. More importantly, cultural awareness promotes effective patient communication. When a health care worker is unsure or unaware of acceptable patterns of behavior for a patient, the recommended action is to "follow the patient's lead." For example, if a patient speaks softly and slowly, speak the same way. If the patient turns to a family member when speaking to you, include the family member in the conversation. If a patient moves closer to you during the conversation, try not to back away from the patient's zone of comfort (Box 1-11 ■). Ways to become more compassionate and culturally competent are to allow patients to teach us, to become active observers of how culturally diverse patients interact with each other, their spouses and family members, and with health professionals. Becoming keen observers of patient preferences, mannerisms, gestures, and facial expressions, reading about cultural groups, watching films and videos, reading novels about cultures different from one's own, and reading newspapers published by cultural groups will make health care workers more informed, empathetic, and better at what they do.[2]

Box 1-11   My Space/Your Space Exercise—Finding Your Comfort Zone

Having respect for an individual's personal space, or zone of comfort, is part of being a compassionate health care worker. The comfort zone of each person varies with gender, culture, and situation. However, most people feel uneasy when strangers are touching them or are "too close for comfort." An example of this uncomfortable sensation is standing in a crowded elevator. People take great measures to move so that they are not touching strangers, and, as people exit the elevator, the remaining people move and shift to provide more space around themselves. This same sense of uneasiness is felt by patients who are approached by unfamiliar health care workers.

To simulate a real patient–health care worker interaction, practice the following exercise with a coworker who is not a close friend. Eye contact should be made during this exercise.

1. Lie on a bed as if you are a patient.
2. Have the coworker slowly approach you. He or she should begin 10 feet away and pause between steps.
3. Note at what distance you begin to feel awkward or uncomfortable. (Usually, this distance is about 2 to 4 feet from the bed.) This distance is the boundary of your zone of comfort.
4. Repeat the exercise with the same coworker. You will probably require a smaller zone of comfort because a person becomes a little more at ease after initial contact with an unfamiliar person.

NEGATIVE BODY LANGUAGE AND DISTRACTING BEHAVIORS

Wandering Eyes

When people roll their eyes upward, they convey the sense of being bored, inattentive, or unwilling to perform a duty. The same can be said about gazing out the window or looking up at the ceiling. If a phlebotomist enters a patient's room and begins addressing the patient while looking out the window, the patient will feel neglected, and the phlebotomist will appear unconcerned. However, a friendly comment about the weather outside might be appropriate; then the phlebotomy procedure can be continued when full attention can be given to the patient. The objective is to make the patient feel at ease through good communication techniques so that the procedure can be successful.

Nervous Behaviors

Behaviors such as squirming or tapping a pencil or a foot can be very distracting. They can make a patient feel nervous, hurried, or anxious about the venipuncture. On the other hand, it is helpful to recognize these behaviors in patients too, especially children, so that efforts can be made to reduce fear. Allowing a few extra moments of conversation or preparation may help.

Breathing Pattern

A deep sigh can convey a feeling of boredom or a reluctance to do the job. Likewise, if a patient sighs deeply or moans at the mere sight of the phlebotomist, this should be a cue that a little extra attention, conversation, or a smile might ease the patient's reluctance for the procedure.

Other Distracting Behaviors

Many other actions can convey negative or defensive emotions from the perspective of the health care worker or the patient. Among these are crossed arms, a wrinkled forehead, frequent glances at a clock or watch, rapid thumbing through papers, chewing gum, yawning, or stretching. Health care workers should realize that these behaviors can detract from their professional image when they are communicating with patients, families, visitors, coworkers, and supervisors.

Active Listening

Another component of effective communication is the art of listening. **Active listening** helps close the communication loop by ensuring that the message sent can indeed be repeated and understood. Listening skills do not depend on intellect or educational background; they can be learned and practiced. Table 1-5 ■ provides tips for becoming an active listener in your professional and personal life. Because individuals can mentally process words faster than they can speak them, a good listener must focus on the speaker to keep his or her mind from wandering.

Listening carefully to the patient can have important ramifications in the test results. For example, the inpatient may have been instructed that he or she will be fasting or will have "nothing by mouth" until after the early morning blood collections. The phlebotomist should listen to patients' comments, such as, "I didn't have breakfast yet," and "they won't

Table 1-5	Steps for Active Listening
Get ready	Concentrate on the speaker by "getting ready" to listen. Take a moment to clear your mind of distracting thoughts. Begin the interaction with an open, objective mind. Taking a deep breath may help clear your mind and prepare it to receive information.
Pause occasionally	Use silent pauses in the conversation wisely to mentally review what has been said.
Verify that you are listening	Let the speaker know you are listening by using phrases, such as "I see," "Oh," "Very interesting," and "How about that."
Avoid making hasty judgments	Keep personal judgments to yourself until the speaker finishes relaying his or her idea. Listen for true meaning in the message, not just the literal words.
Provide feedback	Verify the conversation with feedback to make sure that everything was clear to the receiver. Ask for more explanation if necessary. Mentally review the key words to summarize the overall idea being communicated. Paraphrase the conversation to ensure complete understanding.
Notice body language	Pay attention to body language and ask for clarification. Simple prompts, such as "You look sad," and "You seem upset or nervous," can add more meaning to the conversation and encourage the speaker to verbalize feelings.
Maintain eye contact	Eye contact communicates interest or concern.
Use encouragement	Encourage the listener to expand his or her thoughts by using simple phrases, such as "Let's discuss it further," "Tell me more about it," and "Really?"
Practice, practice	Practice active listening at work and at home.

feed me." Even a question or comment about food may inspire a response to confirm that the patient was truly fasting. When in doubt, the phlebotomist can confirm that the patient has been fasting by simply asking the patient if he or she has eaten or had anything to drink other than water.

Telephone and Email Communications

Because the telephone is a vital communication tool for all health care facilities, it is important to follow the rules of good communication for incoming or outgoing calls. Some facilities have procedures for telephone communication such as those listed in Box 1-12 ■. In addition, regarding the use of personal cellular phones while at work, most health care facilities discourage the use of cellular phones (talking or texting) except during authorized meals or other short breaks.

Email communications are considered legal documents and are admissible in court cases, so it must be used in a highly professional manner. Follow the facility's policies for the authorized use of email related to transmission of patient data, departmental information, etc. In general, however, it is important to reply to email in a timely manner with accurate information and with the utmost concern for patient confidentiality. Avoid language that is offensive, obscene, or not factual, and avoid use of excessive symbols (e.g., !!!!!, ????, %$#!!).

Box 1-12	Guidelines for Telephone Communications

Incoming calls

1. Answer on the first ring if possible and no later than the third ring.
2. Try to smile as you answer, to reflect a positive tone of voice.
3. Speak clearly and courteously.
4. Identify the department or doctor's office: "Good morning, Dr. Jones's office."
5. Identify yourself by stating your name and/or title: "This is Ann, the phlebotomist."
6. Ask how you may help the caller: "How may I help you?" (Always use the word *may* instead of *can*.)
7. Acquire information from the caller using proper etiquette and record the date and time:
    a. "May I have your name, please?"
    b. "Could you please spell that?"
    c. "Could you repeat that, please?"
8. If you cannot provide the proper response, ask for assistance.
9. Before putting the caller on hold, give the caller an option to hold or leave a message. Ask the caller, "May I put you on hold for a few moments while I get the information?"
10. Do not keep the caller on hold for more than 30 seconds, or check back with the caller to see if he or she wants to continue holding.
11. Read the message back to the caller to ensure that you have the correct information. Double-check spellings, phone numbers (with area codes), and other pertinent information.
12. End the call in a professional manner with "Thank you." or "Good-bye.", do not use the phrase "No problem." Allow the caller to hang up first, just in case he or she may want to add something at the last minute.

Outgoing calls

1. Be prepared: have pencils, message pads, telephone set-up, and all information available prior to calling.
2. Do not call to socialize, and remember to use discretion with confidential information.
3. State your name, where you are calling from, and the purpose of your call.
4. Leave preferred times and phone numbers where you can be reached if a follow-up call is necessary.
5. Thank the receiver for taking your message.

Quality Assessment

QUALITY BASICS

The quality of phlebotomy services can encompass many factors that involve organizational structures, processes, outcomes, and customer satisfaction. The area where individual phlebotomists have the greatest impact is on constantly improving the services that are provided to stakeholders or customers. Quality improvement efforts for phlebotomy services often involve evaluating the following:

■ The health care worker's technique
■ Complications, such as hematomas

- Recollection rates resulting from contamination
- Multiple sticks on the same patient
- Turn around times (the time it takes from when the laboratory test is ordered to the time the final result is reported)

All these issues have the potential to result in a negative outcome for the patient. Thus, continuous improvement in minimizing these problems would be most beneficial to the patient and the health care worker.

EXAMPLES OF STAKEHOLDERS (CUSTOMERS) IN HEALTH CARE

Stakeholders are also considered to be "customers." External stakeholders are individuals or groups outside the organization; internal stakeholders are individuals or groups within a health care organization itself.

External Stakeholders:

- Local community
- Insurance companies and employers that pay for services
- Grant agencies and/or foundations that provide funding
- Federal or state agencies
- Accrediting agencies (such as The Joint Commission)
- Advocacy groups (such as AARP)

Internal Stakeholders (within the health care organization and/or specimen collection services):

- Inpatients and outpatients
- Patients's families and friends and support groups
- Clinical laboratory staff
- Pathologists and other medical doctors
- Students, research staff, and/or volunteers

A QUALITY PLAN FOR PHLEBOTOMY SERVICES

Quality assessment for phlebotomy involves reviewing structures, processes, outcomes, and customer satisfaction.

Assessments of structure—Physical or organizational properties of the settings where care is provided. Assessments of structural components include:

Physical structure—Facilities where services are provided, adequacy of supplies and equipment, safety devices, safety procedures, and availability and condition of equipment, such as computers, sterilizers, refrigerators, thermometers, centrifuges, autoclaves, and glucose-monitoring devices.

Personnel structure—Adequate numbers of personnel and support staff, ratios of staff to patients, qualifications of staff, and availability of the medical director or supervisors.

Management or administrative structure—Updated, available procedure manuals, adequacy of systems for secure record keeping, and open lines of communication throughout the organization.

Quality assessments of structural components may reveal potential problems that other assessments cannot. For example, the use of outdated blood collection tubes may cause faulty laboratory test results, even though the blood collection, testing, and reporting processes are perfect and the treatment plan for the patient is appropriate.

Assessment of processes—What is done to the patient or client. Process assessments are common throughout the specimen collection and clinical testing arenas and include procedures and skill assessment. This is where traditional **quality control** (QC) measures are applicable. Examples of QC measures that phlebotomists may be involved with are checking the expiration dates of supplies such as needles and specimen tubes, monitoring temperatures of specimen refrigerators, performing equipment checks for point-of-care instruments, performing preventive maintenance on centrifuges, and routine cleaning of surfaces where specimens are processed.

In addition to the normal laboratory data collection routines, however, other methods are effective for monitoring processes. These include evaluation of patient records for complications, correct technical skills, and correct documentation procedures; direct observation of practices; videotaping of health care interactions and practices; patient interviews; and questionnaires.

Assessments of outcomes—What is accomplished for the patient. Most outcomes assessments rely on information in the patient's medical record. Chart reviews usually evaluate the health status after services are provided. Timing is usually an important component of these measures. Outcomes assessments are typically the most difficult to measure and often relate to recovery rates, infection rates, incidence of **iatrogenic anemia** (anemia caused by the medical treatment, in this case by excessive blood removal), return to normal functions, and so on. Poor patient outcomes have been described as the "5 Ds": death, disease, disability, discomfort, and dissatisfaction.

Customer satisfaction—Knowing why customers are dissatisfied and which customers are unhappy. The study of satisfaction among patients is accomplished by using questionnaires, surveys, and telephone or personal interviews.

Clinical Alert ❗

Unfortunately, phlebotomists can have a negative impact on quality (the 5 Ds). For example, misidentification of a patient can result in an erroneous cross-match and blood transfusion, which could be fatal to a patient (death). Inappropriate cleansing techniques or hand hygiene could result in transmitting nosocomial infections (hospital-acquired disease). Repeated blood collections or drawing too much blood at one time can result in iatrogenic anemia. Poor venipuncture techniques, such as improper needle insertion or excessive probing, could result in nerve damage (disability) or severe pain (discomfort). And, lengthy waiting times, rude behavior, or messy work sites can contribute to a patient's negative feelings (dissatisfaction).

TOOLS AND PRACTICE EXERCISE FOR PERFORMANCE ASSESSMENT

In a laboratory, check sheets, run charts, and statistical tests can be used to review both the analytic and nonanalytic parts of the laboratory. The phlebotomist should be a routine part of quality and performance assessments.

Tools for implementing **continuous quality improvement (CQI)** include the following:[3]

- **Flow charts.**   Useful for breaking a process into its components so that people can understand how it works (Figure 1-12 ■).

- **Pareto charts.**   Bar charts that show the frequency of problematic events; the Pareto principle says that "80 percent of the trouble comes from 20 percent of the problems" (Figure 1-13 ■).

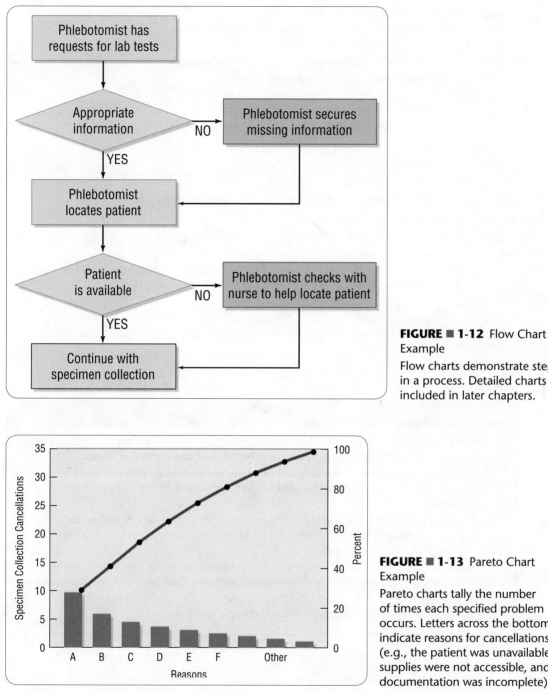

FIGURE ■ 1-12 Flow Chart Example

Flow charts demonstrate steps in a process. Detailed charts are included in later chapters.

FIGURE ■ 1-13 Pareto Chart Example

Pareto charts tally the number of times each specified problem occurs. Letters across the bottom indicate reasons for cancellations (e.g., the patient was unavailable, supplies were not accessible, and documentation was incomplete).

- **Cause-and-effect (Ishikawa) diagrams.**   Diagrams that identify interactions between equipment, methods, people, supplies, and reagents (Figure 1-14 ■).
- **Plan-Do-Check-Act cycle (PDCA).**   A cycle for assessing and making positive changes, then reassessing the effects of the change.
- **Line graphs, histograms, scatter diagrams.**   Pictorial images representing performance trends.
- **Brainstorming.**   Method used to stimulate creative solutions in a group (Box 1-13 ■).

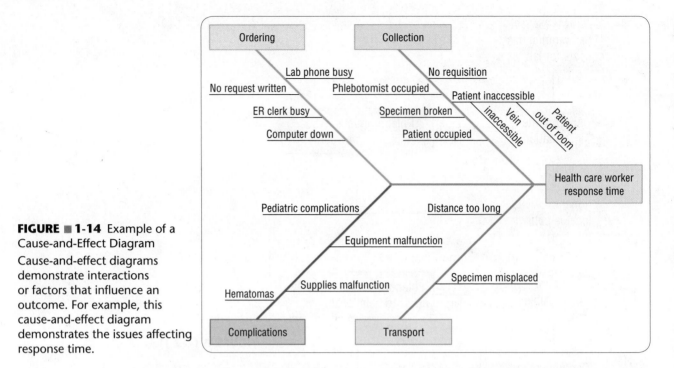

FIGURE ■ 1-14 Example of a Cause-and-Effect Diagram

Cause-and-effect diagrams demonstrate interactions or factors that influence an outcome. For example, this cause-and-effect diagram demonstrates the issues affecting response time.

Box 1-13	Brainstorming Exercise

1. Break into groups of no more than three or four people. Groups are preferred because they tend to come up with a greater number of, and more creative, ideas.
2. One group should take the viewpoint of a new phlebotomist, and the other group should take the viewpoint of the patient. (In brainstorming, there are no "wrong" answers!)
3. Consider the idea of "excellence" or "perfection" in a phlebotomy encounter. What quality factors are important from your point of view? List/discuss as many ideas as you can in about 10 minutes.
4. Come to a consensus about the order of importance of the factors. Make sure everyone in the group has a chance to participate and give their opinions about the order of importance.
5. Compare and discuss the lists from each group's viewpoint.

QUALITY IN SPECIMEN COLLECTION SERVICES

Phlebotomists can consider the clinical laboratory testing process in several phases, such as preanalytical, analytical, and postanalytical. These phases in specimen collection, processing, and testing are part of every laboratory's operation. For purposes of this text, the quality assessment discussion focuses on the preanalytical phases, where the phlebotomist has the most impact. Refer to Box 1-14 ■ to review examples of aspects of quality assessment for phlebotomy services. Box 1-15 ■ lists the basic requirements for a quality specimen. A periodic review of the laboratory's collection procedures and policies is recommended to reduce collection errors.

Box 1-14	Quality Assessments for Specimen Collection Services

- Worker response time (for inpatients)
- Patient waiting time (for outpatients)
- Time required for completion of the phlebotomy procedure
- Percentage of successful blood collections on the first attempt
- Number of successful blood collections on the second attempt
- Daily blood loss per patient due to venipunctures
- Number and size of hematomas
- Number of patients who faint
- Amount of time spent and number of telephone calls needed to acquire appropriate identification
- Number of redraws due to inadequate specimens
- Turnaround times of designated laboratory tests
- Frequency of incomplete data, documents, logs, and so forth
- Number of therapeutic drug-monitoring tests with incorrect timing documentation
- Number of specimens received in incorrect tubes
- Contamination rate for blood cultures
- Patient satisfaction questionnaires
- Frequency of complaints

Box 1-15	Basic Requirements for a Quality Specimen

Aspire to provide the highest quality patient specimens in a professional and safe environment 100 percent of the time. Be familiar with the following requirements:

1. Using standard precautions, identify, assess, and properly prepare the patient, and avoid medication interference if possible.
2. Collect specimens from the correct patients and label appropriately.
3. Use correct anticoagulants and preservatives and collect a sufficient amount of blood. Use devices that minimize accidental needlesticks.
4. Handle specimens carefully to prevent damage and/or hemolysis.
5. Collect fasting specimens in a timely fashion and verify that they are actually fasting samples. If they are not, note the condition.
6. Collect timed specimens at the right time and document accurately.
7. Allow specimens without anticoagulants to stand a minimum of 30 minutes, so that clot formation can be completed. (Some tubes, depending on the manufacturer, may shorten the time of clot formation.)
8. Transport specimens to the clinical laboratory in a timely fashion (within 45 minutes), and it is recommended that the blood cells be separated from serum or plasma within 2 hours. Document a list of the specimens that are delivered after the designated time limits, to help detect the source of the problem if necessary.

IMPORTANT FACTORS AFFECTING QUALITY

Anticoagulants and Preservatives

■ Phlebotomists use anticoagulants and preservatives in the collection of blood specimens. (A more thorough discussion is presented in Chapter 6.) Phlebotomists are responsible for filling the tubes in the correct order, so that carryover of anticoagulants to other tubes will not occur, and for mixing the specimens with the anticoagulant promptly after blood is drawn.

- When restocking the supply of collection tubes, phlebotomists should place the tubes with a shelf life (**expiration date**) nearest the current date at the front of the shelf so that these tubes are used first. The phlebotomist should be cognizant of expiration dates on any item used in specimen collection.

- Phlebotomists should know how to store or preserve specimen tubes if the blood specimen is not to be tested immediately.

Number of Blood Collection Attempts

- Many laboratories periodically monitor the number of unsuccessful blood collection attempts (i.e., the number of times a patient is stuck unsuccessfully). If a phlebotomist has had consecutively unsuccessful phlebotomy attempts on different patients, his or her blood collection technique must be reviewed, modified, and improved.

Blood Loss Due to Phlebotomy

- For adults, blood loss due to venipuncture is usually well tolerated physiologically because the volume constitutes a small percentage of the total blood volume in the body. However, in some cases, if patients are very ill, more laboratory tests are ordered, which results in more total blood collected. The same is true for neonates and infants. When too much blood is taken for laboratory analysis, the patient may become anemic, so blood conservation becomes a priority.

Clinical Alert !

If too much blood is withdrawn in a short period of time, a patient may become anemic and require a blood transfusion. This type of induced blood-loss resulting in anemia is called iatrogenic anemia. It is important to monitor daily blood loss if patients are neonates, have poor prognoses, or are being tested frequently. In these cases, the use of smaller test tubes and/or microcollection techniques is warranted.[4]

Self Study

Study Questions

The following questions may have more than one answer.

1. Examples of nonverbal, distracting behaviors include which of the following:

   a. tapping a pencil

   b. gazing outside the window

   c. direct eye contact

   d. glancing at the clock

2. Which of the following statements is/are inappropriate during a phlebotomy procedure?

   a. "This won't hurt a bit!"

   b. "Your name is Mrs. Jones, isn't it?"

   c. "You are required to cooperate with this."

   d. "Could you please spell your name for me?"

3. Which of the following are key elements in effective communication?

   a. active listening

   b. nonverbal cues

   c. verbal skills

   d. point-of-care procedures

4. Which of the following is the main area of responsibility for every phlebotomist?

   a. analytical testing

   b. data collection

   c. reporting results

   d. preanalytical processes

5. What feelings does one experience when a stranger gets "too close for comfort"?

   a. anxiety

   b. fear

   c. confidence

   d. security

For the following questions, select the one best answer.

6. What are "competency statements" for phlebotomists?

   a. verbal cues for patients

   b. entry-level skills, tasks, roles

   c. identification policies

   d. certification exam questions

7. Veracity is an essential character trait for a phlebotomist. Select the most appropriate example of what it means.

   a. being an impeccable dresser

   b. ability to tell a good story

   c. telling the truth

   d. performing well in harsh situations

8. How should a phlebotomist treat a patient who may have deafness?

   a. speak in a very loud voice

   b. ask the patient whether you should repeat the steps before proceeding

   c. tell the patient not to worry about anything

   d. assure the patient that "it won't hurt"

9. Why is eye contact helpful during a phlebotomist–patient interaction?

   a. it promotes a sense of trust

   b. it is an expression of authority

   c. it helps the patient focus on the phlebotomist's instructions

   d. it helps the phlebotomist read the patient's lips

10. Select the best example of internal stakeholders for clinical laboratory services.

   a. doctors and nurses

   b. health insurance companies

   c. advocacy groups

   d. accrediting agencies

Case Study

Mrs. Gonzales is an alert, ambulatory, 84-year-old patient who speaks English with a heavy Spanish accent. You observe that she argues about everything and does not seem to like anyone. Many of your coworkers are afraid to approach her, and you are assigned to collect her blood for laboratory analysis.

Questions

1. Describe what you would do or say to communicate with Mrs. Gonzales.

2. Identify factors that may be contributing to her anger or anxiety.

3. Describe what you might tell your coworkers about cultural issues affecting communication with Mrs. Gonzales.

Advocating Patient Safety Case Study

Positive and professional communication is essential in all aspects of health care. Mistakes can easily be made by simple misunderstandings. For example, phone communications for phlebotomy services are used for a variety of tasks for patients such as laboratory testing requests, coordinating timed specimens, laboratory results reporting, etc.

Question

List at least 3 examples of unprofessional or poor communication on a phone conversation and how these mistakes might jeopardize a patient's safety.

Competency Assessment

Check Yourself: Readiness for Phlebotomy Practice

1. Examine your lifestyle and character traits. List the values, beliefs, and traditions that are important to you. Think about how these might relate to your work as a phlebotomist. Which traits might be most beneficial in the work place (e.g., compassion, integrity)?

2. Based on your own experiences having blood specimens collected, can you think of ways to help improve the phlebotomy experience? Describe your impressions during a phlebotomy procedure.

3. Imagine yourself in 5 years. What do you expect to learn from being a phlebotomist?

4. Describe examples of communication styles (gentle, compassionate, assertive, aggressive, straight-to-the-point, etc.) that you like and dislike. Think about how you would change the negative styles to make them more positive. Which style of communication do you use the most?

Competency Checklist: Communication

This checklist can be completed in a classroom setting using a make-believe scenario or in the clinical setting during a patient interaction. The phlebotomist should do the following:

(1) Completed (2) Needs to improve/Repeat lesson and checklist

_____ 1. Demonstrate empathy for the patient.

_____ 2. Demonstrate respect for the patient's privacy, for their condition, for their family members.

_____ 3. Build trust by maintaining confidentiality and telling the truth.

_____ 4. Explain procedures clearly using simple terms appropriate to the age of the patient.

_____ 5. Establish rapport by being courteous and showing interest.

_____ 6. Listen actively by facing the patient, maintaining a nonauthoritative posture, establishing eye contact, and listening intently.

_____ 7. Provide specific feedback to the patient when appropriate.

Competency Checklist: Quality Basics

The phlebotomist should have an understanding of some fundamental factors related to providing quality services. The phlebotomist should do the following:

(1) Completed (2) Needs to improve/Repeat lesson and checklist

_____ 1. Provide 5 examples of stakeholders (customers).

_____ 2. Give one example of how a phlebotomist may have a negative effect on quality.

_____ 3. List 5 examples of quality improvement assessments that could be monitored for phlebotomy services.

_____ 4. Describe at least 3 examples of preanalytical factors that affect phlebotomy services.

References

1. Clinical and Laboratory Standards Institute (CLSI): Procedures for the Handling and Processing of Blood Specimens for Common Laboratory Tests; Approved Guideline—4th edition, Document H18-A4, CLSI, Wayne, PA, 2010.

2. Luckman J: *Transcultural Communication in Health Care.* Albany, NY: Delmar, 2000.

3. Graham NO: *Quality in Health Care: Theory, Applications, and Evolution.* Gaithersburg, MD: Aspen Publishers, 1995.

4. McPherson RA: Blood sample volumes: Emerging trends in clinical practice and laboratory medicine. *Clin Leader Manage Rev,* Jan/Feb 2001:3–10.

PEARSON
myhealthprofessionskit™

Go to www.myhealthprofessionskit.com to access the Companion Website created for this textbook. Simply select "Clinical Laboratory Science" from the choice of disciplines. Find this book and log in using your username and password to access interactive learning games, assessment questions, and more.

Chapter 2

Ethical, Legal, and Regulatory Issues

KEY TERMS

assault

battery

Clinical Laboratory
Improvement
Amendments (CLIA)

defendant

ethics

Health Insurance
Portability and
Accountability Act
(HIPAA)

informed consent

implied consent

liable

litigation process

malpractice

medical records

negligence

patient's confidentiality

plaintiff

CHAPTER OBJECTIVES

Upon completion of Chapter 2, the learner
should be able to do the following:

1. Explain how ethics and laws differ and
   describe their importance to health care
   providers.
2. Describe the basic functions of the
   medical record.
3. Define *informed consent* and *implied
   consent* and how they differ.
4. Describe how to avoid blood collection
   lawsuits.
5. Identify key components of the *Health
   Insurance Portability and Accountability
   Act (HIPAA)* and *Clinical Laboratory
   Improvement Amendments (CLIA)*.
6. Identify methods to maintain
   confidentiality of privileged information
   on patients.
7. Define the medicolegal terms related
   to phlebotomy procedures, policies,
   and protocols designed to avoid
   medicolegal problems.

Ethics and Laws

All health care workers are faced with ethical decisions at one time or another. **Ethics** are a set of principles or values based on religious and moral teachings. These ethics provide a standard of conduct by which a health care worker involved in blood collection guides his or her own actions and judges those of others (refer to Box 2-1 ■). Fairness and honesty are linked closely to the ethical values needed in the phlebotomy profession. But how do ethics and laws compare? Laws are a collection of rules to enforce order in a community, state, or other group. Laws have been developed for the community and society. An action can be moral but not legal, and vice versa. For example, an elderly paralyzed woman who is in a rehabilitation center stops breathing, and the health care professional does not attempt to take action so that the patient will start breathing again. This action is probably ethical if, on previous occasions, the patient had expressed a desire to die, but it could be questioned whether the action is legal.

To evaluate a difficult situation as a health care professional, the following questions should come to mind:

- Is this action legal?
- Does it foster a "win-win" situation with the patient and my supervisor?
- How would I feel about myself if I read this decision in the newspaper?
- Can I live with myself after making this decision, and is it right?

Basic Legal Issues

Patients know more about health care these days because of the Internet, the newspaper, and other sources. Thus, they are much more willing to sue anyone whom their lawyer believes has caused them harm in providing health care, including health care workers who are collecting blood specimens. Consider the following scenarios and ask yourself whether the health care worker has truly made an error and should be sued for the error due to malpractice.

Scenario 1: When a child refused to have his blood collection, the health care worker locked the child in the blood collection room, and the child was forced to have his blood collected.

Scenario 2: Two phlebotomists using a laboratory computer have accessed the electronic medical records of a friend and are discussing the friend's (patient's) medical condition.

Scenario 3: A health care worker performing bedside glucose testing misread the point-of-care (POC) glucose testing meter and wrote the wrong glucose results on the test reporting slip.

BOX 2-1   Example of Ethical Behavior for a Health Care Worker

If the health care worker realizes that he or she has made a mistake in identifying a patient and specimens, he or she faces an ethical decision about whether to report the mistake. Reporting it may result in disciplinary action against him or her.

- Each health care worker should go through the ethics check questions to see that the right ethical decision is to report his or her own mistake as soon as possible in order to avoid any medical treatment based on the wrong test results.

- This is the right decision because it creates a "win-win" situation for the patient and doctor, and, above all, it is simply the right thing to do. In addition, a lawsuit is less likely for the phlebotomist and the health care facility if the error is corrected and documented.

LEGAL TERMINOLOGY

If a health care worker understands words used for legal activities, this understanding can help to determine whether he or she is legally in trouble for activities that may occur in this field of health care. Such understanding can reduce the risk of legal action in health care activities.

It has been estimated that 44,000 to 98,000 Americans die each year as a result of medical errors.[1] Liability for causing harm or loss due to the lack of proper health care may be enforced on any health care worker, including health care institutions, physicians, nurses, laboratorians, patient care technicians, and phlebotomists. The number of lawsuits against health care workers as a result of improper care has grown in recent years as patients have become more sensitive to possible harmful effects of health care treatments.

Because the legal system is becoming more involved in health care, the health care worker should have some knowledge of basic legal terminology. A few major definitions with health care examples can be found in Box 2-2 ■.

NEGLIGENCE

In the past decade, the number of legal cases in which blood collectors have been directly or indirectly involved has increased noticeably and they have been related to negligence.[2] **Negligence** is "failure to provide proper care, resulting in injury to others."

Many things could be considered negligence if health care workers are not extremely careful. For example, there have been legal cases in which the confusion of patient samples led to a patient's death.[3]

MALPRACTICE

Malpractice, or professional negligence, is defined as improper care of a patient by a health care professional, resulting in injury to the patient. If the physician is the medical director overseeing clinical laboratory testing, in most cases he or she is responsible, under the law,

---

BOX 2-2 Legal Terminology

- **Assault.** Without permission, the attempt to touch a person or the threat to do so in such circumstances as to cause the other to believe that it will be carried out or to cause fear. An assault may be permissible if proper consent has been given (e.g., consent to obtain a blood specimen).
- **Battery.** The intentional touching of another person without permission (consent); also, the unlawful beating of another or carrying out of threatened physical harm. Because battery always includes an assault, the two are commonly combined in the phrase assault and battery. Liability of hospitals, physicians, and other health care workers for acts of battery is most common in situations involving lack of or improper consent to medical procedures, such as blood collection. For example, a small boy who refused to have his blood collected was locked in the blood collection room by the health care worker and was forced to have his blood collected by the health care worker. The patient's parents sued and won the lawsuit against the phlebotomist for this assault and battery.
- **Defendant.** The health care worker and/or institution against whom the action or lawsuit is filed.
- **Litigation process.** The process of legal action to determine a decision in court. Many malpractice cases are settled out of court.
- **Plaintiff.** The party (claimant) who brings a legal action (lawsuit).
- **Standard of care.** All health care workers must conform to a specific standard of care to protect patients. It is a measuring stick that represents the conduct of the average health care worker in the community. The community has become a "national" standard.

for all aspects of laboratory testing. Therefore, the health care worker collecting blood for laboratory tests could place both the physician and him- or herself at risk.

PATIENT'S CONFIDENTIALITY

Negligence cases can also occur when a health care worker abuses a **patient's confidentiality.** "No one except the patient may release patient results without a clinical need to know." Patient or employee laboratory test results must be considered strictly confidential. For example, negligence can be claimed if employees' or patients' drug abuse test results are released to anyone other than the attending physician or other authorized individuals. This is particularly true regarding employee or athlete drug or alcohol abuse screening and human immunodeficiency virus (HIV) testing. Confidential materials include communications between the physician and the patient, the patient's verbal statements, medical computer entries on patients, and nonverbal communications, such as laboratory test results.

CONFIDENTIALITY AND HIV EXPOSURE

An increasing concern for health care workers collecting blood from patients who are homebound is the health care worker's rights in relation to accidental exposure to blood or body fluids, whether by a needlestick or some other means. In some states, laws allow health care workers to know the identity of a patient who has acquired immunodeficiency syndrome (AIDS) or who is HIV positive. Many states, however, do not allow this sensitive patient information. A home health care worker who routinely collects blood specimens from homebound patients should obtain information about the state's law regarding confidentiality and HIV status.[4] It can be obtained from the health care worker's employer, from lawyers, or from a national or state health professional organization.

It is important to use the proper blood collection techniques with safety steps and required infection control procedures for homebound patients. If exposure to the blood occurs through a needlestick, a lancet, or another means, the home health care worker needs to obtain the patient's HIV status and information about other potential infectious diseases (e.g., hepatitis C), to ensure that the proper immediate and long-term self-protective procedural steps can be taken.

If employed by a health care facility, the health care worker should follow the guidelines established by the facility. If self-employed, it is important to see a health care provider for a postexposure protocol and follow-up. Also, counseling should be sought to obtain emotional support during this stressful time.

INFORMED CONSENT AND IMPLIED CONSENT

Informed consent is voluntary permission given by a patient to allow touching, examination, and/or treatment by health care providers. It allows patients to decide what will be performed on or done to their bodies. Without informed consent, intentional touching can be considered a criminal offense. Patients must be told about the possible positive and negative outcomes of having or not having particular medical treatments. An informed consent form is then signed by the patient to approve the medical treatment(s), including blood collection. Also, the form must have a witness signature (Figure 2-1 ■). Often in the doctor's office, the physician will want blood to be collected from the patient for diagnostic testing. If the patient agrees to allow the blood collection by the phlebotomist, the patient is giving the phlebotomist **implied consent** for the procedure. Essential to consent is the patient's belief that the health care worker to whom the consent is given has the knowledge and technical ability to properly perform the tasks. Thus, the patient can expect the blood collector to know the proper blood collection techniques and procedures. The patient does have the right to refuse the blood collection or any procedure. If that occurs, the phlebotomist needs to contact his/her supervisor or the physician regarding the patient's decision.

MEMORIAL HEALTH

COMPLETE ORIGINAL IN INK FOR HOSPITAL CHART
PATIENT MUST BE AWAKE, ALERT AND ORIENTED WHEN SIGNING

DATE: _____ TIME: _____ ☐ AM ☐ PM

I AUTHORIZE THE PERFORMANCE UPON _____
OF THE FOLLOWING OPERATION (state nature and extent): _____
_____
_____

TO BE PERFORMED UNDER THE DIRECTION OF DR. _____

1. I HAVE BEEN ADVISED THAT THERE IS A FAVORABLE LIKELIHOOD OF SUCCESS, BUT I UNDERSTAND THAT A COMPLETELY SUCCESSFUL OUTCOME MAY NOT BE ACHIEVABLE, AND THERE ARE NO GUARANTEES REGARDING THE OUTCOME. I ALSO UNDERSTAND THAT CERTAIN ADVERSE EVENTS COULD OCCUR AS A RESULT OF THE PERFORMANCE OF THE PROCEDURE OR TREATMENT, INCLUDING PAIN, INFECTION, LACERATION OR PUNCTURE OF INTERNAL ORGANS, BLEEDING, NERVE DAMAGE OR EVEN IN RARE CASES, DEATH. I UNDERSTAND THAT HOSPITALIZATION OR OTHER INSTITUTIONAL CARE, HOME CARE OR CARE BY HEALTH PROFESSIONALS MAY BE NEEDED FOLLOWING THE PROCEDURE OR TREATMENT, RELATED TO FULL RECOVERY, RECUPERATION OR CONVALESCENCE. I UNDERSTAND THE ALTERNATIVES TO THIS PROCEDURE, INCLUDING MY RIGHT TO REFUSE TO CONSENT TO IT, AND I NEVERTHELESS HAVE DECIDED TO CONSENT TO PERFORMANCE OF THE PROCEDURE OR TREATMENT.

2. I CONSENT TO THE PERFORMANCE OF OPERATIONS AND PROCEDURES IN ADDITION TO OR DIFFERENT FROM THOSE NOW CONTEMPLATED, WHETHER OR NOT ARISING FROM PRESENTLY UNFORESEEN CONDITIONS WHICH THE ABOVE NAMED DOCTOR OR HIS/HER ASSOCIATES OR ASSISTANTS MAY CONSIDER NECESSARY OR ADVISABLE IN THE COURSE OF THE OPERATION.

3. I CONSENT TO THE DISPOSAL BY HOSPITAL AUTHORITIES OF ANY TISSUES OR PARTS WHICH MAY BE REMOVED.

4. THE NATURE AND PURPOSE OF THE OPERATION/PROCEDURE, POSSIBLE ALTERNATIVE METHODS OF TREATMENT, THE RISK AND BENEFITS INVOLVED, AND THE COURSE OF RECUPERATION HAVE BEEN FULLY EXPLAINED TO ME. NO GUARANTEE OR ASSURANCE HAS BEEN GIVEN BY ANYONE AS TO THE RESULTS THAT MAY BE OBTAINED.

5. I UNDERSTAND AND AGREE WITH THE ABOVE INFORMATION. I HAVE NO QUESTIONS WHICH HAVE NOT BEEN ANSWERED TO MY FULL SATISFACTION. I UNDERSTAND THAT I HAVE THE RIGHT TO ASK FOR FURTHER INFORMATION BEFORE SIGNING THIS CONSENT.

I have crossed out any paragraph above which does not apply or to which I do not give consent.

PATIENT SIGNATURE: _____ WITNESS SIGNATURE: _____
(OR PARENT OR GUARDIAN IF PATIENT IS UNDER 18 YEARS OF AGE) *(OF PATIENT, PARENT OR GUARDIAN SIGNATURE)*

RELATIONSHIP: _____ WITNESS SIGNATURE: _____
☐ **TELEPHONE CONSENT** *(2ND WITNESS NEEDED FOR TELEPHONE CONSENT)*

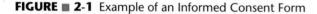

FIGURE ■ 2-1 Example of an Informed Consent Form

Clinical Alert ❗

- Children must have the informed consent of their parents or legal guardians for medical care, including blood collection.
- If a patient does not speak English, a consent form should be available in languages other than English or an interpreter may be necessary so that information for consent may be given in the patient's native language.
- States have laws requiring that informed consent be obtained before most HIV specimen collection and testing is performed. The laws state the type of information that must be given for the patient to be considered informed. This information includes:
  - A description of the laboratory test;
  - Possible uses of the HIV test; and
  - The meaning of the test results.

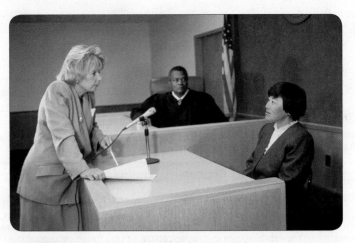

FIGURE ■ 2-2 Giving Testimony in a Lawsuit
Being involved in a lawsuit can be very unsettling for both the plaintiff and defendant
Source: Copyright © Dennis MacDonald/PhotoEdit

ADVICE TO AVOID LAWSUITS

Lawsuits are very expensive. Lawyers' fees typically range from $300 to $900 per hour, and other costs can lead to thousands of dollars in legal fees. In addition, lawsuits are time consuming and, most of all, emotionally draining (Figure 2-2 ■). Thus, to avoid a malpractice lawsuit, the health care provider should heed the advice in Box 2-3 ■.

BOX 2-3 Lawsuit Prevention Tips for Minimizing Risks	
Common Issues in Lawsuits against Health Care Providers	**Prevention Tips for Health Care Providers Involved in Blood Collection**
Documentation	Always document the time, date, and blood collector's initials on the blood collection containers.
Reporting of incidents	Document the information legibly and spell correctly. If an injury occurs to the patient and/or the blood collector before, during, or after blood collection, report the incident to your immediate supervisor and complete the appropriate documentation including the time, date, and place of the incident, the blood collection equipment and technique used, detailed steps that led to the incident and then the follow up that occurred to correct it. Any other details that can assist in this documentation should be included.
Failure to follow health care facility's procedure	Be knowledgeable and up-to-date on the policies and procedures in the health care facility.
Failure to ensure patient's safety	Check to see that the patient is okay during and after blood collection.
	Return bed rails to the raised position if the bed rails were raised before blood collection.
	Secure the patient in the blood collection chair for the complete blood collection procedure.

BOX 2-3	Lawsuit Prevention Tips for Minimizing Risks *(cont.)*

Common Issues in Lawsuits against Health Care Providers	Prevention Tips for Health Care Providers Involved in Blood Collection
	If an outpatient says that he or she faints during blood collection, have the patient lie down to collect blood and make the patient stay in that position for at least 20 minutes after collection before letting him or her stand up and leave the facility.
	Remove all supplies and equipment after the procedure.
Improper treatment and performance of treatment	Use proper techniques and equipment (e.g., gloves) when performing procedures.
	Update your collection skills and techniques through continuing education classes.
Failure to monitor and to report	Report any changes in a patient's condition (e.g., patient continues to bleed from the puncture site after blood collection).
Equipment use	Learn how to use blood collection equipment as designed.
	Use biohazardous waste containers as indicated in procedures.
	If involved in off-site blood collections, carry biohazardous waste containers.
	If involved in off-site collections, have the correct types and amounts of insurance coverage.
Training and continuing education	Document the health care professional training and continuing education that you have completed prior to and after obtaining employment in blood collection. In addition, pursue board certification in phlebotomy as a way to verify your quality assurance in blood collection knowledge.

Medical Records

Medical records are necessary for every patient. A health care worker cannot be expected to remember a patient from whom blood was collected 3 to 4 years ago. The medical records must be neat, legible, and accurate. They are extremely important if a medical malpractice case goes to court (Box 2-4 ■).

Medical records are also used for nonmedical reasons that are not directly tied to medical services, such as billing, utilization review, quality improvement, and so on.

Health care workers and their supervisors have a legal duty to keep records, documentation, and laboratory test results confidential. Medical record documentation is covered in more detail in Chapter 5.

BOX 2-4	Purpose of Medical Records

Medical records have four basic purposes:

1. To monitor for continuous patient care;
2. To provide a record of the patient's illness and treatment;
3. To provide a method of communication between the physician and the health care team; and
4. To provide a legal document that can be used by patients and by hospital or health care workers to protect them in a possible lawsuit and for regulatory agency compliance.

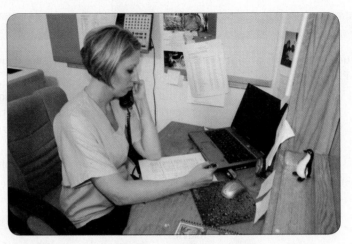

FIGURE ■ 2-3 Proper Documentation
Proper electronic or written documentation of laboratory test
results into medical records is extremely important.

HIPAA

The federal **Health Insurance Portability and Accountability Act (HIPAA)** (Figure
2-3 ■) was created in 1996 to protect the privacy and confidentiality of every patient's medical
information.[5] HIPAA requires that health care providers obtain a patient's written consent
before transferring the patient's medical information for routine uses that include diagnosis,
treatment, and payment. Thus, each laboratory must give patients information about their
rights and about the ways in which their laboratory test results will be used.[6] Health care
workers involved in blood collection must have HIPAA training and then sign an agreement
that indicates that they know that privacy and confidentiality are basic rights in our society
and that these rights must be protected for all patients.

This signature verifies that they will:

- keep the confidentiality of all patients' information, including lab tests to be performed;
- keep the computer password for entering the laboratory patients' database secure
  from others' knowledge; and
- maintain the confidentiality of patients' information when looking at the computer
  database of patients' medical record information.

Some examples of seemingly innocent activities that can lead to lawsuits include:

- Discussing patient information with a patient's family member without the patient's
  permission.
- Throwing laboratory test requests into the regular trash.
- Not logging off the computer after entering blood collection updates.
- Sending a patient's laboratory test requests to be printed and forgetting to take it off
  the printer.

Legal Cases Related to Clinical
Laboratory Activities

Most phlebotomy cases are settled after a lawsuit is filed but before the court passes down
a judgment. The following sections discuss cases that are of interest to health care workers
involved in blood collection.

DELMETREA SALTER v. DEACONESS FAMILY MEDICAL CENTER ET AL

A heated washcloth was placed on the heel of an infant to facilitate collecting blood from his heel. The washcloth was placed in a microwave oven to heat it prior to placing on the infant. The infant sustained second degree burns from the heated cloth. Professional negligence on the part of the health care worker performing the blood collection procedure was the outcome with an award of damages of $125,000 for past pain and suffering.

LAZERNICK v. GENERAL HOSPITAL OF MONROE COUNTY (PA 1977)

A patient who was pregnant for the first time had her blood typed in January 1971. The report sent to her physician indicated that her blood type was A positive. The patient gave birth to her second child in June 1977. The child was brain damaged and paralyzed on the right side of the body as a result of hemolytic blood disease. The laboratory records in 1971 and 1977 showed that the mother's blood type was O negative. In a malpractice suit, the parents charged that the physician's and his employee's negligence caused the child's injuries. The physician, who was chief of the laboratory when the blood test was performed, was found **liable,** as was the health care worker.

HELMANN v. SACRED HEART HOSPITAL

Failure to follow proper isolation techniques, such as proper handwashing and prevention of cross-contamination, is a major area of concern for hospitals. The patient in *Helmann* v. *Sacred Heart Hospital* (62 Wash. 2d 136, 381 P. 2d 605 [1963]) had multiple fractures in the area of the left hip socket. After surgery on his hip, he was returned to a semiprivate room. His roommate complained of a sore under his right arm. After 11 days in the same room, it was determined that the roommate had a highly contagious wound infection caused by *Staphylococcus aureus.* The infected roommate was immediately placed in an isolation unit. For the preceding 11 days, however, the hospital attendants had administered care to both patients without washing their hands between patient care.

   The patient with the hip injury developed a *Staphylococcus aureus* infection at the site of his hip incision. The infection penetrated into the hip socket, destroying tissue and leading to additional surgery and the hip being fused into a nearly immovable position. The patient with the hip injury won a malpractice lawsuit against the health care workers and the hospital for negligent care.

Cases Resulting from Improper Technique and Negligence

Health care workers who collect blood by venipuncture must be thoroughly trained and skilled in proper techniques, safety, and the use of collection equipment. Problems that can arise include:

■ Wristband or identification error

■ Hematoma (hemorrhage from inadequate pressure to the vein after the venipuncture)

■ Abscess at the puncture site

■ Patient falling

■ Patient fainting before, during, or after blood collection procedure

- Nerve damage
- Emotional distress
- Complications from collecting blood from the arm on the same side as a mastectomy (removal of breast)

In one case, settled out of court, a health care worker had not received proper blood collection training. She performed a venipuncture by inserting the needle approximately 2 inches above the antecubital fold. The needle went through the vein, through muscle, and into the nerve, severely injuring the patient's arm, which remained permanently damaged even after three surgeries to repair the damage caused by the resultant hematoma and nerve injury.

Another case involved a medical technologist under pressure to collect specimens from ambulatory patients as quickly as possible. One of the patients stated before blood collection that she had fainted during blood collection at a previous time. The phlebotomist, however, took no precautions to avoid syncope, collected the patient's blood, and allowed the patient to leave immediately. The patient fainted at the elevator and suffered a permanent loss of smell and a permanent "ringing sound" in her ears.

In another case, a health care worker collecting bedside glucose results misread the glucometer and caused the deaths of three patients with diabetes. The errors might have been avoided with better training, supervision, and quality monitoring.

In yet another case, a phlebotomist collected blood at an excessive angle of needle insertion from the patient's basilic vein when the median cubital vein was clearly an option for collection. The blood collection resulted in injury to the patient's median nerve and a malpractice lawsuit. In addition, documentation errors were evident for the collection. In all, the patient was awarded thousands of dollars for the health care worker's violations of proper standards of care.[7]

HIV-Related Issues

If a health care worker becomes infected with HIV during employment at a health care facility, workers' compensation benefits are usually available. The health care worker should follow the guidelines established by the facility. The health care worker must demonstrate a causal connection between his or her HIV infection and his or her employment. This causal connection includes having a documented incident report at the health care facility involving a needlestick injury, a puncture wound, or other exposure to HIV-contaminated blood or body fluids. In addition, the health care worker's lifestyle will be investigated to determine whether the exposure occurred elsewhere. Pre-employment health evaluations may prove to be useful later should the health care worker allege contraction of infection during the time of employment. Employers are legally responsible for monitoring postexposure management and treatment.

If a health care worker resigns because of contracting AIDS, unemployment benefits may be available if the worker can show that he or she believed in good faith that continued employment would jeopardize his or her health.

Malpractice Insurance

The new focus on medical errors and patient safety in the health care facilities has affected the need of health care workers to have malpractice insurance.[8] Because hospitals are places where seriously ill patients are admitted and treated with highly sophisticated medical technology, the likelihood for problems, including medical errors is greater there than in other health care settings. Often, the health care staff in the hospital or clinical laboratory

---

BOX 2-5 Purchasing Malpractice Insurance

If the health care worker decides to purchase malpractice insurance, the following factors should be carefully considered:[10]

1. Does the health care facility carry liability insurance for the health care worker?
2. Is adequate dollar value coverage provided? In recent lawsuits, total damages of $1 million or more have been awarded against physicians.
3. What are the coverage limitations? How much does one have to lose if sued?
4. What are the procedures that must be followed for the policy to provide coverage? The health care worker should not assume that the lawyers representing the hospital, laboratory, or clinic will have his or her best interests at heart. The attorney's first obligation is to serve those who have hired him or her. There have been cases in which the hospital was cleared of all charges but the health care professional was held liable for damages.
5. Is a job change expected soon?
6. Are specimen collecting services provided off-site or in patients' homes?

---

is covered by a blanket malpractice insurance policy. If, however, the health care worker is employed by a physician who has a contract with an institution or owns a clinic, the staff may be protected by the physician's malpractice insurance policy.

Health care workers, in the past, have not been the targets of lawsuits because they do not carry malpractice insurance and do not have as much money as hospitals have. The advances in technology and increased complexity of health care, however, have increased legal exposure for allied health and nursing professionals. The health care worker who routinely deals with the public in patient–health care worker relationships is indeed liable. Therefore, each individual should examine the possibility of malpractice suits and the need for malpractice insurance from a personal standpoint (Box 2-5 ■).[9]

The lawyer's fee and court costs are usually covered if professional liability insurance is bought. Some professional organizations offer professional liability insurance at a reduced rate. A record of continuing education courses, seminars, workshops, and academic credits should be a part of each health care worker's personal file.

Clinical Laboratory Improvement Amendments (CLIA)

In October 1988, the U.S. Congress passed Public Law 100-578, **Clinical Laboratory Improvement Amendments (CLIA).**[11] These regulations are enforced to ensure the quality and accuracy of laboratory testing. CLIA '88 essentially applies to every clinical laboratory testing facility in the United States and requires laboratory certification by the federal government. The certification requires an inspection by federal and/or state agencies to determine whether the laboratory testing facility uses methods to test patients' specimens that lead to accurate, reliable, and good-quality test results. The blood collection procedures area is a major part of CLIA inspections, because it has been found that most laboratory errors occur during the preanalytical (specimen collection and handling) phase of testing.

Self Study

Study Questions

For the following questions, select the one best answer.

1. A blood collector was performing a venipuncture on a prison inmate in the state hospital when the prisoner (patient) suddenly pulled the needle and adapter from his arm and jabbed the blood collector in the arm. When should the blood collector report this incident?
   a. after seeing the employee health physician
   b. after 24 hours to see whether the needlestick is healing
   c. immediately
   d. at the end of the work shift

2. A legal term for allowing the phlebotomist to touch the patient for blood collection after the patient agrees to the blood collection is:
   a. assault and battery
   b. battery
   c. implied consent
   d. negligence

3. Specimen collection and handling is referred to as
   a. analytical phase
   b. preexamination phase
   c. postexamination phase
   d. analytical prephase

4. The federal law that regulates the quality and accuracy of laboratory testing (including blood collection) through certification inspections is referred to as
   a. CLIA '88
   b. FDA
   c. EPA
   d. CMS

5. Malpractice in blood collection is the same as
   a. professional negligence
   b. informed consent
   c. battery
   d. criminal action

6. The measuring stick representing the conduct of the average health care worker is the
   a. community where the health care provider works
   b. community where the health care provider lives
   c. national community
   d. international community

7. A phlebotomist wanted to look up her friend's laboratory tests' results on the laboratory computer and used a colleague's password to enter the laboratory access files to access the tests' results. What law has she violated?
   a. OSHA
   b. HIPAA
   c. no law has been violated, because she was checking on blood tests for a patient
   d. CLIA

8. For potential lawsuits that may occur in the health care facility, which of the following must be maintained in the health care worker's employee file?
   a. number of patients from whom the health care worker has collected blood during the preceding year
   b. names of patients from whom the health care worker has collected blood during the preceding year
   c. record of continuing education courses
   d. whether the health care worker has additional jobs other than the one at the health care facility

9. The intentional touching of another person without permission is considered to be
   a. assault
   b. battery
   c. malpractice
   d. negligence

10. Before a patient's laboratory test results can legally be released, the patient must
   a. tell his or her physician that it is okay
   b. express verbal permission to the laboratory receptionist
   c. provide written consent
   d. provide written consent from his or her lawyer

Case Study

The health care worker, Ms. Garner, was in the ambulatory clinic and was going to collect blood from Ms. Ann Cardo for a prothrombin time (PT) and chemistry profile. After Ms. Garner prepped the arm for the venipuncture, she inserted the needle into the arm; as she did, Ms. Cardo screamed and jumped with apparent pain. Apparently, because of the needle insertion at the time of the patient's jump, the needle went through the vein and deeper into the arm. The patient screamed again, and then Ms. Garner released the tourniquet and pulled the needle back out of the arm. She placed gauze on the venipuncture site and also applied pressure with her fingers to the site as she raised the patient's arm. After a few minutes, she checked the venipuncture site and a large hematoma (mass of clotted blood under the skin) had developed.

Questions
1. What should Ms. Garner do next?
2. What corrective actions, if any, should be taken?
3. What legal situations might arise from this situation?

Advocating Patient Safety Case Study

A phlebotomist became infected with HIV from a needlestick injury. After aggressive treatment at the health care institution where she obtained the needlestick injury, she requested to go back to work as a phlebotomist.

Question
What are the legal issues involved in her returning to work?

Competency Assessment

Check Yourself: Ready to Collect Blood

1. Review in your mind the blood collection steps to follow each time you approach a patient to collect blood, and recall the prevention tips for minimizing risks for patient injury and lawsuits as you prepare for the next blood collection.

2. You are having a quick coffee break with your new coworker in the hospital cafeteria where both of you work. Your coworker starts the conversation with the topic of the Hepatitis C positive patient in Room 617 that he had to collect blood from this morning. Describe what you should say at this point in the conversation.

Competency Checklist: Ethical, Legal, and Regulatory Issues

This checklist can be completed as a group or individually.

(1) Completed (2) Needs to improve/Repeat lesson and checklist

_____ 1. List four common issues in lawsuits against health care providers.

_____ 2. List four problems that have occurred in patients as a result of negligence on the part of the phlebotomist.

_____ 3. List two differences between ethics and laws.

References

1. Kohn L, Corrigan J, Donaldson M, eds. *To Err Is Human: Building a Safer Health System.* Washington, DC: National Academics Press, 2000.

2. Kozier B, Erb G, Berman A, Snyder S: *Fundamentals of Nursing–Chapter Four: Legal Aspects of Nursing.* Upper Saddle River, NJ: Prentice Hall Publishers, 2004.

3. *Parker* v. *Port Huron Hospital,* 105, N.W. 2d 854, 1981.

4. Brent NJ: Confidentiality and HIV status: The nurse's right to know. *Home Healthcare Nurse* 1990; 8(3): 6–8.

5. U.S. Congress. *Health Insurance Portability and Accountability Act of 1996,* 18th Cong., 2nd sess. Rep. 64.

6. Travis J: Complying with HIPAA: Are you ready? *ADVANCE Med Lab Professionals* 2003; 15(4): 16–18, 25.

7. Ernst D: Phlebotomy on trial. *MLO* April 1999: 46–50.

8. Mello M: *Understanding medical malpractice insurance: A primer,* Robert Wood Johnson Foundation Research Synthesis Report #3, January, 2000, pp. 7–8.

9. Pozgar GD: *Legal Aspects of Health Care Administration.* Gaithersburg, MD: Aspen Publishers, 1993.

10. Markus K: Your legal risk in giving advice or care. *Healthweek* October 6, 1997: 5.

11. Clinical Laboratory Improvement Amendments of 1988 (CLIA): Final Rule for the Centers for Medicare & Medicaid Services CMS-2226F. *Fed. Register* January 24, 2003. Available at: http://www.cms.hhs.gov/CLIA/.

PEARSON
myhealthprofessionskit™

Go to www.myhealthprofessionskit.com to access the Companion Website created for this textbook. Simply select "Clinical Laboratory Science" from the choice of disciplines. Find this book and log in using your username and password to access interactive learning games, assessment questions, and more.

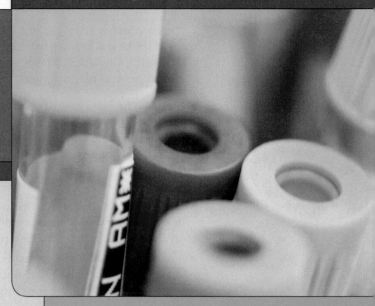

Chapter 3

Basic Medical Terminology, the Human Body, and the Cardiovascular System

KEY TERMS

antecubital
anterior
aorta
arteriole
artery
atria
blood cells
blood volume
capillary
cerebrospinal fluid
cv system
distal
dorsal
hematology
hematopoiesis
hemostasis
homeostasis
iatrogenic anemia
immunology
invasive
lateral
lipemic

medial
microbiology
osteoporosis
pathogenesis
pathology
phlebotomy
pleural fluid
posterior
proximal
pulmonary arteries/
    veins
steady state
superficial
synovial fluid
turbid
vascular
veins
vena cavae
ventral
ventricle
venules

CHAPTER OBJECTIVES

Upon completion of Chapter 3, the learner should be able to do the following:

1. Define word elements such as roots, prefixes, and suffixes.
2. Combine elements to make words and divide complex words into these elements.
3. Define basic terms used in the laboratory.
4. Describe the basic functions of the cardiovascular system.
5. Identify chambers of the heart and major heart blood vessels.
6. Distinguish the characteristics of arterial, venous, and capillary blood.
7. Locate the veins most commonly used for phlebotomy.
8. Define *hemostasis* and list five basic steps in the coagulation (blood clotting) sequence.

Basic Medical Terminology

To be an effective member of a health care team, one must learn how to pronounce basic medical terms and know what they mean. Medical terminology becomes easier with practice and by using fundamental tools to understand how words are formed. Medical terms/words consist of several parts:

■ **Root**—The main part of the word that describes what the word is about; for example, *cardio-* is the word root for heart, so every time a medical term contains cardio-, it means it has something to do with the heart, and *phleb-* is a word root relating to vein. Thus, the root provides the medical meaning. Knowing the meaning of roots allows knowledge about the word without having to look it up each time you see it in a medical term.

■ **Prefix**—A word element that is added *before* the root, at the *beginning of the word*. It makes the word more specific; for example, *endo-* is the prefix meaning inside. Not every medical term contains a prefix.

■ **Suffix**—A word element that is added *after* the root, at the *end of the word*. It also adds to the meaning of the root; for example, *-itis* is the suffix for inflammation, and *-tomy* is the suffix for cut or incision. Most medical terms contain a suffix.

■ **Combining vowel**—Sometimes a vowel (usually i, o, u, or y) is added to make a word easier to pronounce.

Combining the examples used above would result in the words:

endocarditis (endo/card/itis), which means an inflammation of the inside lining of the heart. In this example, there was no need to add a combining vowel.

phlebotomy (phleb/o/tomy), which means a cut or incision into the vein. In this example, the *o* in the middle helps make the pronunciation easier.

When different prefixes or suffixes are added to the word root, the meaning changes. You can build a huge medical vocabulary by learning the meanings of word parts and how to combine them (Figure 3-1 ■ and Tables 3-1 ■, 3-2 ■, and 3-3 ■).

Tables 3-1 and 3-3 list selected prefixes and suffixes and their meanings that you will use as you build medical terms. The word roots listed in Table 3-2 are used to build medical terms that relate to the cardiovascular system.

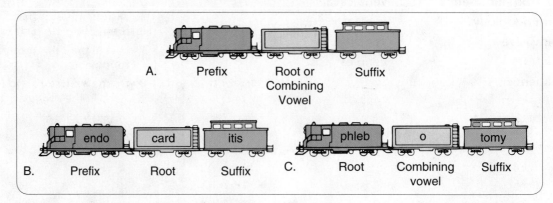

FIGURE ■ 3-1 Word Elements in Medical Terminology

Table 3-1	**Primary Word Elements: Prefixes**	
Prefixes That Pertain to Position, Location, Direction, or Placement		
ab away from	**epi** upon, above	**intra** within
ad toward	**ex** out, away from	**meso** middle
ana up	**extra** outside, beyond	**para** beside
ante before	**hyper** above, excessive	**retro** backward
cata down	**hypo** below, deficient	**sub** below, under
circum, peri around	**infra** below	**supra** above, beyond
endo within, innermost	**inter** between	**trans** across, through
Prefixes That Pertain to Numbers, Amounts, or Speed		
ambi both	**hyper** above, more than normal	**primi** first
bi two, double		**quadri** four
brady slow	**hypo** below, deficient	**quint** five
centi a hundred	**milli** one-thousandth	**semi, hemi** half
deca ten	**mono** one, single	**tachy** fast
dipl double	**multi** many, much	**tetra** four
di(s) two	**nulli** none	**tri** three
	poly many	**uni** one
Prefixes That Are Descriptive and Are Used in General		
a, an without, lack of	**dys** bad, before, difficult	**micro** small
ante, anti, contra against	**eu** good, normal	**nephr** related to kidney
auto self	**hepat** related to liver	**oligo** scanty, little
brachy short	**hetero** different	**pan** all
brady slow	**homeo** similar, same	**pseudo** false
cac, mal bad	**hydro** water	**re** again and again
de reversal of, without	**mal** bad, inadequate	**sym, syn** together
dia through	**mega** large, great	

Adapted from S. Turley, *Medical Language* 2nd ed. Upper Saddle River, NJ: Pearson, 2011.

Table 3-2	**Primary Word Roots Related to the Cardiovascular System***		
Root	**Meaning**	**Root**	**Meaning**
ang/i, angi/o, vas/o	vessel	**infarct**	infarct (necrosis of an area)
angin	to choke	**lipid**	fat
arter	artery	**logos**	study
arteri/o	artery	**man/o**	thin
ather/o	fatty substance or deposit	**my/o**	muscle
capillus	hairlike	**phleb**	vein
card	heart	**phleb/o**	vein
card/i, cardi/o	heart	**pulmonar**	lung

continued

Table 3-2	Primary Word Roots Related to the Cardiovascular System (*cont.*)		
Root	**Meaning**	**Root**	**Meaning**
cubitum	elbow, forearm	**rrhyth**	rhythm
cyte	cell	**scler**	hardening
derm	skin	**sera**	serum
diastol/o	dilating	**sphygm/o**	pulse
electr/o	electricity	**steth/o**	chest
embol	to cast, to throw	**systol/o**	contracting
erg/o	work	**tens**	tension
erythr/o	red	**thromb**	clot
hem/o	blood	**ven/i**	vein

Adapted from S. Turley, *Medical Language* 2nd ed. Upper Saddle River, NJ: Pearson, 2011.
*For simplicity and better learning, sometimes a combining vowel is included with the root.

Table 3-3	Primary Word Elements: Suffixes

Suffixes That Pertain to Pathologic Conditions

-algia, dynia pain	**-plegia** paralysis, stroke	**-ptysis** spitting
-cele hernia, tumor, swelling	**-ptosis** drooping	**-rrhage** bursting forth
-emesis vomiting	**-oma** tumor	**-rrhagia** bursting forth
-itis inflammation	**-osis** condition of	**-rrhea** flow, discharge
-lysis destruction, separation	**-pathy** disease	**-rrhexis** rupture
-megaly enlargement, large	**-penia** deficiency	
-oid resemble	**-phobia** fear	

Suffixes Used in Diagnostic and Surgical Procedures

-centesis surgical puncture	**-opsy** to view	**-stasis** control, stopping
-desis binding	**-plasty** surgical repair	**-stomy** surgically created opening
-ectomy surgical excision	**-plexy** surgical fixation	
-gram a weight, or picture	**-rrhaphy** suture	**-therapy** treatment
-graph to write, record	**-scope** instrument	**-tome** instrument to cut
-meter, metry measure	**-scopy** to view	**-tomy** incision

Suffixes That Are Used in General

-blast immature cell, germ cell	**-phasia** to speak	**-pnea** breathing
-cyte cell	**-philia** attraction	**-poiesis** formation
-ist one who specializes, agent	**-phraxis** to obstruct development	**-therapy** treatment
-logy study of		**-trophy** nourishment, development
-lysis breaking, destroying	**-physis** growth	
-phagia to eat	**-plasia** formation, produce	**-uria** urine

Adapted from S. Turley, *Medical Language* 2nd ed. Upper Saddle River, NJ: Pearson, 2011.

BASIC RULES FOR COMBINING WORD ELEMENTS

Medical terms are different from everyday English language because they sound different, they come primarily from Greek or Latin origins, there can be more than one word element for a particular meaning, and changing a simple prefix or suffix can change the entire meaning (Box 3-1 ■). Many terms for the body's organs or structures originate from Latin; for example, *vessel* comes from the Latin word *vascillum,* or little vessel; and **capillary** originates from *capillus,* or hairlike. Most of the terms that describe diseases originate from

Box 3-1	Using Common Suffixes

Following are some examples of the usage of common suffixes. The suffix *-logy* is commonly used in health care and means "the study of" and *-itis* means "inflammation of the."

Term	The Study of:
Cardiology	Diseases of the heart, arteries, veins, and capillaries
Cytology	Cellular structure and functions
Dermatology	Skin
Endocrinology	Diseases of the endocrine (glands and hormones) system
Gastroenterology	Diseases of the intestinal or digestive system
Gynecology	Diseases of the female reproductive system
Hematology	Blood
Histology	Microscopic structures of tissues
Immunology	Diseases of the immune system
Microbiology	Microbes
Nephrology	Diseases of the kidney and urinary system
Neurology	Diseases of the nervous system
Oncology	Tumors and cancer therapy
Parasitology	Parasites
Pathology	Pathogens or disease causing agents
Serology	Antibodies in the serum
Urology	Urinary system
Virology	Viruses

Term	Inflammation of the:
Appendicitis	Appendix
Dermatitis	Skin
Hepatitis	Liver
Meningitis	Meninges
Osteomyelitis	Bone

Greek: for example, *lipo-* means fat and *-oma* means tumor, so *lipoma* means a fatty tumor; *hepat-* means liver and *-itis* means inflammation, so *hepatitis* means inflammation of the liver.[1] A few basic rules make medical terminology easier to learn and use and help us to avoid mistakes.

- Practice using medical terminology with someone who is familiar with the correct pronunciation. A study partner can give you tips about the sound of the word so that confusion is avoided. It is even recommended that you read this section out loud. Following are some basic tips on pronunciation:
  - *ch* sounds like *k;* for example, chronic (kro-nic)
  - *ps* sounds like *s;* for example, psychology (si-kol-o-ji)
  - *pn* sounds like *n;* for example, pneumonia (nu-mo-ni-a)
  - *c* sounds like an *s* when it comes before e, i, and y; for example, cytoplasm (si-to-plazm), centrifuge (sen-tri-fuj)
  - *g* sounds like *j* when it comes before e, i, and y; for example, generic (jen-er-ik)
  - *i* sounds like *eye* when added to the end of a word to form a plural; for example, bacilli (ba-sil-li), bronchi (bron-ki)
- The combining vowel is most often an *o.* For example, **osteoporosis** (oste/o/por/osis) is a condition in which the bone becomes porous. It is easier to say with the addition of the *o* than to say "osteporosis."
- When changing a word from singular to plural, substitute the plural endings as follows:
  - *-ax* as in thorax to *-aces* as in thoraces
  - *-nx* as in phalanx to *-ges* as in phalanges
  - *-en* as in foramen to *-ina* as in foramina
  - *-is* as in crisis to *-es* as in crises
  - *-ix* as in appendix to *-ices* as in appendices
  - *-on* as in spermatozoon to *-a* as in spermatozoa
  - *-um* as in ovum to *-a* as in ova
  - *-us* as in nucleus to *-i* as in nuclei
  - *-y* as in **artery** to *-i* and add *-es* as in arteries or phlebotomy to phlebotomies

Terms for Anatomical Direction and Position

Anatomical terms provide a description of the body's landmarks. These terms are helpful during an assessment of a patient to make the patient's condition understandable to others. The following terms may be useful when describing or evaluating a venipuncture complication, an interfering surgical wound site, the location of a vein or artery, or a potential venipuncture site (see Figure 3-2 ■ and Box 3-2 ■).

- **Anterior**—The front of the body (example: I will draw blood from the *anterior* side of the arm.)
- **Posterior**—Toward the back of the body (example: There is a large bandage on the *posterior* side of the arm.)
- **Medial**—Toward the midline; opposite of a lateral direction (example: The heart is *medial* to the right shoulder.)
- **Lateral**—Toward the sides of the body; opposite of medial direction (example: The hip is *lateral* to the navel.)

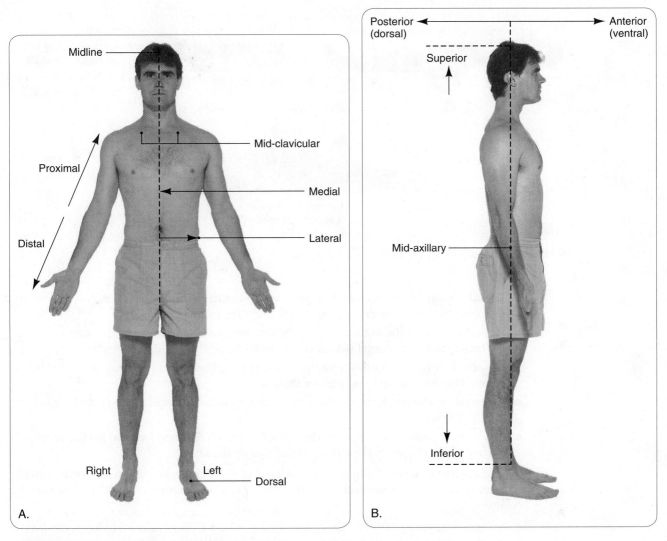

FIGURE ■ 3-2 Terms Related to Body Orientation

Body movements and locations can be described in terms related to imaginary planes that divide the body. A. The sagittal plane (midline) divides the body into two halves. B. The plane that divides the body into front and back is referred to as the superior/inferior plane or cranial/caudal plane.

Box 3-2	Right and Left Sides: The Patient's or the Health Care Worker's?

When speaking with patients, health care workers should refer to the *patient's right* and the *patient's left* sides. This comes up when the health care worker asks to see a patient's right or left arm prior to vein selection for venipuncture. Even though the task seems easy, some health care workers confuse right and left arms when they are face to face with a patient. Practice by facing a friend and pointing to the friend's right and left side until it is done correctly each time. Do not confuse your own right and left side with the patient's right or left side. This task becomes important when there are specific instructions to collect a blood specimen from only one side of a patient because of a clinical condition.

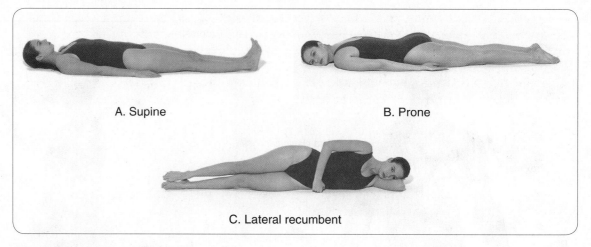

A. Supine

B. Prone

C. Lateral recumbent

FIGURE ■ 3-3 Anatomical Positions

- **Distal**—Away from the center or point of attachment (example: The rash was spreading distal to the elbow and all the way to her fingers.)
- **Proximal**—Near the center or point of attachment; opposite of distal (example: Her leg broke on the proximal side of the knee.)
- **External or Superficial**—Near the surface of the body (example: *Superficial* veins are easily missed unless you feel for them.)
- **Internal or Deep**—Far from the surface of the body (example: Major arteries are in the *deep* tissues.)
- Other terms sometimes used are **dorsal** for the back side and **ventral** for the front side (example: The lesion was on the *ventral* side of the knee.)

Terms that describe body positioning can help you communicate details related to the patient prior to, during, or after a phlebotomy procedure (Figure 3-3 ■). These include the following:

- Normal anatomic position—Erect, standing position with arms at rest and palms forward (never perform a venipuncture on a patient who is standing because of the risk of fainting or falling)
- Supine position—Lying or reclining face-up on his or her back (the best position for performing phlebotomy on patients who are in bed)
- Prone position—Lying with face toward the bed, on his or her stomach (not a recommended position for venipuncture because of awkward orientation of the arms)
- Lateral recumbent position—Lying on left or right side (not a recommended position for venipuncture because the patient can easily roll over, increasing the risk of harmful needle insertion)

The Human Body

HOMEOSTASIS

The design of the human body is elaborate and sophisticated. Trillions of cells make up each individual. Similar groups of cells are combined into tissues, such as muscles or nerves, and tissues are combined into organ systems, such as the circulatory or reproductive system. These organ systems work simultaneously to serve the needs of the body for survival. No one system works independently of the others. The body strives for a **steady state,** or

homeostasis. Literally, homeostasis means "remaining the same." It is a condition in which a healthy body, although constantly changing and functioning, remains in a normal, healthy condition. Homeostasis, or a steady state condition, allows the normal body to stay in balance by compensating with changes. For example, if the body is taking in too much water, it responds to this imbalance by excreting water from the kidneys (urine), skin (perspiration), intestines (feces), and lungs (water in one's breath). A healthy body maintains constancy of its chemical components and processes in order to survive. Each organ system and body structure plays a part maintaining homeostasis. Health care workers can assess homeostasis, or normal functioning, by taking "vital signs"; for example, temperature, pulse rate, respiration rate (together known as TPR), and blood pressure. Another way to monitor normal functioning is to perform laboratory analyses on blood specimens (Box 3-3 ■). Refer to Figure 3-4 ■ to learn more about each organ system and the types of laboratory tests that are useful in evaluating each system.

Cardiovascular System

All body systems are linked by the **cardiovascular system,** a transport network that affects every part of the body within seconds (see Table 3-4 ■). To maintain homeostasis, the cardiovascular system must provide rapid transport of water, nutrients, electrolytes, hormones, enzymes, antibodies, cells, and gases (oxygen and carbon dioxide) to all cells. In addition, the cardiovascular system helps bodily defenses, controls the blood coagulation process, and controls body temperature. The term *cardiovascular* refers to the cardiac muscle (i.e., the heart, refer to Figure 3-5 ■), the **vascular** system (i.e., a network of blood vessels that includes **veins,** arteries, and capillaries), and the circulating blood (refer to Box 3-4 ■).

Box 3-3	**Laboratory Specimens and How They Are Used**

Laboratory test results provide information about an individual's organ systems. In general, laboratory results are used for the following reasons:

1. Diagnosis—(e.g., heart enzyme levels help establish the diagnosis of a heart attack)
2. Monitoring—(e.g., glucose levels are used to monitor treatment of diabetes)
3. Therapy—(e.g., drug levels can help determine effective dosage and prevent toxicity)
4. Screening—(e.g., tests such as prostatic specific antigen can help in the detection of prostate cancer)

The most common body samples used for clinical laboratory analysis are blood and urine. However, other specimens, such as bone marrow, **cerebrospinal fluid** (CSF, from around the spinal cord), **synovial fluid** (joint fluid), **pleural fluid** (from around the lungs), biopsy tissue, semen, and others, can be microscopically analyzed, assayed, and cultured to determine **pathogenesis** (the origin of the disease). Health care workers who collect blood specimens may also have a part in the collection, transportation, processing, or testing of all types of body specimens. Many of these (e.g., bone marrow, CSF, biopsy tissue, and synovial or pleural fluids) are acquired from the patient by the physician and a team of assistants through the use of **invasive** procedures (those requiring that a medical instrument be inserted directly into the body cavity or organ). These specimens must be handled and transported in a similar manner to blood specimens, with the utmost care and efficiency. Health facilities often have special procedures for handling/transporting these types of specimens. Health care workers must understand that these specimens are much more costly and difficult to acquire than blood samples in terms of discomfort to the patient and the health care resources needed to acquire them. Thus, even if it is possible to get a repeat specimen, it is extremely uncomfortable for the patient, inefficient, and costly.

FIGURE ■ 3-4 Organ Systems of the Body

Organ System	Major Functions	Common Disorders*	Common Laboratory Tests*
Integumentary system	Protection, temperature regulator, and sensory receptor.	Infections, cancers	Skin scrapings potassium hydroxide (KOH) preparation Biopsy staining procedures
Skeletal system	*Framework and Movement:* Shape, support, protection, and storage place for minerals. Movement is made possible through joints.	Arthritis, gout, tumors, infections, developmental conditions, eg., dwarfism	Calcium, phosphate, alkaline phosphatase uric acid, Vitamin D, blood cell counts, cultures, cytogenetic analysis
Muscular system	*Framework and Movement:* Muscles produce movement, maintain posture, and produce heat.	Muscular dystrophy, multiple sclerosis tendinitis, infections	Muscle enzymes, eg., creatine phosphokinase (CK), lactate dehydrogenase
Nervous system	*Communication and Control:* Transmits impulses, responds to change, is responsible for communication, and exercises control over all parts of the body.	Infections, eg., meningitis, encephalitis, tumors, epilepsy, Parkinson's disease amyotrophic lateral sclerosis (ALS)	Hormone, protein, and enzyme analysis microbial cultures
Endocrine system	*Communication and Control:* The glands of the endocrine system produce hormones, chemical messengers, that provide for communication and control over various parts of the body.	Addison's disease, Cushing's Syndrome, diabetes, hyper or hypothyroidism, goiter	Hormone analysis, thyroid function tests
Cardiovascular system	*Transportation and Immunity:* Transports oxygen and carbon dioxide, delivers nutrients and hormones, regulates blood clotting and removes waste products.	Tumors, heart disease, hemophilia	Heart enzymes, hemoglobin, hematocrit (H&H), cell counts, platelet function tests, coagulation factors, bone marrow analysis, cytogenetic analysis
Lymphatic system	*Transportation and Immunity:* The lymphatic system stimulates immune response, protects the body, and transports proteins and fluids.	Tumors, eg., lymphoma, Hodgkin's disease, immune disorders, infections	Bone marrow analysis, immune function tests
Respiratory system	*Distribution and Elimination:* Furnishes oxygen for use by individual tissue cells and removes their gaseous waste products, carbon dioxide.	Infections, eg., pneumonia, tuberculosis, sore throats, laryngitis, coughs, colds, influenza	Blood gases, eg., CO_2, & O_2, blood pH, electrolytes (sodium, chloride, potassium), bicarbonate, microbial cultures
Digestive system	*Distribution and Elimination:* Digestion, absorption, and elimination.	Peridontal disease, stomach disorders, eg., ulcers, acid reflux, hernias, intestinal disorders, eg., appendicitis	Occult blood test, microbial cultures, and parasitic analysis
Urinary system	*Distribution and Elimination:* Produces urine, transports urine, and eliminates urine. The kidneys help maintain electrolyte, water, and acid–base balance of the body.	Acidosis and alkalosis	Protein, glucose, ammonia, creatinine, blood urea nitrogen, electrolytes
Reproductive system	*Cycle of Life:* Responsible for sexual characteristics of the male and/or female. Proper functioning ensures survival of the human race.	Tumors, infertility, cysts, cancer, sexually transmitted diseases (STD)	Cytogenetic analysis, semen analysis, biopsies, hormone analysis, prostatic specific antigen (PSA)

* Disorders and laboratory tests listed are only a few examples. The lists are not comprehensive.

Table 3-4 The Cardiovascular System	
Organ/Structure	**Primary Functions**
Heart	■ Muscular organ about the size of an adult's closed fist ■ Contractions push blood throughout the body ■ Average heart beats 60 to 80 times per minute ■ **Aorta** is the largest artery of the body, supplies oxygenated blood to the circulatory system; it exits the heart from the left ventricle and runs downward (in front of the spine). ■ **Atria** and **ventricles** are the two upper and two lower chambers of the heart, respectively, and contract to push blood through the heart. They are described as the right and left atria, and the right and left ventricles. ■ **Vena cavae** are the largest veins of the body carrying deoxygenated blood into the heart. The inferior vena cava carries blood from the lower body and the superior vena cava carries blood from the head and upper body. ■ **Pulmonary arteries/veins**-the right ventricle of the heart pumps blood into the pulmonary arterial branches that go into the right and left lungs; then they branch into arterioles and capillaries to exchange O_2 and CO_2; the capillaries then flow into venules and back into two pulmonary veins (right and left) that return blood to the heart through the left atrium. (Note that pulmonary veins are different in that they are the only veins that contain a high O_2 content. All other veins carry blood with a low O_2 content. Likewise, pulmonary arteries are the only ones that contain a low O_2 content.)
Arteries	■ Transport blood from the right and left chambers of the heart to the entire body ■ Large arteries branch into **arterioles** the farther they are from the heart ■ Carry oxygenated blood that is bright red in color ■ Have thicker elastic walls than veins do ■ Have a pulse ■ Are located deep in muscles/tissues
Veins	■ Transport blood from peripheral tissues back to the heart and lungs ■ Large veins branch into **venules** in the peripheral tissues ■ Carry deoxygenated blood back to the lungs to release carbon dioxide ■ Carry blood that is normally dark red in color ■ Have thinner walls than arteries and appear bluish ■ Have valves to prevent backflow of blood ■ Are located both deep and superficially (close to the surface of the skin)
Capillaries	■ Connect arterioles with venules via microscopic vessels ■ Exchange oxygen and carbon dioxide, nutrients, and fluids in tissue capillaries ■ Pass waste products from tissue cells into capillary blood, then on to removal from the body ■ Carry blood that is a mixture of arterial blood and venous blood
Circulating Blood	■ Transports oxygen and carbon dioxide, nutrients, and fluids ■ Removes waste products ■ Disburses nutrients ■ Regulates body temperature and electrolytes ■ Regulates the blood clotting system

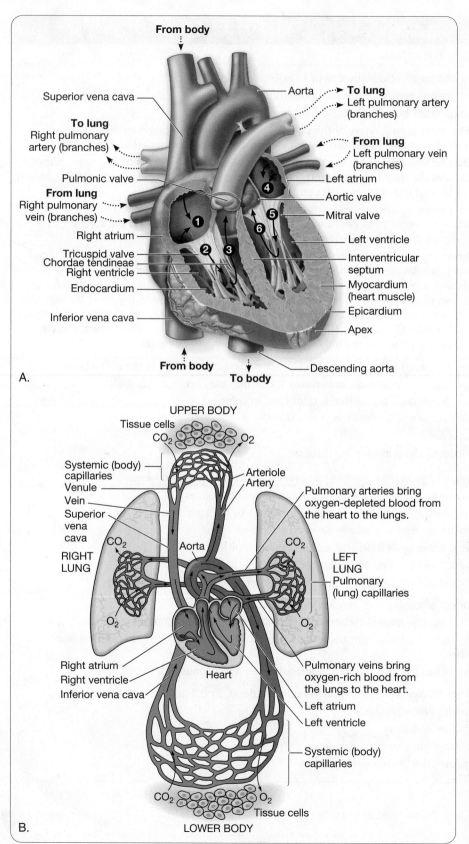

From body

Superior vena cava

Aorta

To lung
Left pulmonary artery
(branches)

To lung
Right pulmonary
artery (branches)

From lung
Left pulmonary vein
(branches)

Pulmonic valve

Left atrium

From lung
Right pulmonary
vein (branches)

Aortic valve

Mitral valve

❶

❹

❺

❻

Right atrium

Left ventricle

❷ ❸

Tricuspid valve
Chordae tendineae
Right ventricle

Interventricular
septum

Endocardium

Myocardium
(heart muscle)

Inferior vena cava

Epicardium

Apex

A.

From body
To body

Descending aorta

UPPER BODY

Tissue cells

CO_2 O_2

Systemic (body)
capillaries

Arteriole
Artery

Venule

Vein

Pulmonary arteries bring
oxygen-depleted blood from
the heart to the lungs.

Superior
vena
cava

CO_2

CO_2

LEFT
LUNG

RIGHT
LUNG

Aorta

Pulmonary
(lung) capillaries

O_2

O_2

Right atrium

Right ventricle

Heart

Pulmonary veins bring
oxygen-rich blood from
the lungs to the heart.

Inferior vena cava

Left atrium

Left ventricle

Systemic (body)
capillaries

CO_2 O_2

Tissue cells

B.

LOWER BODY

FIGURE ■ 3-5 Internal Anatomy
of the Heart and Path of Blood
Circulation

A. This is a diagrammatic frontal
section of the heart showing the
major structures. Numbers indicate
the path of blood flow through
the heart. B. The path of blood
flow throughout the body. Arteries
(red color) carry oxygen-rich blood
(oxygenated) from the lungs and
heart to the upper and lower
body. Most veins carry oxygen-
poor (deoxygenated) blood from
the upper and lower body back
to the heart and lungs to pick up
more oxygen. However, pulmonary veins carry O_2-rich blood back
to the heart from the lungs. Also,
only the pulmonary arteries carry
O_2-poor blood from the heart
directly to the lungs.

Box 3-4 | **Study Your Veins**

Take a look at the superficial veins in one of your hands or in the hands of a friend. Try to find veins that are prominent and easy to see. (Remember that arteries are located deeper in the tissues and are not visible.) Study the characteristics:

Bluish color—Caused by the low oxygen/high carbon dioxide content

Direction of blood flow—Venous blood flow is from the tips of fingers toward the heart, because veins are taking blood back to the heart and lungs to get more oxygen. This can be visible by hanging your hand down low for a minute so that, due to gravity, venous blood pools in the veins. Take note of how they become more prominent. Next, raise your hand up: the venous blood empties and veins become less visible.

Firmness—Some veins feel rather soft, whereas others are slightly firm. Try to compare the feeling of veins from different people of different ages. The more practice you have feeling (not seeing) veins, the better your venipuncture outcomes will be (Figure 3-6 ■).

Become familiar with the principal veins of the arms and legs (Figures 3-7 ■, 3-8 ■, 3-9 ■, and 3-10 ■). Although every individual has a slightly different venous pattern, always rely on feeling the "best" vein for a venipuncture.

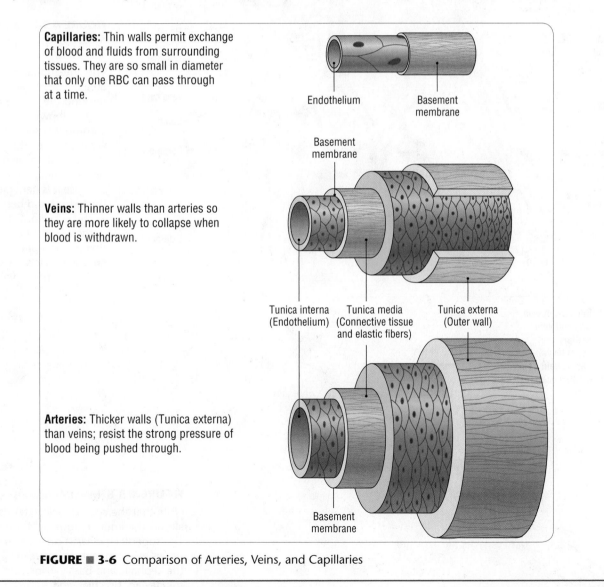

Capillaries: Thin walls permit exchange of blood and fluids from surrounding tissues. They are so small in diameter that only one RBC can pass through at a time.

Endothelium   Basement membrane

Basement membrane

Veins: Thinner walls than arteries so they are more likely to collapse when blood is withdrawn.

Tunica interna (Endothelium)   Tunica media (Connective tissue and elastic fibers)   Tunica externa (Outer wall)

Arteries: Thicker walls (Tunica externa) than veins; resist the strong pressure of blood being pushed through.

Basement membrane

FIGURE ■ 3-6 Comparison of Arteries, Veins, and Capillaries

continued

Box 3-4 Study Your Veins *(cont.)*

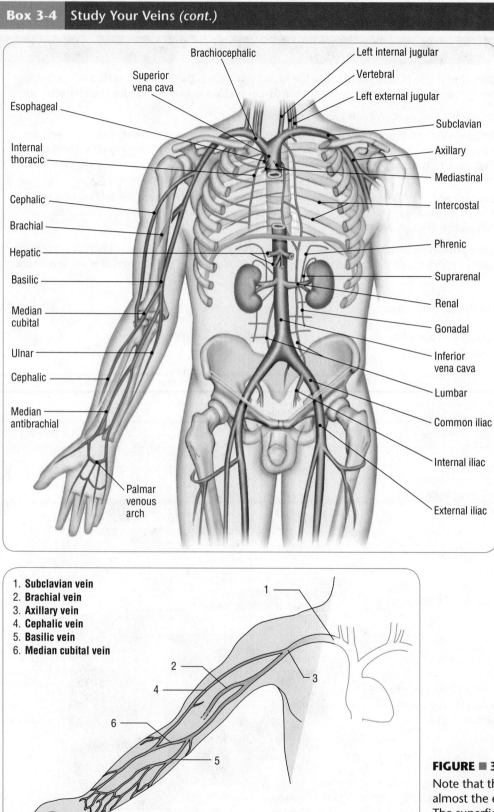

FIGURE ■ 3-7 Venous System of the Upper Torso and Arm

The antecubital area of the forearm (around the crease of the elbow) is most commonly used for venipuncture. The median cubital vein is best for venipuncture because it is generally the largest and best anchored vein. Others in the antecubital area that are acceptable are the basilic vein and the cephalic vein.

Labels in Figure 3-7:
Brachiocephalic, Superior vena cava, Esophageal, Internal thoracic, Cephalic, Brachial, Hepatic, Basilic, Median cubital, Ulnar, Cephalic, Median antibrachial, Palmar venous arch, Left internal jugular, Vertebral, Left external jugular, Subclavian, Axillary, Mediastinal, Intercostal, Phrenic, Suprarenal, Renal, Gonadal, Inferior vena cava, Lumbar, Common iliac, Internal iliac, External iliac

1. **Subclavian vein**
2. **Brachial vein**
3. **Axillary vein**
4. **Cephalic vein**
5. **Basilic vein**
6. **Median cubital vein**

FIGURE ■ 3-8 Major Arm Veins

Note that the *cephalic vein* extends almost the entire length of the arm. The superficial *median cubital vein* serves as a connection between the cephalic and basilic veins. The subclavian, brachial, and axillary veins are deeper veins.

Box 3-4 Study Your Veins *(cont.)*

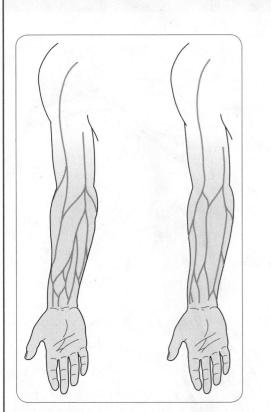

FIGURE ■ 3-9 Variations in Venous Patterns

Because all individuals are unique, the exact location of veins may vary from one person to another. This figure depicts variations in venous patterns in the arms of two individuals.

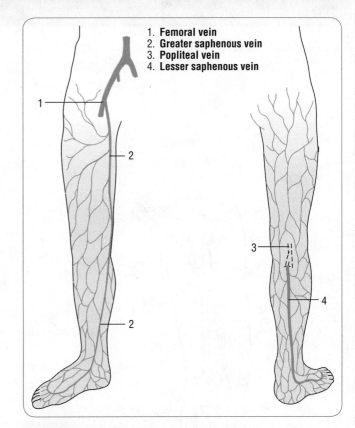

1. Femoral vein
2. Greater saphenous vein
3. Popliteal vein
4. Lesser saphenous vein

FIGURE ■ 3-10 Major Veins of the Leg

The *femoral vein* (1) is a deep vein. Note that the *greater saphenous vein* (2) is the longest vein in the body. It ascends up the medial side of the leg and the medial thigh and empties into the femoral vein in the groin area. The *lesser saphenous vein* (4) comes up the lateral side of the ankle and enters the deeper *popliteal vein* (3) behind the knee.

Also refer to Figure 3-11 ■ that shows the positions of nerves of the arm. Note that veins, arteries, and nerves are all in close proximity to each other, so if a venipuncture procedure is not performed correctly, nerve damage (and severe pain) can result, and/or an artery can be punctured accidentally. The **antecubital** area (anterior side, near the bend) of the arm is preferred for venipuncture. However, in some circumstances when the veins of the antecubital area are not accessible, the puncture site must be on the back or posterior side of the hand (Figure 3-12 ■). *Never use the anterior or palm side of the wrist or hand* to collect a blood specimen because the risk of hitting a nerve is very high due to superficial nerve locations near the skin's surface.

continued

BLOOD

Circulating blood is essential to homeostasis and to sustaining life. Any region of the body that is deprived of blood may die within minutes. Humans contain approximately 5 quarts (4.73 liters) of whole blood that is composed of water, solutes (dissolved substances), and cells. The volume of blood in an individual varies according to body weight; for example, men have 5 to 6 liters of whole blood, adult women usually have 4 to 5 liters, whereas infants who weigh about 3kg or 6.6 pounds may have between

Box 3-4 **Study Your Veins** *(cont.)*

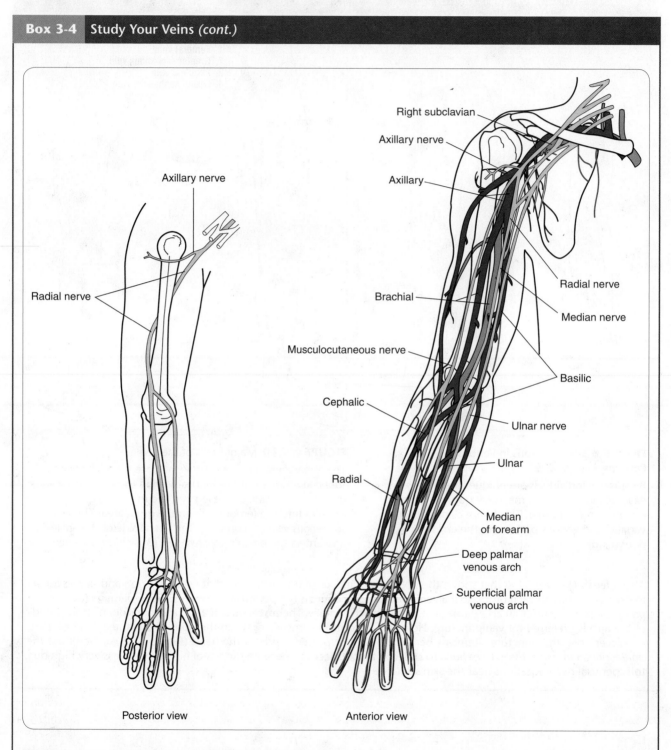

FIGURE ■ 3-11 Posterior and Anterior View of the Arm

Nerves are shown in yellow, veins in blue, and arteries in red. Note that in the area where venipunctures are typically performed (the antecubital area or anterior side of the arm near the crease of the elbow), nerves, veins, and arteries are located within a few centimeters of each other. This can pose a risk of accidental needle puncture to a nerve or artery. Extra care must be taken to position the patient properly, and during venipuncture site selection and needle insertion. (Covered in greater detail in Chapter 8.)

Box 3-4 **Study Your Veins** *(cont.)*

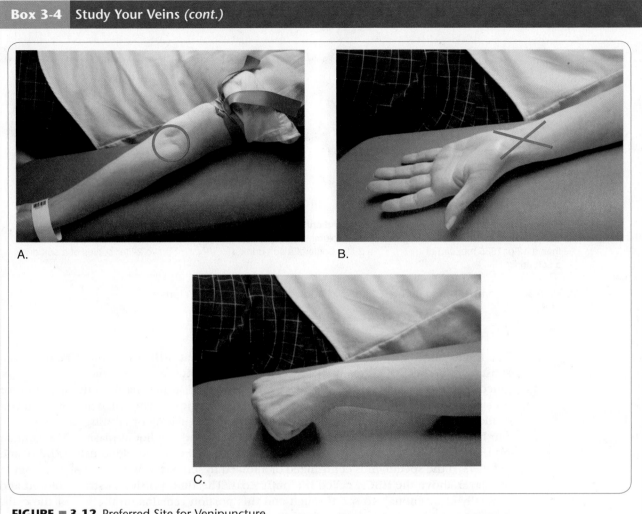

A.

B.

C.

FIGURE ■ 3-12 Preferred Site for Venipuncture
A. The preferred site for venipuncture is the antecubital area of the arm. B. Do not use the wrist area for venipuncture. C. If other preferred sites are not available, use the back (posterior) side of the hand.

240 and 340 milliliters of total **blood volume** (Figure 3-13 ■). When an adequate blood volume is not maintained (due to blood loss during traumatic accidents, complications during surgery, or anemia) a patient may require a blood transfusion. Phlebotomists must understand that the consequences of excessive blood withdrawal for laboratory testing purposes can also cause **iatrogenic anemia,** i.e., anemia caused by the medical treatment itself, in this case, by taking large volumes of blood during venipuncture procedures. Most health care facilities have guidelines about monitoring blood volumes, especially for pediatric patients.

Blood is made up of the liquid portion (plasma) and the cells. There are three main types of circulating **blood cells** that are summarized in Table 3-5 ■ and Figures 3-14 ■ and 3-15 ■. **Hematopoiesis** is the body's mechanism for forming all of the cellular elements in blood. It occurs in the bone marrow and every type of blood cell begins in the bone marrow as a very immature cell called a stem cell (Figure 3-16 ■).

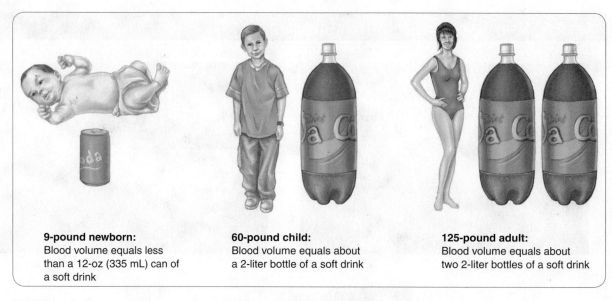

9-pound newborn:
Blood volume equals less
than a 12-oz (335 mL) can of
a soft drink

60-pound child:
Blood volume equals about
a 2-liter bottle of a soft drink

125-pound adult:
Blood volume equals about
two 2-liter bottles of a soft drink

FIGURE ■ 3-13 Comparison of Infant, Child, and Adolescent/Adult Blood Volumes

PLASMA

The liquid portion of blood is called plasma. It is about 90% water and 10% dissolved substances and cells. Normally, blood cells, gases (oxygen or carbon dioxide), proteins, glucose, and other chemical substances are suspended in plasma. It is the medium for transporting constituents in the bloodstream. If a chemical agent called an anticoagulant is added to the blood specimen to prevent it from coagulating or clotting, the specimen can be centrifuged and will result in a layer of cells and the liquid plasma. The cellular portion of the specimen contains white blood cells (WBCs), red blood cells (RBCs), and platelets. If the specimen is centrifuged or allowed to settle, the WBCs and platelets settle in a layer above the RBCs, called the buffy coat. The fluid portion is straw-colored and normally clear enough to see through and this portion remains on the top of the cells. It contains fibrinogen, a clotting factor, and other chemical substances. However, if the sample is mixed, the cells will again become suspended in the plasma and it will again look like normal blood (Figure 3-17 ■).

Table 3-5	Blood Cells			
Cells	**Number/Size**	**Function**	**Formation**	**Destruction**
Erythrocytes (RBCs)	4–6 million/μl(mm³); size 6–7 μm	Transport O_2 and CO_2	Bone marrow	Fragmentation and removal in spleen, liver, and bone marrow; life span: 120 days
Leukocytes (WBCs)	5000–9000/ μl(mm³); size 9–16 μm	Defense	Granulocytes in bone marrow; nongranular WBCs in all lymphatic tissue	Removed in spleen, liver, bone marrow; life span: 1 day to 1 year
Thrombocytes (platelets)	250,000–450,000/ μl(mm³); size 1–4 μm	Clotting	Bone marrow	Removed in spleen; life span: 9–12 days
RBCs, red blood cells; WBCs, white blood cells; O_2, oxygen; CO_2, carbon dioxide				

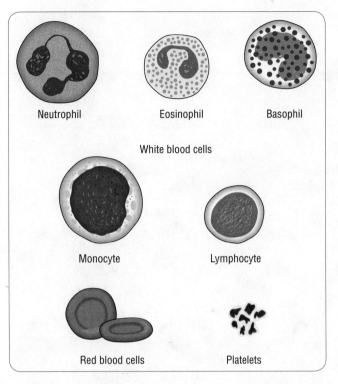

Neutrophil   Eosinophil   Basophil

White blood cells

Monocyte   Lymphocyte

Red blood cells   Platelets

FIGURE ■ 3-14 Human Blood Cells

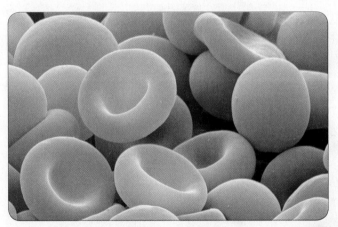

FIGURE ■ 3-15 Erythrocytes or Red Blood Cells (RBCs)
Note the characteristic red color and their unique
"donut" shape. Each RBC has a depressed center and,
when cells from normal circulating blood are analyzed,
no cell nucleus is present.
Source: Andrew Syred / Photo Researchers, Inc.

SERUM

If the blood specimen is allowed to clot, the resulting liquid portion changes from plasma
to serum (also straw-colored and normally clear enough to see through) plus blood cells
meshed in a fibrin clot. Serum contains essentially the same chemical constituents as plasma,
except that the clotting factors (fibrinogen) and the blood cells are contained within the
fibrin clot (Figures 3-17 and 3-18 ■). Sometimes serum may appear **turbid** (cloudy or
opaque) and/or **lipemic** (milky appearance) as a result of several conditions such as high
lipid levels (from eating fatty substances that lead to high cholesterol and triglyceride levels)
or from bacterial contamination. In these cases, the appearance of the serum should be
documented accordingly.

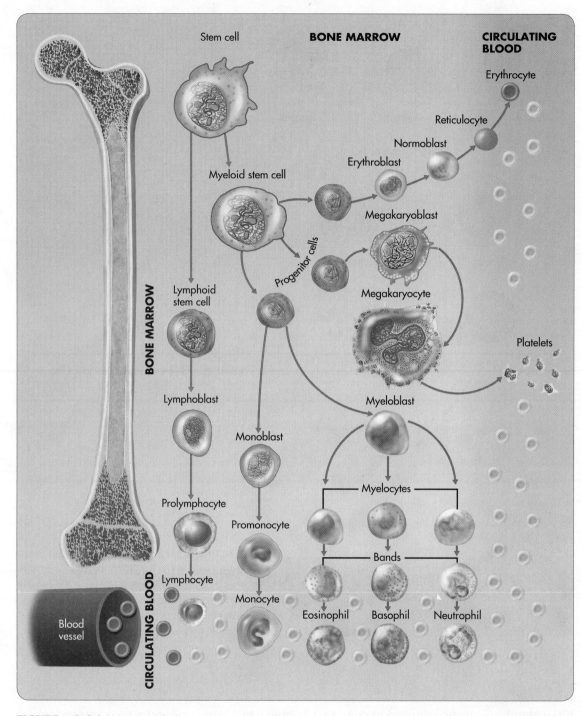

FIGURE ■ 3-16 Hematopoiesis

All cellular elements of the circulating blood found in veins, arteries, and capillaries begin in the bone marrow. Blood cells are considered immature when they are in the bone marrow and mature when they reach the circulating blood, i.e., mature cells can carry out their intended functions of carrying O_2 or CO_2 (RBCs), providing immunity/defense (WBCs), or helping in blood clotting (platelets). Note that the pink background area represents the circulating blood. Hematologic analysis in the laboratory can reveal cellular abnormalities if there are too many of any one cell type, or too few, or if they are immature, or if they are abnormally shaped, etc.

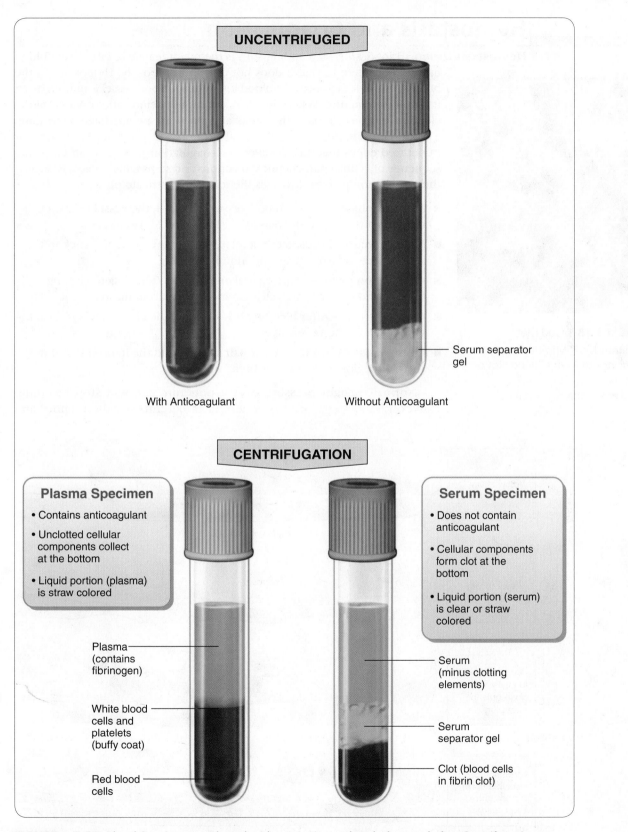

FIGURE ■ 3-17 Blood Specimens with and without Anticoagulant before and after Centrifugation

Hemostasis and Coagulation

Hemostasis (*hemo* = blood, *stasis* = standing still) is the maintenance of circulating blood in the liquid state so that it does not clot spontaneously. Hemostasis is the body's mechanism to prevent blood loss when a blood vessel is injured by an incision or puncture. When this does occur, the hemostatic process (blood clotting response) repairs the break and stops the hemorrhage by forming a blood clot (Figure 3-19 ■). Essentially, the blood clot bridges the torn or punctured edges together. This entire coagulation process is an elaborate sequence of cellular and chemical reactions and steps taking place. Basically, the coagulation process involves the following intricate phases:

- Vascular phase—Once a blood vessel is injured, the vessel constricts (vasoconstriction) to decrease the blood flow to the area.

- Platelet phase—Platelets degranulate, clump together, and stick to the injured site to form a plug and inhibit bleeding.

- Coagulation phase—Many coagulation factors (fibrinogen, clotting factors, and calcium) are released and form a fibrin mesh or clot.

- Clot retraction—After bleeding has stopped, the clot retracts to heal the torn edges of the vessel.

- Fibrinolysis—When the final repair is made and the injured vessel heals, the clot begins to dissolve or break up (lysis).

Normally, slight pressure over a puncture site will stop bleeding. However, laboratory analysis is helpful in determining the number and

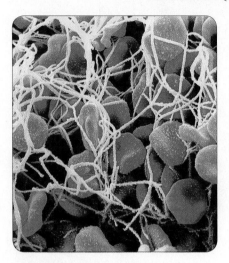

FIGURE ■ 3-18 Blood Clot

These strands of fibrin trap many erythrocytes to form a blood clot or thrombus.

Source: Susumu Nishinaga / Photo Researchers, Inc.

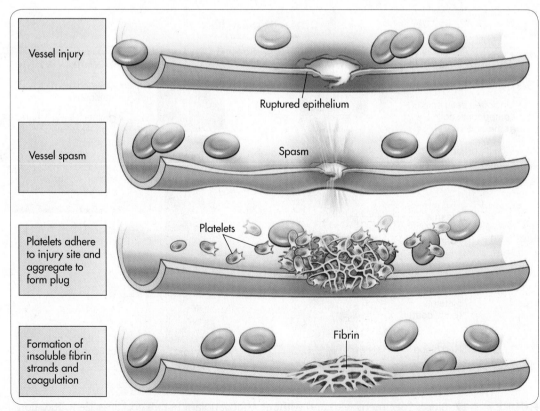

FIGURE ■ 3-19 Hemostasis Overview

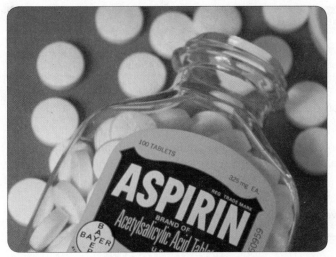

FIGURE ■ 3-20 Some Medications Prolong Bleeding after Venipuncture

functionality of platelets, the presence or absence of clotting factors, or the interference of drugs in the coagulation process. Some drugs called blood thinners are used to treat patients with a history of stroke, irregular heartbeat, artificial heart valves, or a heart attack. These include aspirin (Figure 3-20 ■), heparin, coumadin (warfarin), and clopidogrel (Plavix) and while they are useful in prevention, they also cause a patient to bleed for a longer period of time because they slow down the coagulation process. Phlebotomists must always assure that bleeding has stopped before leaving a patient.

Health care workers regularly deal with patients who are bleeding. External bleeding is described according to the type of blood vessel injured and the color of the blood:

Arterial Bleeding

- Bright red in color (because of the high oxygen content)
- Bleeding is quicker, more abundant (because of higher pressure), and in spurts (with each heartbeat)
- Harder to control and requires special attention from a nurse and/or doctor
- If an artery is accidentally punctured, take immediate steps to terminate the procedure, apply pressure to the site for at least 5 minutes, and seek assistance
- Report accidental arterial punctures immediately to a supervisor

Clinical Alert !

Bleeding should be anticipated during or after a venipuncture. Therefore, always use precautions, including gloves, to avoid direct exposure. A mask, protective eyewear, a face shield, or a gown should be worn if there is a chance of blood splatters or if the patient is coughing up blood. Remember that some patients may be on blood thinners and will bleed more freely and longer than normal.

Also, rarely during a venipuncture procedure, an artery may be accidently punctured instead of a vein. This is a serious error and the procedure should be discontinued immediately by removing the needle device. Bleeding will be more abundant, of longer duration, and in spurts. Direct pressure should be applied with gauze pads until it has stopped. Report the incident to a supervisor.

Always ensure that bleeding has stopped before leaving the patient. If bleeding does not stop after a reasonable time or if it is excessive, call for help. Detailed procedures are covered in Chapter 8.

Box 3-5	**Be Careful with Your Choice of Words**

As you become more proficient with the use of medical terms, remember that some words sound or look similar but have very different meanings. Here are some examples:

Homeostasis	a steady state in the human body
Hemostasis	the blood coagulation system
Hematopoiesis	the process that makes blood cells
Palpation	relates to examining by touching or feeling using fingers or hands (e.g., searching for a superficial vein in the antecubital area)
Palpitation	relates to a rapid heartbeat (e.g., when patients are stressed, they have perceptible heart palpitations)

Venous Bleeding

- Blood is dark red in color (because it lacks oxygen)
- Occurs in a steady flow
- Normal bleeding is easily stopped by applying pressure (because venous pressure is lower than arterial pressure)

Capillary Bleeding

- Occurs slowly and evenly because of smaller size of vessels and lower pressure
- Easily controlled with slight pressure; sometimes stops without intervention
- Blood is a color between the bright red of arterial blood and dark red of venous blood

Self Study

Study Questions

For the following questions, select the one best answer.

1. Homeostasis refers to which of the following?
   a. chemical imbalance
   b. steady state condition
   c. balanced chemistry
   d. thousands of genes

2. The term *superficial vein* means which of the following?
   a. deep vein
   b. vein that has a blockage
   c. vein that is close to the skin surface
   d. vein that is cut open and bleeding

3. What is the best position for a patient to be in when the health care worker performs a phlebotomy procedure?
   a. prone position
   b. standing position
   c. supine position
   d. ventral position

4. Which fact about arteries is correct?
   a. arteries have thin walls
   b. arteries do not have a pulse
   c. blood from arteries appears dark red
   d. blood from arteries appears bright red

5. Capillary blood contains the following?
   a. cells, plasma, arterial blood, venous blood
   b. plasma and cells
   c. only arterialized blood
   d. only venous blood

6. A patient has a severe burn on his left wrist. Select the best description of its location relative to his fingers. The burn is:
   a. proximal to his fingers
   b. distal to his fingers
   c. lateral to his elbow
   d. posterior to his elbow

7. Venous blood is:
   a. blue
   b. dark red
   c. bright red
   d. straw-colored

8. What volume of blood (in liters) does a normal adult have?
   a. 0.5–1.0
   b. 2–3
   c. 4–5
   d. 6–7

9. A patient is taking aspirin. How might this affect a venipuncture?
   a. blood will appear thicker
   b. blood will appear darker than usual
   c. bleeding may be excessive or prolonged
   d. aspirin does not affect the venipuncture at all

10. Hemostasis refers to:
    a. steady state condition
    b. anticoagulant therapy
    c. blood leakage into tissues
    d. control of blood clotting

Case Study

A young man who was from China was scheduled to have laboratory work done in the University Health Clinic. The health care worker was visiting with him prior to the procedure. He asked "Why do my veins look blue? Please explain this to me before you stick a needle in me."

Question
What should the health care worker say to the patient?

Advocating Patient Safety Case Study

A thin, middle-aged woman came to the clinic to have blood specimens collected for laboratory analysis. The process was going smoothly until the phlebotomist began searching for a superficial vein for the venipuncture site. The woman did not have any visible veins in her arm except around the wrist area where they were very prominent. The patient stated that most of her veins were very small and many health care workers in the past had not taken time to search for a good vein. She said lots of times people try to draw blood from her wrist and on one occasion she experienced shooting pain during the procedure. She added that she knew she had a good vein on her right arm.

Questions
1. How should the phlebotomist proceed?
2. Describe (using medical terminology) the preferred area for venipunctures.
3. Describe the reasons that venipunctures are not safe for the patient if they are collected from the anterior side of the wrist.

Competency Assessment

Check Yourself: Basic Medical Terminology

1. In the space provided, write the definition of these prefixes, roots, and suffixes. Do not refer back to the chapter, and leave the space blank for the words that you do not know.

2. After answering as many as you can, go back to the list to check your work. Note the ones that you missed.

Competency Checklist: Prefixes

Write the definitions of the following prefixes:

1. a _____
2. ab _____
3. ad _____
4. ambi _____
5. an _____
6. ana _____
7. ante _____
8. anti _____
9. auto _____
10. bi _____
11. brachy _____
12. brady _____
13. cac _____
14. cata _____
15. centi _____
16. circum _____
17. contra _____
18. deca _____
19. dia _____
20. dipl _____
21. di(s) _____
22. dys _____
23. endo _____
24. epi _____
25. eu _____
26. ex _____
27. extra _____
28. hemi _____
29. hetero _____
30. homeo _____
31. hydro _____

32. hyper _____
33. hypo _____
34. infra _____
35. inter _____
36. intra _____
37. mal _____
38. mega _____
39. meso _____
40. micro _____
41. milli _____
42. multi _____
43. nulli _____
44. oligo _____
45. pan _____
46. para _____
47. peri _____
48. poly _____
49. primi _____
50. pseudo _____
51. quadri _____
52. quint _____
53. retro _____
54. semi _____
55. sub _____
56. supra _____
57. sym _____
58. syn _____
59. tetra _____
60. tri _____
61. uni _____

Competency Checklist: Root Words

Write the definitions of the following roots:

1. angio _____
2. angin _____
3. arter _____
4. arterio _____
5. athero _____
6. capillus _____
7. card _____
8. cardi _____
9. cardio _____

10. cubitum _____
11. cyte _____
12. derm _____
13. electro _____
14. embol _____
15. ergo _____
16. erythro _____
17. hemo _____
18. infarct _____

19. lipid _____
20. logos _____
21. mano _____
22. myo _____
23. phleb _____
24. phlebo _____
25. pulmonar _____
26. rrhyth _____

27. scler _____
28. sera _____
29. sphygmo _____
30. stetho _____
31. tens _____
32. thromb _____
33. vaso _____
34. veni _____

Competency Checklist: Suffixes

Write the definitions of the following suffixes:

1. algia _____
2. blast _____
3. cele _____
4. centesis _____
5. cyte _____
6. desis _____
7. dynia _____
8. ectomy _____
9. emesis _____
10. gram _____
11. graph _____
12. ist _____
13. itis _____
14. logy _____
15. lysis _____
16. megaly _____
17. meter _____
18. oid _____
19. oma _____
20. opsy _____
21. osis _____
22. pathy _____
23. penia _____
24. pexy _____
25. phagia _____
26. phasia _____

27. philia _____
28. phobia _____
29. phraxis _____
30. physis _____
31. plasia _____
32. plasty _____
33. plegia _____
34. pnea _____
35. poiesis _____
36. ptosis _____
37. ptysis _____
38. rrhage _____
39. rrhagia _____
40. rrhaphy _____
41. rrhea _____
42. rrhexis _____
43. scope _____
44. scopy _____
45. stasis _____
46. stomy _____
47. therapy _____
48. tome _____
49. tomy _____
50. trophy _____
51. uria _____

Competency Checklist: Identifying Medical Terms

Write the medical terms for the following definitions:

1. _____ Process of forming a blood clot
2. _____ Substance used in blood specimens to prevent blood clotting
3. _____ The study of diseases of the blood
4. _____ Excess sugar in the blood
5. _____ White blood cell

6. _____ Red blood cell
7. _____ Study of diseases
8. _____ Front area of the elbow
9. _____ Decrease in white blood cells
10. _____ Hardening of the arteries

Competency Checklist: Spelling

In the spaces provided, write the correct spelling of these misspelled terms:

1. imumology _____
2. phlebtomy _____
3. hemmorage _____
4. hemacrit _____
5. leukema _____

6. erthocyte _____
7. homatology _____
8. embollis _____
9. thrombes _____
10. millemeter _____

Competency Checklist: Cardiovascular System

Match the appropriate lettered meaning to the numbered word:

1. Erythrocyte
2. Leukocyte
3. Arteries
4. Venules
5. Capillary
6. Veins
7. Plasma
8. Serum
9. Antecubital
10. Median cubital vein
11. Basilic vein
12. Saphenous vein
13. Fibrinogen
14. Femoral artery
15. Platelets
16. CO₂
17. Hemostasis
18. Homeostasis
19. Deoxygenated blood
20. Cardiac muscle

A. steady state condition of the body
B. heart
C. carbon dioxide
D. blood clotting mechanism in the body
E. a blood clotting factor
F. deep vessel in the leg
G. thrombocytes
H. RBC
I. WBC
J. near the bend of the elbow
K. thick-walled vessels
L. thin-walled vessels
M. branching vessels that flow back to the heart
N. contains a mixture of arterial and venous blood
O. blood specimen that does not contain anticoagulant
P. blood specimen that does contain an anticoagulant
Q. best vein to use for venipuncture
R. alternate vein to use for venipuncture
S. blood that is carried in the veins
T. the longest vessel in the body

References

Turley, S: *Medical Language,* 2nd edition, Upper Saddle River, NJ, Pearson, 2011.

Resources

www.medterms.com Provides easy-to-understand descriptions of medical terms.

www.familydoctor.org Provides a dictionary of common medical terms.

www.medilexicon.com Provides medical terminology definitions.

Chapter 4

Safety and Infection Control

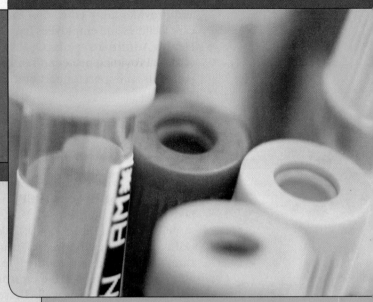

KEY TERMS

antiseptics

aseptic

bloodborne pathogens (BBP)

Centers for Disease Control and Prevention (CDC)

chain of infection

disinfectants

double bagging

Environmental Protection Agency (EPA)

fomites

health care–associated (nosocomial) infections

infection control programs

isolation procedures

mode of transmission

National Fire Protection Association (NFPA)

Occupational Safety and Health Administration (OSHA)

personal protective equipment (PPE)

protective environment (reverse isolation)

source

standard precautions

susceptible host

transmission-based precautions

universal precautions

CHAPTER OBJECTIVES

Upon completion of Chapter 4, the learner should be able to do the following:

1. Explain the safety policies and procedures that must be followed in specimen collection and transportation.

2. Define the term *health care–associated (nosocomial) infection.*

3. Identify the basics of safety, infection control, and isolation procedures.

4. Explain the proper techniques for handwashing, gowning, gloving, masking, double bagging, and entering and exiting the various isolation areas.

5. Identify steps to avoid transmission of bloodborne pathogens (BBP) and reduce risks for BBP accidental needlesticks.

6. Explain the measures that should be taken for fire, electrical, radiation, and chemical safety in a health care facility.

7. Describe the essential elements of a disaster emergency plan for a health care facility.

8. List three precautions that can reduce the risk of injury to patients.

The goal of safety for health care facilities is to get rid of hazards for patients and employees and provide safety education for health care workers. Safe working guidelines for health care facilities and employees have been developed by the federal **Occupational Safety and Health Administration (OSHA)** and the **Centers for Disease Control and Prevention (CDC).** Providing protection from hazardous events in the health care environment for the patient is an important part of the health care worker's everyday responsibilities.

Personal Safety from Infection During Specimen Handling

Patients' specimens should be handled with caution to prevent the possibility of acquiring **bloodborne pathogens (BBP),** which are infectious organisms found in blood and other body fluids (e.g., hepatitis A, B, C, D, and E viruses; human immunodeficiency virus [HIV], syphilis, malaria (Table 4-1 ■)). This preventive approach is called **universal precautions.**[1] OSHA requires health care facilities to protect workers exposed to biological hazards. Health care workers who are routinely exposed to blood and body fluids must wear gloves and other **personal protective equipment (PPE)** (facial shields, gowns, etc.) to protect themselves from infection as well. These requirements have occurred because of the 1991 OSHA standards for occupational exposure to bloodborne pathogens (29 CFR 1930.1030) and the Needlestick Safety and Prevention Act (2001).[2] These federal regulations require that, in most cases, warning labels be placed on containers (refrigerators, freezers, infectious waste, etc.)

Table 4-1 Bloodborne Pathogens
Examples of Body Fluids that Can Potentially Carry the HIV and Hepatitis B Virus and Other BBP
■ Blood ■ Saliva involved in dental procedures ■ Cerebrospinal fluid ■ Cell cultures ■ Human tissue ■ Semen and vaginal secretions ■ All body fluids containing blood
Transmission Routes
■ Exposure to broken skin ■ Risk increases if contact involves a large area of skin or BBP contact is prolonged. ■ Increased BBP levels leads to increased risk ■ Misuse of sharps (e.g., eyes, nose, and/or mouth splashed by infected body fluid)
Engineering Controls
■ Leakproof containers ■ Sharps containers ■ Needleless devices (e.g., retractable syringes, self-sheathing needles)
Personal Protective Equipment
■ Gloves ■ Lab coats, scrub suits, gowns ■ Goggles, safety glasses

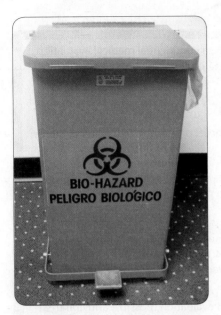

FIGURE ■ 4-1 Label for Biohazard
Source: Centers for Disease Control and Prevention (CDC)

FIGURE ■ 4-2 Label for Biohazard
Source: Centers for Disease Control and Prevention (CDC)

that contain blood or other potentially infectious materials. The labels required are fluorescent orange or orange-red and feature the biohazard alerts shown in Figure 4-1 ■ and Figure 4-2 ■.

EXPOSURE CONTROL

If an accident such as a needlestick occurs, the injured health care worker should immediately cleanse the area with isopropyl alcohol and apply an adhesive bandage. Any incident of exposure to potentially harmful bloodborne pathogens or other infectious body fluids should be reported immediately to the supervisor.[3,4] Each health care worker should know who to contact, where to go, and what to do if exposed to harmful pathogens. The report must include the blood collection device that did not work effectively to protect the health care worker during blood collection. If exposures are not reported, it is difficult to prove, retrospectively, that an exposure to an infection was caused by working conditions.

HEALTH CARE–ASSOCIATED (NOSOCOMIAL) INFECTIONS

Health care–associated (nosocomial) infections are those that are acquired by a patient after admission to a health care facility, such as a hospital, clinic, or nursing home. In an attempt to control them, **infection control programs** have been developed. Using guidelines established by the CDC, The Joint Commission, and state regulatory agencies, managers of health care institutions address the issues of proper **aseptic** technique (i.e., maintaining conditions to prevent growth of microorganisms), **isolation procedures,** education, and management of health care–associated infections. The cornerstones of infection protection for patients and health care workers are aseptic techniques, which include the following:

■ Frequent handwashing (hand hygiene)
■ Use of barrier garments and personal protective equipment (PPE)
■ Waste management of contaminated materials
■ Use of proper cleaning solutions
■ Following standard precautions
■ Using sterile procedures when necessary

Clinical Alert !

OSHA requires managers at health care facilities to provide a confidential medical evaluation, treatment, and follow-up for any employee who has had a bloodborne exposure incident (e.g., needlestick). Immediately after an exposure incident, the employee must:

- decontaminate the needlestick site or other sharps injury (e.g., shards of glass) with soap and water or an appropriate antiseptic (e.g., iodine) for 30 seconds.
- flush the exposed mucous membrane site (e.g., eyes, nose, or mouth) with water or sterile saline for 10–15 minutes. Use an eyewash station if available to flush the site. Contact lenses must be removed immediately and disinfected before reuse or discarded.
- report the incident to his or her supervisor, who will direct the employee to the appropriate clinic for medical evaluation, treatment, and counseling.

The medical evaluation involves the following steps:

1. The exposed health care worker (HCW) is identified in a confidential manner and tested for HIV, hepatitis B virus (HBV), and hepatitis C virus (HCV) with permission from the health care worker. Hopefully, the HCW has previously received the HBV vaccine, as required for working in a health care environment.

2. The exposed HCW should receive counseling, medical evaluation, possible antiviral treatment and postexposure testing immediately. The scheduled protocol for follow-up treatment, testing, and counseling is dependent upon the severity of the exposure.

3. The exposed HCW is counseled to be alert for acute viral symptoms within 12 weeks of exposure. This entire medical evaluation must be completely confidential.

These protective procedures must become part of a health care worker's routine procedures and standards for practice. Because each health care facility has its own infection control program and policy manual, the health care worker should read and be familiar with both.

Chain of Infection

Nosocomial (health care–associated) infections result when the **chain of infection** is complete (Table 4-2 ■).

The three components that make up the chain are the (1) **source,** (2) **mode of transmission,** and (3) **susceptible host.** Infection control programs aim at breaking the infection chain at one or more links, as shown in Figure 4-3 ■.

Table 4-2   Chain of Infection
A *pathogen* must be present
A *source* of disease, including patients who have a disease and human carriers of disease (e.g., health care provider and patient's family members) who are unaware they have the disease but can still transmit it to another
A *mode of transmission* for the pathogen to pass directly from the source to the new host (e.g., touching infected individuals, individuals spreading infection through coughing or sneezing, inadequate ventilation, and invasive medical instruments)
A *susceptible host* (e.g., hospital patient) that cannot fight off the pathogen (e.g., elderly persons and patients with cancer)

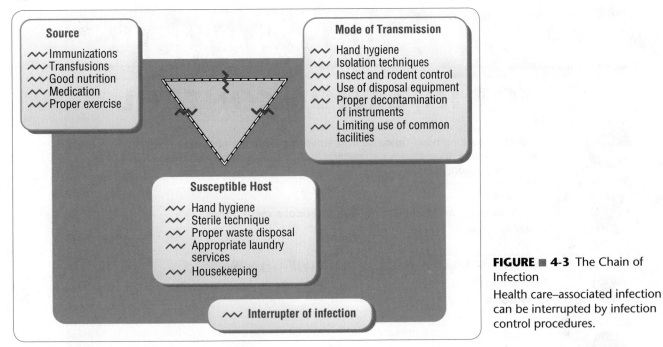

Source
~~ Immunizations
~~ Transfusions
~~ Good nutrition
~~ Medication
~~ Proper exercise

Mode of Transmission
~~ Hand hygiene
~~ Isolation techniques
~~ Insect and rodent control
~~ Use of disposal equipment
~~ Proper decontamination of instruments
~~ Limiting use of common facilities

Susceptible Host
~~ Hand hygiene
~~ Sterile technique
~~ Proper waste disposal
~~ Appropriate laundry services
~~ Housekeeping

~~ **Interrupter of infection**

FIGURE ■ 4-3 The Chain of Infection
Health care–associated infection can be interrupted by infection control procedures.

Hand hygiene procedures for sterile technique, proper waste disposal, appropriate laundry services, and housekeeping are ways of controlling the sources. Isolation techniques, control of insects and rodents, and the use of disposable equipment and supplies help interrupt the modes of transmission. Host susceptibility is controlled by speeding the patient's recovery. Immunizations, transfusions, proper nutrition, medication, and adequate exercise all help the patient to become healthy.

Standard Precautions

Standard precautions (Figure 4-4 ■) have been designed through the CDC to decrease the risk of transmission of microorganisms from both recognized and unrecognized sources of infection in hospitals. Standard precautions include *universal precautions* that are designed to prevent transmission of all infectious agents in the health care setting. They provide protection from contact with blood, all body fluids, mucous membranes, and nonintact skin. **Transmission-based precautions** are used in addition to standard precautions for patients with known or suspected infections that are spread in one of three ways; by (1) airborne transmission; (2) droplet transmission; or (3) contact transmission.[5,6,7]

- *Airborne precautions* decrease the spread of airborne droplet transmission of infectious diseases such as rubeola, varicella, and tuberculosis.[7]

- *Droplet precautions* are used to decrease the transmission of diseases such as pertussis (whooping cough) and pneumonia. These diseases can be transmitted through contact with eye, mouth, or nose secretions from sneezing, coughing, or talking.

- *Contact precautions* decrease the risk of infection to other patients and health care workers from diseases such as herpes simplex that can occur through direct or indirect contact.

STANDARD PRECAUTIONS

FOR INFECTION CONTROL

Hand Hygiene

Wash after touching **body fluids**, after **removing gloves**, and between **patient contacts**. If hands are not visibly soiled, use an alcohol-based hand rub for routinely decontaminating hands.

Gloves

Wear **Gloves** before touching **body fluids**, **mucous membranes**, and **nonintact skin**.

Mask & Eye Protection or Face Shield

Protect eyes, nose, mouth during procedures that cause **splashes** or **sprays** of **body fluids**.

Gown

Wear **Gown** during procedures that may cause **splashes** or **sprays** of **body fluids**.

Patient-Care Equipment

Handle soiled equipment so as to prevent personal contamination and transfer to other patients.

Environmental Control

Follow hospital procedures for cleaning beds, equipment, and frequently touched surfaces.

Linen

Handle linen soiled with **body fluids** so as to prevent personal contamination and transfer to other patients.

Occupational Health & Bloodborne Pathogens

Prevent injuries from needles, scalpels, and other sharp devices.
Never recap needles using both hands.
Place sharps in puncture-proof sharps containers.
Use **Resuscitation Devices** as an alternative to mouth-to-mouth resuscitation.

Patient Placement

Use a Private Room for a patient who contaminates the environment.

"Body Fluids" include **blood**, **secretions**, and **excretions**.

Condensed Version

Form No. **SPR-C**   BREVIS CORP., 225 West 2855 South, SLC, Utah 84115 www.brevis.com   © 2004 Brevis Corp.

FIGURE ■ **4-4** Infection Control
Source: Courtesy of BREVIS Corp.

All three types of precautions may be used at one time when multiple infectious micro-organisms are suspected in a patient. These precautions are *always* used with standard precautions. Table 4-3 ■ provides detailed recommendations by the Department of Health and Human Services, CDC, for using these isolation precautions.

Table 4-3	HICPAC* Recommendations for Transmission-Based Precautions		
	Contact	**Droplet**	**Airborne**
Purpose	• Prevent transmission of known or suspected infected or colonized microorganisms by direct or indirect hand or skin-to-skin contact that occurs when providing direct or indirect patient care. Conditions for which contact precautions are required: diphtheria, herpes simplex, scabies, staphyloccus infection, hepatitis A, and respiratory syncytial virus wound or skin infection	• Prevent transmission of large-particle droplets, larger than 5 microns (μm) (e.g., diphtheria, pertussis, streptococcal pharyngitis, pneumonia, scarlet fever, meningitis, rubella)	• Prevent transmission of small-particle residue of 5 microns (μm) or smaller droplets (e.g., measles, varicella, tuberculosis)
Patient	• Private room	• Private room	• Private room
Placement	• Can be placed in room of patient with same microorganism	• Can be placed in room of patient with same diagnosis	• Can be placed in room of patient with same diagnosis • Monitor negative air pressure • Keep door closed • Keep patient in room
Respiratory Protection	• Mask not necessary (Respiratory hygiene/cough etiquette) Instruct symptomatic persons (i.e., patients, visitors, health care workers) to cover their mouth and nose when sneezing/coughing; use tissues and dispose in no-touch receptable	• Use mask when working within 3 feet of patient	• Respiratory protective equipment • Do not enter room of patients with rubeola or varicella if susceptible to these infections. Follow health care institution's policy for possible cases of multi-drug resistant TB, SARS, influenza, and other highly contagious respiratory diseases.
Gloves and Gown	• Wear gloves when entering room • Change gloves after contact with infective material, such as wound drainage or fecal material • Wash hands immediately after removing gloves	• Follow standard precautions	• Follow standard precautions

continued

Table 4-3	HICPAC* Recommendations for Transmission-Based Precautions (*cont.*)		
	Contact	**Droplet**	**Airborne**
	• Wear gown when working with patients with diarrhea, ostomies, or wound drainage not contained in dressing • Wear gown if contact with patient or environment will occur		
Patient Transport	• Transport only if essential • Ensure precautions are maintained to minimize risk of transmission	• Transport only if essential • Place mask on patient when outside room	• Transport only if essential • Place mask on patient when outside room
Patient Care Items	• Patient care items and environmental surfaces are cleaned daily • Dedicate equipment to single patient use (e.g., stethoscope, thermometer)		

*Hospital Infection Control Practices Advisory Committee.

Adapted from Department of Health and Human Services: CDC, *Federal Register* "Guidelines for Isolation Precautions in Hospitals"; and CDC Guideline for Isolation Precautions: Preventing Transmission of Infectious Agents in Healthcare Settings 2007 authored by Siegel JD, Rhinehart E, Jackson M, Chiarello L, and the Healthcare Infection Control Practices Advisory Committee. http://www.cdc.gov/ncidod/dhqp/pdf/isolation2007.pdf

Clinical Alert !

Respiratory Hygiene and Cough Etiquette

The CDC has designed measures to minimize the transmission of respiratory diseases via droplet or airborne routes in health care settings. The keys of Respiratory Hygiene/Cough Etiquette are: 1) covering the mouth and nose during coughing and sneezing, 2) using tissues to avoid spreading respiratory secretions to others with immediate disposal into a no-touch receptacle, 3) offering a mask to persons who are coughing to decrease contamination of the surrounding environment, and 4) turning the head away from others and maintaining separation, ideally greater than 3 feet, when coughing. These measures should be followed by all individuals with symptoms of respiratory infection.[8]

USE OF STANDARD PRECAUTIONS

Health care workers should follow these guidelines when collecting blood from a patient in order to reduce the possibility of becoming infected by a patient.

1. Use personal protective equipment (PPE) (i.e., gloves, facial masks, shields, gowns, respirators) to prevent skin and mucous membrane exposure when contact with blood or other body fluids of any patient is anticipated. This will prevent transmission by **fomites** (objects that transmit infection, such as door knobs, telephones, countertops, etc.).

a. Gloves should be worn for

   i. Handling objects or surfaces soiled with blood or body fluids; and

   ii. Performing venipunctures, skin punctures, and intravenous (IV) line collections.

b. Gloves should be changed after contact with each patient and wash the hands or use alcohol hand sanitizers after glove removal and before donning new gloves.

c. Masks and protective eyewear or face shields should be worn to prevent exposure of mucous membranes of the mouth, nose, and eyes during procedures that are likely to cause droplets or splashes of blood or other body fluids.

d. A personal respirator should be used if the risk of tuberculosis is present.

e. Footwear (i.e., covers for the entire foot) should be worn that protects against broken glass possibly contaminated with blood or other body fluids (flip flops, sandals, and clogs are *not* recommended).

2. Hand hygiene includes both handwashing with either plain or antiseptic-containing soap and water, and use of alcohol-based products (e.g., gels, foams) (Figure 4-5 ■) that do not require the use of water. Hands and other skin surfaces should be washed immediately and thoroughly if contaminated with blood or other body fluids. Hands should be washed immediately after gloves are removed! Proper handwashing technique is shown in Procedure 4-1 ■. Although alcohol-based hand antiseptics are not appropriate for use when hands are visibly dirty or contaminated, alcohols are more effective than plain or antimicrobioal soap for standard handwashing or hand antisepsis by health care providers.[9]

   It is important to always wash your hands after contact with blood, body fluids, or contaminated objects, whether or not gloves are worn. Placing gloves on dirty hands can transfer microorganisms after the gloves are taken off. Proper donning and removing of gloves is shown in Procedure 4-2 ■.

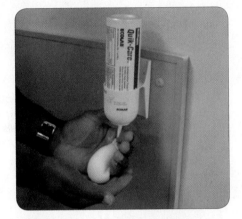

FIGURE ■ 4-5 Alcohol-based hand antiseptic kills 99.9% of the most common microorganisms in 15 seconds.

> **Clinical Alert !**
>
> - Do not wear artificial fingernails or extenders because of the possible spread of pathogenic infections and fungus to patients.
> - Remove gloves after collecting blood from a patient. DO NOT wear the same pair of gloves for the blood collection of more than one patient.
> - Wash or decontaminate hands with alcohol-based rub before placing new gloves on hands.

3. Take precautions to prevent injuries caused by needles and other sharp instruments or devices

a. During blood collection procedures

b. During the disposal of used needles, lancets, etc.

c. When handling any sharp instruments after procedures

4. To prevent infections from BBPs as a result of needlestick injuries, health care workers should

a. Only use safety engineered needle and sharps devices.

b. *Not* recap needles, purposely bend or break them by hand, remove them from disposable syringes or holders, or handle them for any reason.

    c. Immediately dispose of the blood tube holder and safety needle as a single unit after blood collection.

    d. Place disposable syringes and needles, lancets, and other sharp items, after they are used, in puncture-resistant containers for transport to the biohazardous waste center.

Procedure 4-1

Handwashing Technique

RATIONALE
To perform proper handwashing technique.

PROCEDURE

(1) Remove rings (with the exception of wedding bands) and stand at the sink without allowing clothing to touch the sink. Wet hands with water. Foot pedals are preferable for controlling the flow of water but they are not available in all health care facilities (Figure 4-6 ■).

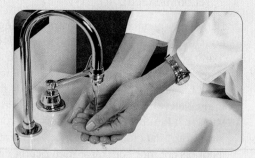

Figure ■ 4-6

(2) Dispense a small amount of soap to the hands (1–2 teaspoonfuls or the amount recommended by the manufacturer) (Figure 4-7 ■). If using bar soap, keep the bar in hands and use enough soap to form a lather by moving your hands over each other and between the fingers of each hand.

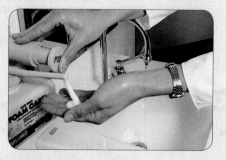

Figure ■ 4-7

(3) Rub hands together vigorously for at least 15 seconds, covering all surfaces of the hands and fingers (Figure 4-8 ■).

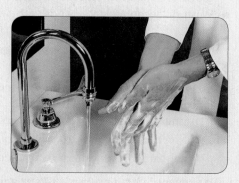

Figure ■ 4-8

(4) Rinse hands in a downward motion with water (Figure 4-9 ■) and dry thoroughly with a clean disposable towel. Multiple-use cloth towels of the hanging or roll type are not acceptable for use in health care settings, because they can transmit microorganisms.

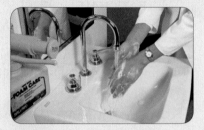

Figure ■ 4-9

(5) Turn off the faucet with a dry disposable towel if not using a foot pedal (Figure 4-10 ■).

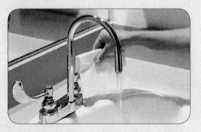

Figure ■ 4-10

Clinical Alert !

- Standard precautions have been designed to be used for patients, health care providers, and visitors in health care facilities.
- Standard precautions reduce the risk of infections being transmitted from health care workers to patients, patients to patients, patients to health care workers, and health care workers to other health care workers or visitors.
- These precautions apply in the following situations:
    - Contact with blood
    - Contact with body fluids
    - Contact with mucous membranes and wounds

ISOLATION FOR HOSPITAL OUTBREAKS

Occasionally, outbreaks of particular infections occur in one or more hospital areas. To control the outbreak, the need for special precautions and isolation procedures might occur. Any health care worker entering or exiting these areas should be made aware of the special circumstances.

Procedure 4-2

Donning and Removing Gloves

RATIONALE

To place gloves on properly for blood collection and remove properly after procedure is performed.

EQUIPMENT

■ Clean gloves (clean, nonsterile gloves are appropriate for most blood collection procedures)
■ Trash container

PROCEDURE

(1) Complete handwashing prior to donning gloves (Figure 4-11 ■).

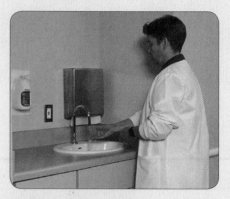

Figure ■ 4-11

(2) Remove gloves from glove dispenser (Figure 4-12 ■).

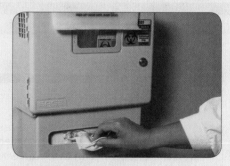

Figure ■ 4-12

(3) Slip your fingers into the openings of the glove as you hold the glove at the wrist edge with your other hand. Then pull the glove up to your wrist (Figure 4-13 ■).

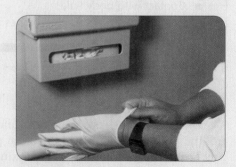

Figure ■ 4-13

4. With your gloved hand, place your fingers under the wrist edge of the second glove and slip your fingers into the openings (Figure 4-14 ■).

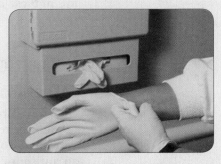

Figure ■ 4-14

5. For glove removal, grasp the wrist of one glove at the cuff by the other gloved hand and pull it off of your hand as the glove turns inside out (Figure 4-15 ■).

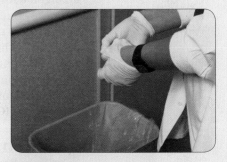

Figure ■ 4-15

6. After placing the rolled-up glove in the palm of the gloved hand, remove the second glove by slipping one finger under the glove edge and pulling it inside out as the glove goes down the hand. This glove will roll over the other glove with no exterior glove exposure from either glove (Figure 4-16 ■).

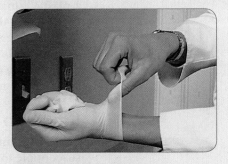

Figure ■ 4-16

7. Dispose of these contaminated gloves in the proper container, not at the patient's bedside. Then complete hand hygiene (Figure 4-17 ■).

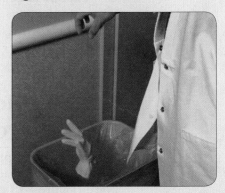

Figure ■ 4-17

PROTECTIVE ENVIRONMENT (REVERSE ISOLATION)

Some hospitals in the United States have **protective environment** facilities for patients who have suppression of their immune system due to stem cell transplantation or other disorders such as cancer. They must live in an environment that is completely sterile. All food and articles are sterilized before they are taken into the patient's room. Some patients must live in these protected environments when they are recovering from, for example, cancer treatments.

INFECTION CONTROL IN SPECIAL HOSPITAL UNITS

Infection Control in a Nursery Unit

Newborns are easy targets for infections of all sorts, because their immune systems are not fully developed at birth. Neonates may pick up pathogens from their mothers, other babies, or hospital personnel. The best way to minimize infection is to use gloves and an antiseptic for handwashing. Special clothing may be worn by nursery personnel, changed daily, and limited to the unit. Bibs should be used and discarded after contact with only one baby. Often, a baby is assigned a single nurse, to limit the possible sources of infection transmission. A major concern in neonatal ICUs and nursery units is the transfer of the highly infectious, methicillin resistant *Staphylococcus aureus* (MRSA) and other antibiotic resistant microorganisms. Many health care institutions have an anteroom (outer room) where the health care worker can perform the infection control procedures of hand hygiene, gowning, gloving and so on prior to entering the nursery or neonatal ICU.

Infection Control in a Burn Unit

Patients with burns are also highly susceptible to infection. Each bed is surrounded by a plastic curtain with sleeves. Hospital personnel use these sleeves to have contact with the patient. All supplies and equipment are kept outside the curtain. In hospitals lacking these facilities, burn patients are housed in private rooms. Gowning, gloving, **double bagging** (described in Procedure 4-5 ■ Disposing of Contaminated Items, page 100), and strict handwashing procedures should be used. All articles in the room, as well as the room itself, should be disinfected or sterilized frequently.

Infection Control in an ICU or Postoperative Care Unit

Patients in intensive care units (ICUs) are more critically ill and, by nature, are more susceptible to infections. In most hospitals, ICUs are open areas, with numerous patients in one large room. Patients with known infections are isolated according to the types of infections they have, and strict handwashing and gloving policies are necessary in all ICUs.

Specific Isolation Techniques and Procedural Steps

In most hospitals, all supplies required for isolation procedures (see Procedures 4-3 ■, 4-4 ■, 4-5 ■, and 4-6 ■) are located in an area or on a cart just outside the patient's room (Figure 4-18 ■). These include:

- Disposable gloves
- Gown
- Mask
- Protective eyewear

The type of PPE used will vary based on the level of precautions required (i.e., standard and contact, droplet, or airborne infection isolation).

ISOLATION ITEM DISPOSAL

The supplies needed for isolation item disposal include:

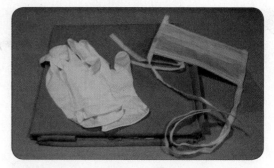

FIGURE ■ 4-18 Supplies for Isolation Procedures

- Garbage bag
- Linen hamper
- Large red isolation bag
- Specimen container
- Plastic bag with biohazard label
- Laundry bag
- Puncture-resistant disposal container for needles and sharps
- Gloves
- Antiseptic agent or antimicrobial agent

Isolation bags for transporting specimens should be turned halfway inside out and left near the door outside the room; someone may be available to hold the bag outside the door. Only the needed supplies should be taken into the room. Phlebotomy requisitions may be

Procedure 4-3

Gowning, Masking, and Gloving

RATIONALE

To prevent the transmission of microorganisms from health care workers to patients, or from patients to health care workers.

EQUIPMENT

- Alcohol-based rub or soap and water
- Gown
- Mask
- Face shield or goggles
- Chemically clean disposable gloves or sterile disposable gloves

(continued)

Procedure 4-3

Gowning, Masking, and Gloving *(continued)*

PROCEDURE

Follow these isolation procedural steps:

(**1**) Complete hand hygiene as described in Procedure 4-1 (Figure 4-19 ■).

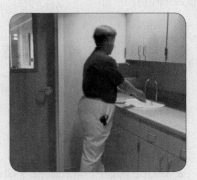

Figure ■ 4-19

(**2**) Use new gowns large enough to cover all clothing (Figure 4-20 ■).

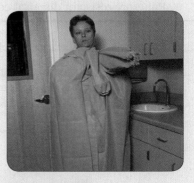

Figure ■ 4-20

(**3**) Touching only its inside surface, place one arm at a time through the gown's sleeves and wrap the gown completely around the body so that the opening is in back. Pull down the sleeves. Then the neck ties or Velcro should be secured around the neck; and the tie strings around the waist need to be tied. Gowns are generally made of cloth and paper (Figure 4-21 ■).

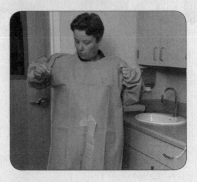

Figure ■ 4-21

④ Don mask if required (Figure 4-22 ■). Masks protect the health care worker from small-particle droplets that may carry pathogens. Often, a small metal band on the mask can be shaped to fit the nose. Two ties are usually made, the first around the upper portion of the head and the second around the upper portion of the neck.

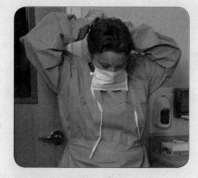

Figure ■ 4-22

⑤ Wear a face shield or goggles during procedures that may possibly generate blood or body fluid droplets (i.e., splashes or sprays), such as from severe patient coughing (Figure 4-23 ■).

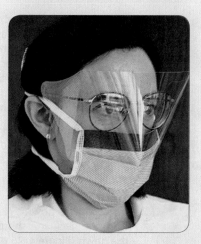

Figure ■ 4-23

⑥ Pull gloves over the ends of gown sleeves to prevent contamination of exposed skin (Figure 4-24 ■). Chemically clean disposable gloves may be used for most isolation procedures. For isolation procedures in which the patient must be protected from any microorganisms, use sterile disposable gloves. Do not wear rings and other pieces of jewelry, because they may puncture a glove during patient contact.

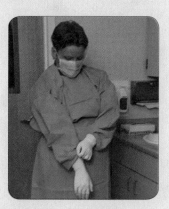

Figure ■ 4-24

Procedure 4-4

Removal of Isolation Gown, Mask, and Gloves

RATIONALE

To prevent the transmission of microorganisms, remove the PPE at the doorway or in the outer room (ante-room), except for the respirator. Remove the respirator after leaving the patient's room and closing the door.

EQUIPMENT

- Large red isolation bag
- Linen hamper
- Special container for disposing masks

PROCEDURE

After the completion of blood collection in an isolation room, follow these steps for removing the isolation gown, mask, and gloves:

(1) Remove the gloves as shown in (Figure 4-25 ■). Pull off the first glove in such a manner as to turn it inside out. Place the rolled-up glove into the palm of the hand that is still gloved. Remove the second glove by slipping the index finger of the ungloved hand between the glove and the hand. Then pull the glove down and off as it turns inside out. Dispose of both gloves in a red garbage bag in the isolation room.

After the removal of gloves, remove the goggles or face shield by touching the head band or ear pieces. (*Do not touch the outside of goggles or face shield because of contamination.*)

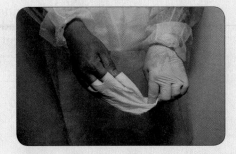

Figure ■ 4-25

(2) Unfasten the gown's ties. Take off the gown by pulling down from the neck and shoulders first and then pull the arms out of the gown (Figure 4-26 ■). Remove the gown and fold it with the contaminated side turned in and with care taken not to touch the outer side.

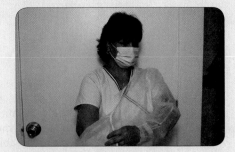

Figure ■ 4-26

(3) Only use gowns once to prevent contamination. Dispose of the gown in the linen hamper or, if disposable, in a garbage bag in the isolation room (Figure 4-27 ■).

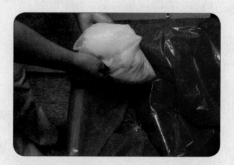

Figure ■ 4-27

(4) Remove the mask by carefully untying the lower tie first, then the upper one (Figure 4-28 ■). Only hold the ends of the ties. Properly dispose of the mask inside the room. In some cases, a special container for masks is placed just outside the room to prevent exposure of hospital personnel to airborne pathogens while inside the isolation room.

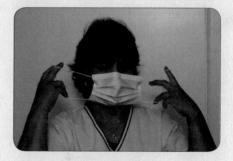

Figure ■ 4-28

(5) Wash hands in the room and again at the nearest sink after exiting the room (Figure 4-29 ■). Use a clean paper towel to open the door. Hold the door open with one foot and discard the used paper towels in the wastebasket directly inside the patient's room.

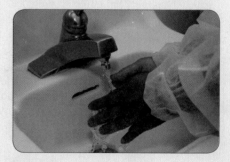

Figure ■ 4-29

Procedure 4-5

Disposing of Contaminated Items

RATIONALE

To properly dispose of contaminated items and prevent the transmission of microorganisms. Trash, linens, and other articles in an isolation room may be removed by using one sturdy biohazard bag or the double-bagging procedure.

EQUIPMENT

- Two large red isolation bags with biohazard written on bags

PROCEDURE

1 Follow dress protocol for entering isolation room, or if already in isolation area, put contaminated material in one bag and seal the bag inside the room as shown in Figure 4-30 ■.

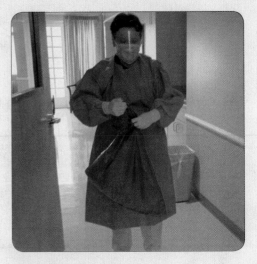

Figure ■ **4-30**

2 Have another person stand outside the room with another opened, clean, impermeable bag (Figure 4-31 ■). The person standing outside the room should have the ends of the bag folded over their hands to shield from possible contamination. Place the sealed bag from the room in the clean bag. The person outside the room can then fold over the edges, expel the air, and seal the outer bag.

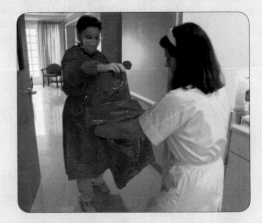

Figure ■ **4-31**

Procedure 4-6

Removal of Patient's Specimen from Isolation Room

RATIONALE

To properly transport a blood specimen or other specimens from a patient in isolation to prevent transmission of microorganisms.

EQUIPMENT

- Blood tube(s)
- Clean biohazard bag

PROCEDURE

1. Follow the required procedure for entering the isolation room.

2. Label blood tube(s) with the patient's name, hospital ID number, and other required identification criteria of the health care facility, and the word "isolation" before entering the isolation room.

3. Collect the blood and place the tube(s) in a clean plastic biohazard bag outside the room (Figure 4-32 ■).

4. Complete hand hygiene.

5. Transport the blood specimen to the laboratory with the appropriate laboratory request form.

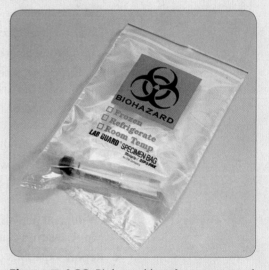

Figure ■ 4-32 Biohazard bag for transport of patient specimens from isolation room.

left outside the room on the isolation cart. If collecting a blood specimen, the health care provider may use a tourniquet in the room or leave the one brought in. The specimen should be labeled at the bedside and the pen left in the room. Used needles, swabs, and so forth should be put in appropriate containers inside the room. Any blood on the outside of the specimen container should be removed with a paper towel. While standing in the doorway and touching only the inside of the isolation bag, the health care worker should place the specimen inside the bag. Gloved hands should be washed in the room. The faucet may be turned off with a paper towel.

INFECTION CONTROL AND SAFETY IN THE CLINICAL LABORATORY

The laboratory receives numerous specimens for diagnostic procedures to be performed to determine causes of diseases and disorders. Health care workers in the laboratory must be extremely cautious, because they often handle specimens with infectious agents. The following essentials of standard precautions and safe laboratory work practices should be adhered to when in the laboratory:

- Perform frequent hand hygiene
- Assume all patients are infectious for HIV and other bloodborne pathogens
- Use personal protection equipment
- Use appropriate waste-disposal practices
- Maintain good personal hygiene, including wearing clean clothes, keeping hair clean and tied back if necessary, keeping fingernails clean, and washing hands frequently
- Avoid wearing laboratory coat or other PPE outside of the designated area for use (i.e., no laboratory coats in lunchroom or at home)
- Do not eat, drink, smoke, or apply cosmetics (including lip balm)
- Avoid storing food and drinks in the laboratory refrigerator or freezer used for reagents and specimens
- Do not insert or remove contact lenses
- Avoid biting nails or chewing on pens
- Carefully dispose of safety needles, lancets, and other blood-collection supplies in appropriate biohazardous labeled containers
- Maintain good health by eating balanced meals, getting enough sleep, and getting enough exercise
- Report personal illnesses to supervisors
- Become familiar with and observe *all* isolation policies
- Learn about the job-related aspects of infection control, and share this information with others
- Caution all personnel working with known hazardous material (this can be done with proper warning labels)
- Report violations of the policies
- Cover patients' specimens at all times during transportation and centrifugation
- Centrifuge specimens within a biohazard safety hood
- Clean phlebotomy trays at least once a week with a 1:10 bleach solution
- Clean the specimen collection area with a decontaminating 1:10 bleach solution

DISINFECTANTS AND ANTISEPTICS

Disinfectants are chemical compounds used to remove or kill pathogenic microorganisms. Chemical disinfectants are regulated by the **Environmental Protection Agency (EPA).** Antiseptics are chemicals used to inhibit the growth and development of microorganisms, but they do not necessarily kill them. **Antiseptics** may be used on human skin, whereas disinfectants are generally used on surfaces and instruments because they are too corrosive for direct use on skin. A disinfectant with a product label claiming that the disinfectant is HIVcidal or tuberculocidal, or a disinfectant having a chlorine bleach dilution of 1:10, should be used to disinfect items contaminated with blood or other body fluids. A more dilute solution of chlorine bleach (1:100) can be used for routine cleaning of surfaces. Gloves and

Table 4-4	Common Antiseptics and Disinfectants for the Health Care Setting
Compound	**Uses and Restrictions**
Alcohols	
Ethyl (70%)	Antiseptic for skin
Isopropyl (70%) (isopropanol)	Antiseptic for skin
Chlorhexidine gluconate	Antiseptic for skin
Chloramine	Disinfectant for wounds
Hypochlorite solutions (bleach)	Disinfectant
Ethylene oxide	Disinfectant (toxic)
Formaldehyde	Disinfectant (noxious fumes)
Glutaraldehyde	Disinfectant (toxic)
Hydrogen peroxide	Antiseptic for skin
Tincture of iodine	Antiseptic for skin (can be irritating)
Benzalkonium chloride	Antiseptic for skin
Iodophors	Antiseptic for skin (less stable)
Phenolic compounds	Disinfectant
1–2% phenols	Disinfectant
Chlorophenol	Disinfectant (toxic)
Hexylresorcinol	Antiseptic for skin
Quaternary ammonium compounds	Antiseptic for skin (ingredient in many soaps)

gowns should be worn when performing decontamination procedures. The minimal contact time for disinfectants to be effective is 10 minutes. Table 4-4 ■ lists some of the more common hospital disinfectants and antiseptics.

Fire Safety

Fire safety is the responsibility of all employees in the health care institution. Fire or explosive hazards may occur in the laboratory or other areas of the health care facility. Health care workers should be familiar with not only the use and location of the fire extinguishers but also the procedures to follow during a fire. They should also be knowledgeable of the exact locations of fire extinguishers and fire blankets. The blankets should be available to smother burning clothes or to use as a fire shield if fire is blocking the exit. Health care institutions usually conduct periodic safety education programs in which the health care worker can participate to become skillful in, and knowledgeable about, the use of fire safety equipment (Figure 4-33 ■).

Health care workers need to learn how to use fire extinguishers.[10] As shown in Figure 4-34 ■, Class A fires require an ABC extinguisher or pressurized water extinguisher for wood, paper, clothing, and trash. The Class B fires need an ABC extinguisher or carbon dioxide (CO_2) extinguisher for liquids, grease, and chemical fires. Class C fires are electrical fires and a CO_2, halon, or ABC extinguisher can be used. The ABC extinguisher is found in most health care facilities, so health care workers need not worry about which extinguisher to use in case of a fire.

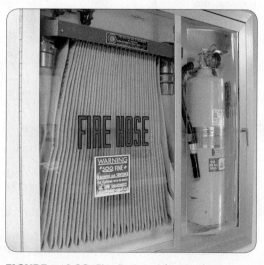

FIGURE ■ **4-33** Fire Extinguisher and Fire Hose

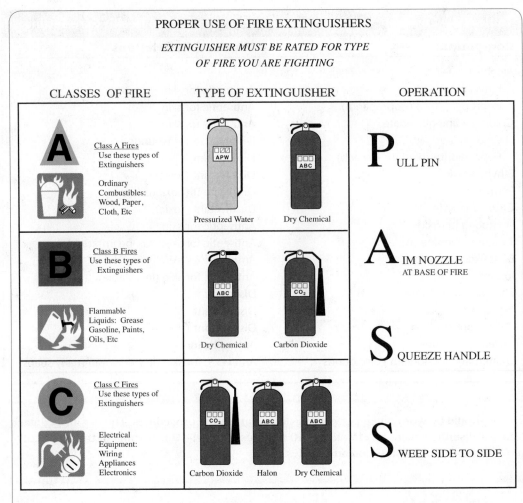

PROPER USE OF FIRE EXTINGUISHERS

EXTINGUISHER MUST BE RATED FOR TYPE
OF FIRE YOU ARE FIGHTING

CLASSES OF FIRE   TYPE OF EXTINGUISHER   OPERATION

A
Class A Fires
Use these types of
Extinguishers

Ordinary
Combustibles:
Wood, Paper,
Cloth, Etc

Pressurized Water   Dry Chemical

B
Class B Fires
Use these types of
Extinguishers

Flammable
Liquids: Grease
Gasoline, Paints,
Oils, Etc

Dry Chemical   Carbon Dioxide

C
Class C Fires
Use these types of
Extinguishers

Electrical
Equipment:
Wiring
Appliances
Electronics

Carbon Dioxide   Halon   Dry Chemical

PULL PIN

AIM NOZZLE
AT BASE OF FIRE

SQUEEZE HANDLE

SWEEP SIDE TO SIDE

BEFORE YOU BEGIN TO FIGHT A SMALL FIRE

ACTIVATE FIRE ALARM
*CALL UTPD (**FROM A SAFE LOCATION**)*
BE SURE FIRE IS CONFINED TO SMALL AREA AND IS NOT SPREADING
BE SURE THAT A SAFE AND UNOBSTRUCTED EXIT IS READILY AVAILABLE
BE SURE YOUR EXTINGUISHER IS THE PROPER SIZE AND TYPE FOR THE CLASS OF FIRE

FIGURE ■ 4-34
Proper Use of Fire
Extinguishers

*Source: Courtesy
Environmental Health &
Safety, The University of
Texas Health Center at
Houston*

EMERGENCY RESPONSE TO POSSIBLE FIRE

If a fire or explosion occurs in the workplace, the health care worker should *not* do the
following:

- Block entrances
- Reenter the building
- Panic
- Run

Instead the health care worker should RACE: *Rescue Alarm Contain Exit*. RACE by doing
the following:

- Pull the nearest fire alarm.
- Call 911 or the hospital's fire emergency number, which should be posted on or near
  the phone.

- Remove patients from danger if on patient floor.
- Close windows and doors to prevent spreading of the fire.
- If the fire is small and isolated from other possible fuel sources, use an ABC extinguisher to fight it:
  1. Pull the plastic pin off of the extinguisher (Figure 4-35 ■).
  2. Aim the extinguisher at the base of the fire and squeeze the handle.
  3. Spray the solution toward the base of the fire but do not point it directly at an individual.
- If the fire threatens to block exits or is not small, leave the area immediately. Take the stairs, not the elevator.
- If clothing is on fire, drop to the ground and roll, preferably in a fire blanket.
- If caught in a fire, crawl to the exit. Because smoke rises, breathing is easier at floor level. Breathing through a wet towel is also helpful.

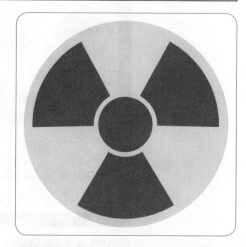

Figure ■ 4-35 Pull pin off fire extinguisher to use it.

Electrical Safety

A major hazard in any area of a health care institution is the possibility of electrical current passing through a person. The important safety points to remember are:

- Do not use power cords that are frayed.
- Avoid using extension cords.
- Unplug electrical equipment before preventative maintenance or any repairs.
- While collecting blood, avoid contact with any electrical equipment, because the electricity may pass through you and the needle and shock the patient.
- Use three-pronged electrical plugs for all equipment (Figure 4-36 ■).

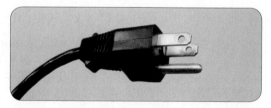

Figure ■ 4-36 Three-Pronged Grounded Plug

Radiation Safety

The three cardinal principles of self-protection from radiation exposure are time, shielding, and distance. Radiation exposure is cumulative; thus, limiting the length of exposure at any one time is a major factor in minimizing the hazard.

Areas where radioactive materials are in use and stored must have warning signs (Figure 4-37 ■) posted on the entrance doors. The health care worker will probably encounter potential hazards from radiation exposure only if he or she must collect specimens from patients in the nuclear medicine or x-ray department or must take specimens to the radioimmunoassay section of a research or a clinical chemistry laboratory. Thus, the health care worker should be cautious when entering an area posted with the radiation hazard sign and should be knowledgeable about the institution's procedures pertaining to radiation safety. If the health care worker must collect specimens in areas where high levels of radioactivity may occur (i.e., nuclear medicine, imaging center), he or she must wear a dosimeter badge to determine the amount

FIGURE ■ 4-37 Radiation Hazard Sign

of radioactivity received. These badges *must* be turned into the health care facility's safety department according to the facility's scheduled intervals to check the radioactivity exposure level. The health care worker must abide by these periodic radioactive badge readings for his or her protection. Health care workers who are pregnant should be aware of the potential hazard of radiation to the fetus.

Chemical Safety

Health care workers who collect blood for diagnostic testing sometimes must transport these specimens to various sections of the clinical laboratory. Usually, in the clinical laboratory are areas where chemicals are used and stored. Thus, he or she should be knowledgeable about chemical safety (Figure 4-38 ■). Labeling may be the single most important step in the proper handling of chemicals. Laboratorians should be able to ascertain from appropriate labels not only the contents of the container but also the nature and extent of hazards posed by the chemicals. Carefully read the label before using any reagents.

The **National Fire Protection Association (NFPA)** developed a labeling system for hazardous chemicals that is frequently used in health care facilities (Figure 4-39 ■). The system uses a diamond-shaped symbol, four colored quadrants, and a hazard rating scale of 0 to 4. The health hazard is shown in the blue quadrant; the flammability hazard is shown in the red quadrant; the instability hazard is indicated in the yellow quadrant; and the specific hazard is shown in the white quadrant. Common laboratory chemicals, such as isopropyl alcohol or diluted bleach (sodium hypochlorite) in squirt bottles, require regulatory labels (Figure 4-40 ■).

SAFETY SHOWERS AND THE EYEWASH STATION

Safety showers should be nearby for use if an accidental chemical spill occurs. Because permanent damage to the skin can result from chemical burns, the victim of a chemical accident must immediately rinse for at least 15 minutes after removing contaminated clothing.

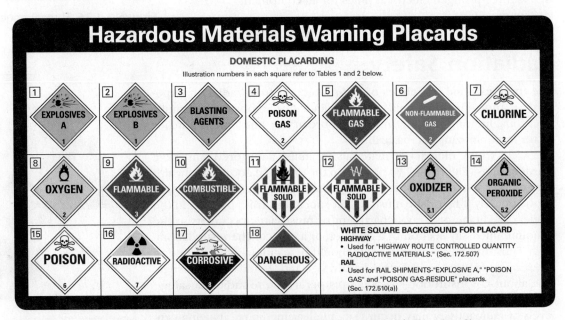

FIGURE ■ 4-38 Department of Transportation (DOT) Hazardous Materials Warning Signs

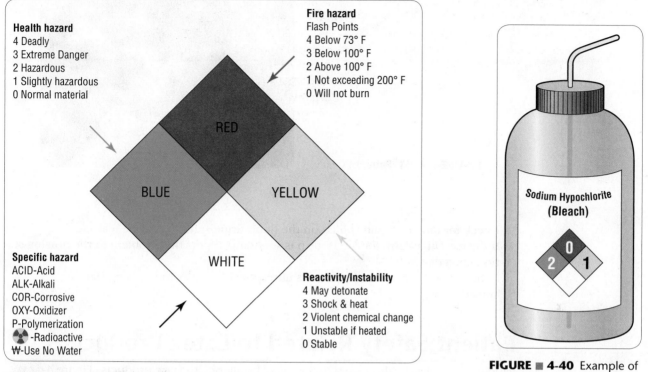

Health hazard
4 Deadly
3 Extreme Danger
2 Hazardous
1 Slightly hazardous
0 Normal material

Fire hazard
Flash Points
4 Below 73° F
3 Below 100° F
2 Above 100° F
1 Not exceeding 200° F
0 Will not burn

RED

BLUE   YELLOW

WHITE

Specific hazard
ACID-Acid
ALK-Alkali
COR-Corrosive
OXY-Oxidizer
P-Polymerization
☢-Radioactive
W̶-Use No Water

Reactivity/Instability
4 May detonate
3 Shock & heat
2 Violent chemical change
1 Unstable if heated
0 Stable

FIGURE ■ 4-39 NFPA Rating System

Sodium Hypochlorite
(Bleach)

2   0   1

FIGURE ■ 4-40 Example of OSHA-Mandated Labeling

In case of a chemical spill in the eye, the victim should rinse his or her eyes at the eyewash station for a minimum of 15 minutes. Contact lenses must be removed before the rinsing in order to thoroughly cleanse the eyes. The victim should not rub the eyes, because doing so may cause further injury. If someone is hurt in a chemical spill, it is preferable to take the victim to the emergency department for treatment after his or her eyes have been rinsed for 15 minutes.

Clinical Alert ❗

When mixing acids with water, *always* add acid to water. *Never* add water to acid because it can explode.

Equipment and Safety in Patients' Rooms

Each member of the health care team is responsible for the safety of the patient. All health care professionals are responsible for patient safety from the time the patient enters the health care setting until his or her departure. First, when collecting blood from a hospitalized patient, provide privacy for the patient during the procedure (Figure 4-41 ■).

As a matter of general patient safety, do the following when in the patient's room:

1. Make certain that all specimen collection supplies, needles, and equipment are either properly disposed of or returned to the specimen collection tray after blood collection.
2. Check to see whether the bed rails are up or down. Always place bed rails up before leaving the patient if they were up when you entered the room.

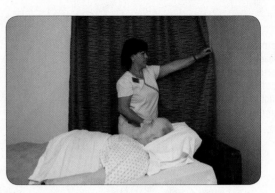

FIGURE ■ 4-41 Patient Privacy

3. Check for food or liquid spilled on the floor, urine spills, or IV line leakage.
4. If the patient's alarm for the IV drip is sounding, report this problem to the nursing station immediately.
5. If the patient is in unusual pain or is unresponsive, notify the nursing station immediately.

Patient Safety Related to Latex Products

Patients, as well as health care workers, may be allergic to latex products (Figure 4-42 ■).

The signs and symptoms of an allergic reaction to latex may include a skin rash, hives, nasal, eye, or sinus irritation, and sometimes, shock. Table 4-5 ■ provides examples of items frequently used in the health care environment that contain latex. Figure 4-43 ■ shows an example of a Latex-Safe Environment sign.

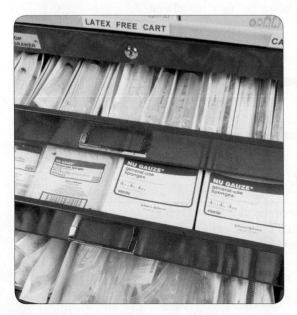

FIGURE ■ 4-42 Latex-Free Cart

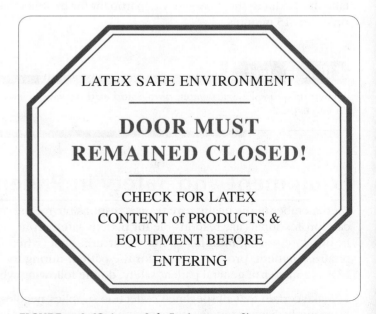

LATEX SAFE ENVIRONMENT

DOOR MUST REMAINED CLOSED!

CHECK FOR LATEX
CONTENT of PRODUCTS &
EQUIPMENT BEFORE
ENTERING

FIGURE ■ 4-43 Latex-Safe Environment Sign

Table 4-5	Products Containing Latex		
Medical Equipment	**Personal Protective Equipment**	**Office Supplies**	**Medical Supplies**
Tourniquets	Gloves	Adhesive tape	Condom-style urinary collection device
Syringes	Goggles	Erasers	Enema tubing tips
Stethoscopes	Rubber aprons	Rubber bands	Injection ports
Oral and nasal airways	Surgical masks		Rubber tops of stoppers on multidose vials
IV tubing			
Disposable gloves			Urinary catheter
Breathing circuits			Wound drains
Blood pressure cuffs			

Source: Reprinted from Preventing Allergic Reactions to Natural Rubber Latex in the Workplace. *National Institute for Occupational Safety and Health Alert, June 1997. Atlanta, GA: The Centers for Disease Control and Prevention.*

Disaster Emergency Plan

Many health care institutions have developed procedures to be followed in case of a hurricane, flooding, earthquake, bomb threat, and other disasters. The health care worker should become familiar with these procedures, because he or she must be prepared to take immediate action whenever conditions warrant such action (Figure 4-44 ■).

Clinical Alert !

If someone telephones and threatens to bomb the health care facility:

- Listen to the person and keep him or her talking.
- Listen for background noises to identify the caller's location.
- Listen for the caller's accent, language, and voice characteristics.
- Ask the caller where the bomb is located and what time it will go off.
- Write down everything the caller states.
- Notify the health care facility's security officer.

If a bomb threat procedure is in place, it must be used by all health care workers.

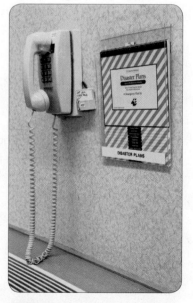

FIGURE ■ 4-44 Disaster Plans and Phone

Self Study

Study Questions

For the following questions, select the one best answer.

1. HBV and HIV transmission occurs most commonly through
   a. large air particles
   b. moisture droplets
   c. blood and body fluids
   d. hand shaking

2. The chain of infection includes all of the following except
   a. mode of transmission
   b. susceptible host
   c. source
   d. handwashing

3. What are the major principles of self-protection from radiation exposure?
   a. time, distance, and shielding
   b. distance, shielding, and combustibility
   c. combustibility, anticorrosiveness, and time
   d. shielding, distance, and anticorrosiveness

4. The health care worker was asked to bring a chemical into the chemistry laboratory. The health care worker noticed that a blue quadrant of a diamond on the chemical's label showed 1. This blue quadrant of the diamond, according to NFPA, indicates a:
   a. flammability hazard
   b. health hazard
   c. instability hazard
   d. specific hazard

5. The most important medically aseptic step in preventing the transmission of infection is
   a. disinfecting door knobs in the clinical laboratory
   b. wearing sterile gloves
   c. hand hygiene
   d. cleaning the countertops with a moist cloth

6. If an accident such as a needlestick occurs, the injured health care worker should first and immediately:
   a. call his or her immediate supervisor from the location of the needlestick accident
   b. cleanse the area with isopropyl alcohol and apply an adhesive bandage
   c. fill out the incident report form
   d. take the needle back to the clinical laboratory for verification of the accident

7. Antiseptics for skin include:
   a. formaldehyde
   b. iodine
   c. ethylene oxide
   d. hypochlorite solution

8. In a health care facility, which is a typical fomite?
   a. 95% isopropyl alcohol
   b. iodine
   c. computer keyboard
   d. facial shield

9. Which of the following isolation techniques is used to decrease the spread of whooping cough?
   a. droplet precautions
   b. contact precautions
   c. airborne precautions
   d. enteric precautions

10. Reverse isolation is the same as:
    a. protective environment
    b. enteric isolation
    c. airborne precautions
    d. contact precautions

Case Study

Ron is a Certified Nursing Assistant who has also been trained to be a phlebotomist in a rural health clinic. His supervisor has asked him to start home health care visits so that he can take history and physical assessments and perform any needed blood collection procedures. On his first assignment, he is sent to three patients' homes that are approximately 40 miles from the clinic to collect *fasting* (has not eaten for 8 to 12 hours) blood samples for glucose testing needed to regulate their insulin injections. When he arrives at the first home, he gathers all of his blood collection equipment and enters the home for the collection. As soon as he opens the blood collection container, he realizes that he does not have gloves for the blood collection. However, because of time commitments, he collects the blood from this patient and the other patients in their homes. He figures that if he washes his hands after collecting the blood from each patient, he will be okay. But upon the last patient's collection, he realizes that he has an open abrasion on his ring finger.

Questions
1. What should he do immediately?
2. What should Ron do when he goes back to the clinic?

Advocating Patient Safety Case Study

Patricia and Danielle, two phlebotomists from the clinical laboratory specimen collection area, are collecting on the same patient floor. Patricia notices that Danielle comes out of one patient's room with gloves on her hands and enters another patient's room with the same gloves.

Question
What should Patricia do as a co-worker with Danielle?

Competency Assessment

Check Yourself: Infection Control Procedures and Safety

1. When you have completed a phlebotomy procedure, what should you always think of doing before going on to the next patient?

2. If you obtain a skin rash on your hands after working as a phlebotomist over a 3-month period, what could possibly be a cause of the rash?

3. Describe what should occur if a small amount of blood is accidently spilled in the clinical laboratory specimen collection area.

Competency Checklist: Infection Control and Safety

This checklist can be completed in a classroom setting using a make believe health care facility or in the clinical setting.

(1) Completed (2) Needs to improve/Repeat lesson and checklist

_____ 1. Looking at the type ABC extinguisher in the health care facility, what type of fire is this extinguisher used for in emergencies?

_____ 2. If you are performing maintenance checks on the centrifuge used to spin down the blood samples, what is the first thing you should do in the maintenance check?

_____ 3. Describe or show the class three pieces of PPE.

_____ 4. Look at the following chemicals in the classroom and identify whether they are an antiseptic or a disinfectant

    isopropyl alcohol

    iodine

    chloramine

References

1. US Department of Labor and Occupational Safety and Health Administration (OSHA): Occupational exposure to bloodborne pathogens; final rule (29 CFR 1910.1030). *Fed. Register* December 6, 1991, 64004–64182.

2. OSHA Revised Bloodborne Pathogens Standard 1910.1030. Needlestick Safety and Prevention Bill Act; April 18, 2001. http://www.osha.gov/SLTC/bloodbornepathogens/index.html

3. Updated US public health service guidelines for the management of occupational exposures to HBV, HCV, and HIV: Recommendations for postexposure prophylaxis. *MMWR Morb Mortal Wkly Rep* June 29, 2001;50(RR11).

4. Clinical and Laboratory Standards Institute (CLSI). *Protection of Laboratory Workers from Occupationally Acquired Infections; Approved Guideline.* 3rd ed. Wayne, PA: CLSI, 2005.

5. Centers for Disease Control and Prevention: Guidelines for isolation precautions in hospitals, part I: Evolution of isolation practices. *Am J Infect Control* 1996;24(1):24–31.

6. Siegel, JD, Rhinehart, E, Jackson, M, Chiarello, L. Guideline for isolation precautions: Preventing transmission of infectious agents in health care settings. The Health Care Infection Control Practices Advisory Committee. *Infect Control Hosp Epidemiol* 2007; 35(10)Supplement 2: S65–S164.

7. Molinari JA: Infection control: its evolution to the current standard precautions. *J Am Dent Assoc* 2003;134:569–574.

8. Respiratory Hygiene/Cough Etiquette in Healthcare Settings www.cdc.gov/flu/professionals/infectioncontrol/resphygiene.htm).

9. Guideline for Hand Hygiene in Health-Care Setting. *MMWR,* 2002, 51(RR14). http://www.cdc.gov/mmwr/preview/mmwrhtml/rr5114al.htm.

10. National Fire Protection Association (NFPA): *National Fire Codes.* Available at: http://www.NFPA.org.

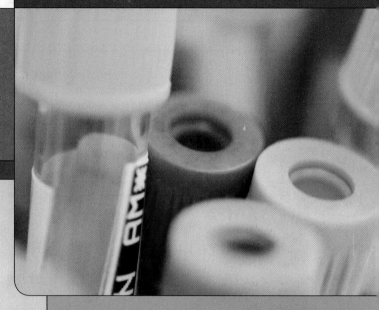

Chapter 5

Documentation, Specimen Handling, and Transportation

KEY TERMS

aliquot

analyte

bar codes

beta-carotene

bilirubin

centrifugation

clinical (or medical) record

confidentiality

constituents

critical value

date of birth (DOB)

diagnostic test results

electronic health (or health care) record (EHR)

electronic medical record (EMR)

percutaneous

photosensitive

plasma

pneumatic tube systems

porphyrins

radio frequency identification (RFID)

requisition form

sample

sample integrity

secondary specimens

serum

specimen collection manual

thermolabile

turn around time (TAT)

CHAPTER OBJECTIVES

Upon completion of Chapter 5, the learner should be able to do the following:

1. Describe the uses of a medical record.
2. Describe the essential elements of a requisition and a final report.
3. List examples of policies and procedures important to phlebotomy.
4. List the basic specimen-handling guidelines for maintaining specimen integrity.
5. Name sources of preexamination error that can occur during blood specimen transportation, processing, or storage.
6. Describe which blood analytes are photosensitive or thermolabile.
7. List reasons for specimen rejection.

Documentation Basics

PATIENTS' RECORDS

All health care organizations provide a legal record for each patient that describes the patient's visit, tests and procedures (including laboratory results), and clinical progress (Box 5-1 ■). The record for each patient is called a **clinical (or medical) record,** or **electronic health (or health care) record (EHR),** or **electronic medical record (EMR),**

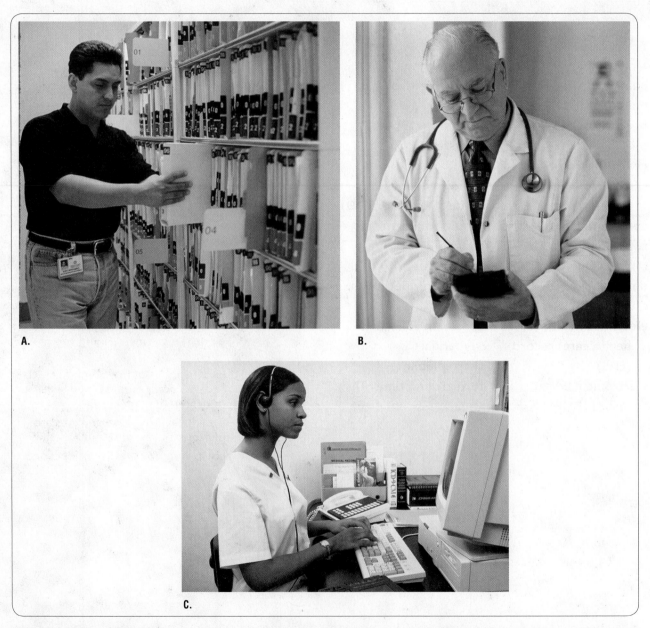

A.

B.

C.

FIGURE ■ 5-1 A. A file room for medical records in a physician's office. *Source: A. Copyright © Michael Newman/PhotoEdit.* B. A physician using a personal digital assistant (PDA) to enter medical information. *Source: B. Masterfile Corporation* C. Entering clinical data into an EMR.

the latter of which are computerized versions (Figure 5-1 ■). Documentation of all clinical events in this record is important for the following reasons (also see Box 5-2 ■):[1]

■ Monitoring the quality of care, goals for the patient, how the patient responds, and maintaining a full account of treatment (what was done and why, or what was withheld and why).

■ Coordination of care among all health care providers involved with the patient

■ Hospital accreditation and clinical research

■ Legal protection. (If something is not documented, it is assumed that it was not done!)

Electronic medical records are beneficial because they allow for the following features:

■ Handwritten errors are eliminated due to electronic entries

■ Times and dates are automatically recorded

■ Electronic orders can be generated for laboratory tests, diagnostic imaging, or other tests

■ Electronic graphs are available for laboratory results, vital signs, etc.

■ Electronic prescription information is readily available for ordering and retrieving

■ Pre-established patient education materials can be specified for an individual patient

■ Digital photos or images can easily be stored

■ Letters, email, and other clinical documents can be quickly found

■ Appointment reminders can be automatically generated

■ Billing is automated and more accurate

Box 5-1 **Common Components of a Medical Record**

All information should be kept confidential to protect the patient's privacy.

Personal information: patient's name, **date of birth (DOB),** social security number (SSN) or other unique identification number, address, marital status, closest relative, known allergies, physician's name, and diagnosis

Personal and family medical history: initial assessment completed by the physician (MD or DO), physician assistant (PA), nurse practitioner (NP), and/or nurse (RN), medical assistant

Ordering documentation: includes MDs and/or other qualified provider's (nurse practitioner's [NP], clinical nurse specialist's [CNS], physician assistant's [PA]) orders for laboratory, radiology, pharmacy, and so on

Informed consent, HIPAA, advanced directives, release forms: treatment consent forms, privacy information forms, authorization forms for release of medical information, and similar documents

Patient's plan of care: MD and nursing care diagnoses, interventions, and patient outcomes

Diagnostic test results: results from all tests performed on the patient

Medication administration record: known allergies, medication dosage and timing, route of administration, site, and date

Progress notes and consultations: patient's progress, interventions used, and treatment effectiveness

Discharge plan/summary: plans for special diets, medications, therapy, home health visits, and follow-up appointments

Financial information: insurance information, insurance company release forms, and correspondence

| **Box 5-2** | **Tips for Documenting Clinical Information** |

Health care workers involved in blood collection can provide useful information by making extra notations of circumstances related to the venipuncture site, timing, fasting status, or STAT (priority) status. Health care facilities have special procedures for situations (incidents related to patient falls, accidental patient injuries such as erroneous arterial puncture, etc.) that need to be documented and for determining who is authorized to make the notations or electronic entries in the medical record. Be sure to follow your health facilities policies.

THE FIVE C'S OF MEDICAL RECORD DOCUMENTATION[1]

- **Concise:** Entries must be factual and to the point; do not include information that is unrelated to the patient's health care.
- **Complete:** Entries must be complete and objective; exclude opinions and judgments.
- **Clear:** If information is handwritten, it should be printed (usually requiring the use of blue or black ink), not in cursive; it should be in an easy-to-read format.
- **Correct:** Medical records should be error-free but errors may result by improper additions and/or omissions (see error documentation below).
- **Chronologic:** Generally speaking, medical records should be in chronologic order with the latest entries on top (if the record is a paper version); however, electronic medical records may vary in their formats even though all entries are chronological and traceable.

If an error is detected in a medical record:

- **Report it immediately** to a supervisor and document it.
- **Include all relevant information in a timely manner.** (For example, if a phlebotomist is unable to identify a patient because of a missing armband, the notation on the correct form should include the *time, date,* and *name* of the nurse who positively identified the patient, and the *phlebotomist's name.*)
- **Document errors according to institutional policies.** If it is a paper copy, note the error by marking a single line through it and writing the word "error" next to it with your signature (first initial and last name, e.g., J. Doe, is sufficient). Do not leave extra space between your notations and your signature. Legally, this "space" on the record becomes your responsibility, so do not leave room for someone else to add information to your notation. If it is an EMR, follow institutional guidelines and software requirements for making corrections or changes in the computer.
- **Be accurate and legible.** Record facts, not opinions. If it is a paper copy, use ink, print clearly, and do not erase or use correction fluid.
- **Correcting errors.** Records should never be changed or falsified to cover a mistake. On a paper document, an error should be noted by marking a single line through it, writing the word "error," and signing your initials next to it.
- **Do not assign blame.**

POLICIES AND PROCEDURES

All health care facilities have manuals that detail operating procedures to be followed (Table 5-1 ■). Depending on the facility, there may be several manuals—safety manual, administrative manual, employee handbook, **specimen collection manual**—or just one manual separated by sections. These may also be accessible electronically. Table 5-1 lists the topics generally covered in procedure manuals; these topics are particularly important to health care workers involved in blood collection. Health care workers may be involved in developing, writing, and practicing these procedures (Figure 5-2 ■).

Clinical Alert !

Remember that it is very tempting to discuss interesting patient situations with peers, friends, or family members. Although patient situations are learning experiences and they may occasionally be discussed with authorized laboratory personnel, this type of information must *not* be shared with anyone else without the prior consent of the patient or prior authorization. This mandate assures compliance with the Health Insurance Portability and Accountability Act (HIPAA) which details patients' rights to protection of their health information. HIPAA prohibits the disclosure of any health information unless written consent has been obtained from a patient.

Table 5-1	Policies and Procedures for Health Care Workers Involved in Phlebotomy
Type	**Procedures Included**
Specimen collection	Patient preparation Type of collection container and amount of specimen required; type and amount of preservative or anticoagulant needed Timing policies (e.g., creatinine clearance, therapeutic drug monitoring, etc.) Special handling or transportation needs (e.g., refrigeration) Proper labeling requirements Priority status (STAT/emergency specimens) Need for additional data when indicated (e.g., fasting vs. nonfasting, etc.) Reporting of **critical values** (abnormally high or low test results) Handling specimens going to or coming from outside organizations Reporting incidents such as patient falls or other patient injuries, and accidental needlesticks
Administrative procedures and/or Employee Handbook	Performance evaluation procedures and job descriptions Disciplinary policies and **confidentiality**/nondisclosure policies Compensatory time, attendance, annual leave, and overtime policies Other human resources procedures (nondiscrimination, benefits, dress code, etc.)
Safety	Fire and radiation safety Internal and external disaster plan Exposure control plan Hazard communication manual
Infection control (IC)	Precautions/isolation procedures Disposal policies Decontamination procedures Hand-hygiene procedures Accidental **percutaneous** (through the skin) needlesticks Postexposure procedures
Quality control (QC) and preventive maintenance (PM)	Maintaining appropriate supplies; proper use, storage, and handling of supplies; supplies and equipment maintenance and inventory procedures Monitoring reagents and equipment Stability of reagents and expiration dates (when the item should no longer be used) Measuring precision and accuracy; acceptable symbols, abbreviations, and units of measure Maintaining confidentiality

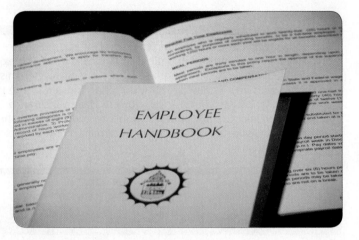

FIGURE ■ 5-2 Employee Handbooks should be updated frequently and made available to each new employee.
Source: Copyright © Tony Freeman / PhotoEdit

Laboratory Test Requisitions and Labels

Regardless of the method used for submitting a laboratory test request or labeling blood samples or specimens (Box 5-3 ■), there are standards for required information that each health care facility must follow. The College of American Pathologists (CAP) and the Clinical and Laboratory Standards Institute, CLSI, have established guidelines or standards for laboratory testing requisitioning and specimen labeling. The primary purpose of these standards is to promote the correct identification of the patient and their respective blood samples from the time they are collected, through the testing of **analytes** (the measurable quantity of a blood component), and through the final reporting of test results. Health care facilities must maintain updated procedures based on these or other standards of practice. However, studies have shown that paper-based and/or handwritten systems for ordering laboratory tests (requisitioning) or for labeling blood specimen tubes are more prone to human error, such as transcription mistakes (misspellings, illegible writing, or transposed numbers, etc.), lost requisitions, and duplicate orders. Use of electronic patient data assists in maintaining accurate patient and specimen identity. Standardizing patient identification methodology through the use of electronic data systems is important in reducing errors.

Box 5-3 Is It a Sample or a Specimen?

The Clinical and Laboratory Standards Institute (CLSI), a global organization, has emphasized standardization of terms for purposes of achieving worldwide uniformity. While many health care workers use the terms blood sample and blood specimen interchangeably, CLSI suggests the following definitions:[2]

Sample—one or more parts (e.g., blood or tissues) taken from a system (the patient's body), and intended to provide information on the system;

Specimen—the discrete portion of a body fluid (e.g., blood or urine) or tissue taken for examination, study, or analysis of one or more characteristics (analytes), to determine the character of the whole.

Thus, an example of the use of these terms would be: "A blood *sample* was taken from a patient and subdivided into multiple *specimens* for testing in different areas of the laboratory."

TRANSMITTAL OF THE TEST REQUEST TO THE LABORATORY

A laboratory test request from a physician or his/her designee (nurse) initiates the preexamination/preanalytical phase of laboratory work through the use of either an interactive computer system; or a manual request system (paper-based, usually a multi-part request form that is color-coded, and is sometimes also used for final test results) (Figure 5-3 ■).

Most hospitals use automated/electronic procedures for test requests and specimen labels. This fosters greater accuracy in patient identification and specimen labeling. Basic guidelines for required information on a laboratory test request are summarized below.[2]

- patient identification (ID) (name, registration or identification number, and location, or unique confidential specimen code that has an audit trail to the patient);
- patient's gender and date of birth (DOB) or age;
- name of physician or legally authorized person ordering the test (the physician's address is needed if it is different than the receiving laboratory);
- tests requested;
- date and, if appropriate, time of sample collection;
- source of sample, when appropriate; and
- other pertinent clinical information when appropriate

In cases of emergency, the test request is called a *STAT request* and should be documented.

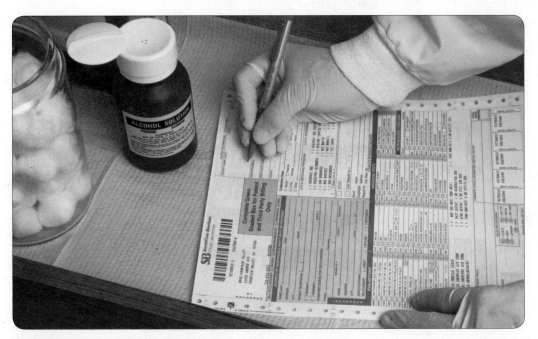

FIGURE ■ 5-3 Example of a Multipart Laboratory Requisition Form

Use of a multiple-part requisition form is common in non-automated systems and can also be used as a temporary request until a formal requisition can be entered into a computer system

Specimen Labels and Blood Collection Lists

Accurate specimen identification is essential and must continue from the time of collection through disposal of the specimen. Identification methods vary from manually copying all patient identification information onto the container to using highly automated, bar-coded labels. Manually labeling specimens can be time-consuming and prone to errors so by using electronic systems to generate labels the problems are eliminated, the correct number of labels for tubes can be generated, and productivity is improved. Labeling systems include those that can imprint a patient identification card or electronically print patient identification information onto the specimen label. CLSI provides requirements for the format and location of every patient specimen label and includes five requirements whether they are hand written or produced by a portable printer at the time of collection:[3]

- patient name
- unique patient identifier
- DOB
- specimen collection time and date
- a designated space for the phlebotomist's identification (a signature, initials, or code)

Furthermore, the CLSI standards provide for each health care facility or laboratory to add individualized information to the label as needed. Additional information could be as follows:

- specific tests requested;
- types of specimen collection tubes required for the requested tests;
- type and volume of specimens to be obtained;
- unique accession numbers (compatible with the laboratory information system, LIS, or sample numbers to be used for that particular collection time);
- special handling requirements such as for pH, temperature, preservatives, routing, test codes, or order status (routine, STAT);
- collection order of the tubes;
- which laboratory section will receive the specimen (hematology, immunology, etc.)
- who to call for a critical result;
- smaller labels may be generated to label **aliquot** tubes (an aliquot is a portion of a blood specimen that is removed, usually after centrifugation, and placed in a separate tube for concurrent testing or for future use; aliquots are chemically identical to the original sample, but should be labeled with information distinct from, but linked to, the original specimen container), pediatric collection tubes, cuvettes, and/or microscope slides; and
- some hospitals may generate a blood drawing list by floor or unit using this same data.

CLSI also provides guidelines for label placement, sizes, and formats so that the patient's name is always placed in the upper left corner of the label and other data elements are consistently placed in the same proximity on the label and the label is oriented the same way on tubes. This reinforces patient-safety practices during specimen accessioning, relabeling, and other workflow tasks.[3]

BAR CODES

Bar-coded labels (similar to the ones used for pricing grocery items or tracking railroad boxcars) are used for identifying patients (on an armband, an ID card, etc.) and blood specimens (Figures 5-3, 5-4 ■, and 5-5). **Bar codes** consist of a series of light and dark bands that relate to specific alphanumeric symbols (i.e., numbers and letters) so when bands are placed together in a series, they can correspond to a name (patient, health care worker, or test) or a number (identification or test code, etc.). Bar codes are available in several formats, one or two dimensional, and an optical reading device is needed at the line-of-sight to scan/read the actual bar code. Bar

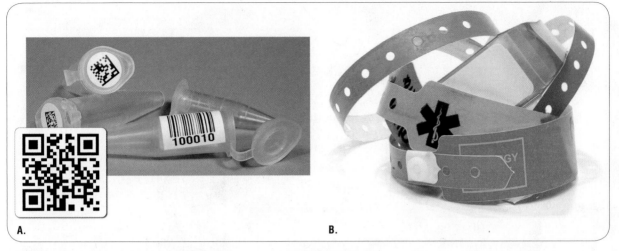

FIGURE ■ 5-4 Examples of Bar Code Labels and Identification Armbands
A. These small labels would be used for specimen aliquots. *Source: Courtesy of Electronic Imaging Materials.* B. There are many styles of patient armbands available. *Source: Rob Byron/Shutterstock.com*

codes have been proven to improve efficiency and accuracy because they are faster (reducing **turn around time, TAT**) due to the elimination of typing or handwriting information.

RADIO FREQUENCY IDENTIFICATION

Radio frequency identification (RFID) is another automated system for identification and tracking of patients or specimens. RFID tags are tiny silicon chips that transmit data to a wireless receiver (such as a computer). In contrast to a bar code, RFID does not require line-of-sight reading with a scanner and can hold more data/information than a bar code. The tag can be detected at various distances by hand-held or stationary readers/computers, depending on the frequency of the tags. RFID tags make it possible to identify and/or track many items simultaneously.

BIOMETRICS

Biometric technology is also being investigated for applications in patient identification and specimen tracking. This type of technology includes: fingerprints, face recognition, voice prints, iris patterns, retinal vascular patterns, and digitized signature verification.[2]

Clinical Alert ❗

Even with the best technology, there are no foolproof methods that prevent all errors. Patient and specimen identification errors can occur at any time during the preexamination and examination (preanalytical and analytical) phases of the laboratory cycle due to human error. As specimens are transported, centrifuged, processed, relabeled, separated into aliquots, etc., there are still opportunities for mistakes. Therefore, labeling procedures for samples must include careful placement and verification at each step. For example, when an aliquot is made and labeled from the primary sample, a step should be included that links identification from the requisition and the primary container to the aliquot tube. This verification step should apply to all **secondary specimens** (serum or plasma that has been removed after centrifugation of the primary tube). The utmost diligence and attention to accuracy is vital for all health care workers involved in phlebotomy practice.

In addition, because many tests are highly automated and the analyzer will read the barcode label directly from the specimen tube, labeling the specimen requires specific alignment of the label on the tube. Failure to do so will result in delays reporting test results and lost efficiency (Figure 5-5 ■).

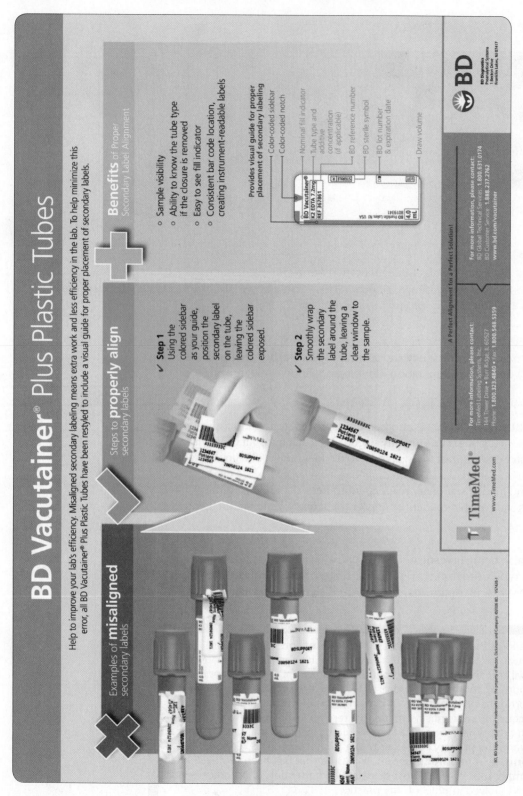

FIGURE ■ 5-5

Alignment of the Tube Label

Source: Courtesy of BD VACUTAINER Systems, Preanalytical Solutions, Franklin Lakes, NJ

Specimen Handling and Transport

Sample integrity (quality or completeness of the blood sample) can be affected by the method of transport, timing delays, temperature, humidity, agitation, exposure to light, and centrifugation methods. Some, but not all, specimens need to be centrifuged before analysis. The CLSI defines basic standards for the handling and processing of blood samples after consideration of numerous variables that might affect laboratory testing during precentrifugation (after the specimen is collected but before centrifugation), **centrifugation** (while the specimen is in the centrifuge), and postcentrifugation (after centrifugation of the specimen but before removal of an aliquot of **serum** or **plasma** for testing).

CLSI committees have studied the research literature that contributes to specific recommendations for specimen handling, storage, and transport. Because there are hundreds of laboratory assays, chemical reagents, and manufacturers' instructions for testing specimens, it is beyond the scope of this text to address them all. It is up to each laboratory to customize their procedures to fit the specific tests they perform, to keep these procedures updated and in accordance with CLSI guidelines, and to provide information and training to phlebotomists as needed.

Table 5-2 ■ summarizes basic CLSI recommendations for the handling and processing of blood specimens. It only provides an overview of essential recommendations adapted from the CLSI approved guideline entitled *Procedures for Handling and Processing of Blood Specimens.*[4] This guideline is much more detailed and provides numerous references and resources for further information. Every laboratory is under pressure to balance transportation, time, test accuracy, and specimen rejection issues, so health care workers must follow their own institution's policies.

SPECIMEN TRANSPORTATION GUIDELINES

Every health care facility has a specific protocol for specimen transportation and processing. Most laboratories require the use of a leak-proof plastic bag for enclosing and transporting the primary specimen tube (i.e., the blood samples taken directly from the patient). This biohazard bag protects the health care worker from exposure to pathogenic (disease-producing) microorganisms from leakage or spillage during specimen transportation. The transport/biohazard bag may have a pouch on the outside for a laboratory request or other documentation, which eliminates the potential for contamination (Figure 5-6 ■).

Table 5-2 Summary of Recommendations for the Handling and Processing of Blood Specimens[4]
Basic Rules of Thumb
Precentrifugation refers to specimen handling and processing after collection and before centrifugation.
■ Not all specimens require centrifugation.
■ Tubes with additives should be gently inverted 5–10 times at the patient's bedside to mix the specimen with the additive as soon as the specimen is withdrawn. Excessive agitation causes hemolysis.
■ Specimens without anticoagulant additives (serum specimens) should be clotted before centrifugation, which usually takes 30 to 60 minutes at room temperature (22°C–25°C).
■ Clotting time is affected (often delayed) by anticoagulant therapy/medications that the patient may be taking.
■ Chilling (2–8°C) the specimen will delay clotting.
■ Clotting may be accelerated with the use of activators/accelerators.
■ Anticoagulated specimens (plasma specimens) can be centrifuged immediately after collection.
■ Serum or plasma should be removed from cells as soon as possible. (In general, this should be no more than 2 hours after the time of collection unless there is documentation that longer contact times do not affect test results.)
■ Some **constituents** are **thermolabile**—that is, they degrade if exposed to warm temperatures, so they need to be chilled immediately.

continued

Table 5-2	Summary of Recommendations for the Handling and Processing of Blood Specimens[4] (cont.)

- Chilling a specimen stabilizes most constituents.
- If potassium (K) is being tested, the specimen cannot be chilled for more than 2 hours, because this causes K to leak out of the cells, causing a false elevation.
- Specimens for testing electrolytes (including potassium) should not be chilled.
- Specimens that require chilling are: (Blood gases are covered in Chapter 11)

ammonia	lactic acid
catecholamines	parathyroid hormone
gastrin	pyruvate

- Tests for RNA-based molecular tests can be temporarily stored at 4°C if they cannot be tested within 48 hours.
- Conversely, some tests require maintenance at normal body temperature (37°C) until tested. These include:
  cold agglutinins and cryofibrinogen
- Some analytes are **photosensitive,** or sensitive to light, and they should be wrapped with aluminum foil or placed in an amber specimen container to shield the specimen from light. Tubes should be kept closed at all times. Photosensitive analytes include:

bilirubin	**beta-carotene**
vitamins A and B_6	**porphyrins**

Centrifugation refers to a specimen handling and processing procedure in which the specimen is spun rapidly to separate cells from the liquid portion of blood.

- The manufacturer's specifications generally indicate the speeds and times of centrifugation.
- Blood specimens should be allowed to clot before centrifugation.
- Tubes should be centrifuged with closures/stoppers in place.
- The centrifuge should have a top that secures appropriately.
- Because centrifuges generate internal heat, they should be temperature controlled at 20–22°C; and for analytes that are temperature sensitive, specimens should be centrifuged in a temperature controlled centrifuge and separated from the cells at 4°C.
- Specimens (especially those for potassium measurement) should not be centrifuged more than once.
- Many types of gel and non-gel devices are available to enable a barrier to form between the serum/plasma and the blood clot/cells during centrifugation. They all have a particular viscosity and specific gravity that is between those of the clot/cells and the serum/plasma. They may be incorporated into the tube as an additive, or they may be added just before centrifugation. Whatever the case, the manufacturer's directions should be followed.

Postcentrifugation refers to specimen handling/processing after centrifugation and prior to removal of serum or plasma.

- Again, serum or plasma should be physically separated from cells as soon as possible.
- Separated serum/plasma should remain at room temperature for no longer than 8 hours; and if testing cannot be completed within 8 hours, it should be refrigerated (2–8°C).
- If testing is not completed within 48 hours, the separated serum/plasma should be frozen at or below –20°C unless the assay-specific directions indicate an alternative method of storage.
- Serum/plasma should not be repeatedly frozen and thawed. When thawed, it should be at room temperature (without the use of heat) and inverted 10–20 times.
- Frost-free freezers are not suitable for storage because of temperature variances.
- Serum/plasma may be left in contact with a gel barrier or separator device as recommended by their respective manufacturers.
- Tubes should be stored in an upright position with an air-tight, secure closure to avoid contamination, evaporation, changes in concentration, accidental spills, and/or the creation of aerosols.
- Plunger-type filters are sometimes used after centrifugation to separate serum/plasma from the clot/cells before or after centrifugation. Use the correct size plunger for the tube size and consult the manufacturer's instructions for details and limitations of use.

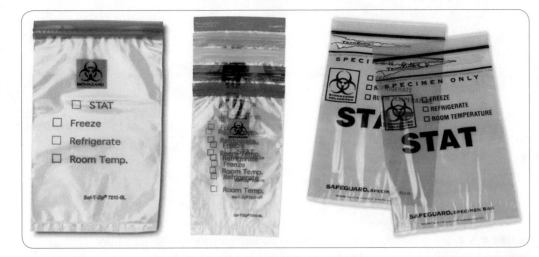

FIGURE ■ 5-6
Specimen Biohazard
Bags
*Source: Courtesy of
MarketLab Inc.
www.marketlabinc.com*

If possible, the blood specimens in evacuated tubes and microcollection tubes should be maintained in a vertical position with the tube cap or closure on top, to promote complete clot formation and to reduce the possibility of agitating the sample which may cause hemolysis. Handling blood specimens in a gentle manner also reduces the chances of hemolyzing the specimens.

For transportation of specimens from remote ambulatory sites, including home health collections, consider the following guidelines:

■ Follow the same handling guidelines set out in standard precautions.

■ Use the same safety equipment that is used in a hospital environment (e.g., closed venipuncture system, gloves, disposable laboratory coat, plastic blood collection tubes, and a biohazardous disposal container).

■ Transport all blood collection equipment and specimens in an enclosed or lockable container to avoid spills in case the transport automobile is in a collision. The container should have a biohazard warning label on it and notification procedures in case of an accident. Cold packs should be used in the container for transport during hot weather, or, conversely, the vehicle should be heated in freezing weather.

■ For home collection, be extra careful to dispose of waste properly and to place blood specimens in leak-proof plastic bags in an upright position inside a labeled transport container.

Clinical Alert !

Glycolytic action (the breakdown of glucose) from the blood cells can interfere with the laboratory analysis of some analytes. Also, rough handling and agitation of the specimen can have an effect on hematology and coagulation. Because of these interfering factors, the blood samples should be transported to the clinical laboratory *as soon as possible* after the time of collection so that the sample can be processed appropriately and serum or plasma can be separated from the blood cells. The serum or plasma that is separated from the cells must be handled according to specified testing procedures, but in general, serum can remain at room temperature (20–25°C) for testing, be refrigerated (2–8°C), be stored in a dark place, or be frozen (at or below −20°C), depending on the prescribed laboratory method.

CHILLED SPECIMENS

As mentioned in Table 5-2, for special types of blood specimens, chilling (2–8°C) is required. The blood sample should be kept cool by using a commercially available cold pack or by being placed in a mixture (slurry) of ice and water (Figure 5-7 ■). Do not use solid chunks

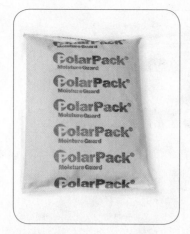

FIGURE ■ 5-7 Some specimens require chilling during transport to the laboratory. Commercially available cold/cool packs are available in a variety of sizes.
Source: Courtesy of MarketLab www.marketlabinc.com

of ice because parts of the specimen may freeze and hemolysis will result. The labeled blood sample tube should be placed in a biohazard bag before being placed in the ice slurry. Again, specimens that may require chilling are:[4]

gastrin

ammonia

lactic acid

catecholamines

parathyroid hormone

pyruvate

Refer to Chapter 11 for discussion of blood gases.

PROTECTING SPECIMENS FROM LIGHT

Some chemical constituents in blood, such as bilirubin, are *photosensitive* (light sensitive) and decompose if exposed to light. Thus, blood collected for light-sensitive chemical analysis should be protected from bright light with an aluminum foil wrapping around the tube (Figure 5-8 ■) or an amber-colored transport bag. Light-sensitive constituents include the following:[4]

Bilirubin (This liver function test is often used in monitoring newborns with jaundice.)

vitamins A and B_6

beta-carotene

porphyrins

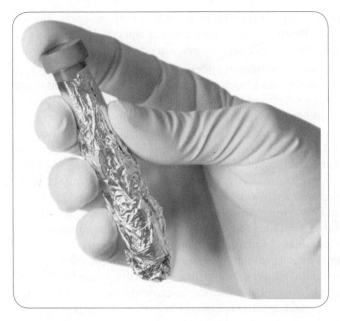

FIGURE ■ 5-8 Specimen wrapped in foil for protection from light. Amber colored bags are also commercially available.
Source: Courtesy of MarketLab Inc.
www.marketlabinc.com

MICROBIOLOGICAL SPECIMENS

Blood, sputum, and urine specimens for microbiological culture need to be transported to the laboratory as quickly as possible so that the specimens can be transferred to culture media and/or the urine analyzed. This enhances the likelihood of detecting pathogenic bacteria. Specimens for blood cultures can also be collected directly into culture media, which minimizes possible contamination and speeds contact with the culture media.

WARMED SPECIMENS

Some specimens require keeping the temperature at 37°C, normal body temperature, until the test is performed. These tests include cold agglutinins and cryofibrinogen. These blood specimens require a regulated heat source (e.g., heating block) for transportation and handling purposes.

Specimen Delivery Methods

In larger facilities, the laboratory is most often the department responsible for the delivery of blood specimens to the location where they will be analyzed. However, other types of specimens, such as CSF, urine, and sputum, are commonly delivered by transportation or nursing staff members. Whatever the site, guidelines should be available for the safe and efficient delivery of specimens; these may include a schedule of pick-ups, how to deliver STAT specimens, where to place specimens, when to "double bag" specimens, how to "log in" specimens, how to store specimens and for how long, and similar procedures. There are a variety of methods to transport specimens:

   Courier services—are used for off-site areas such as reference laboratories, blood drawing stations, or remote clinics. Again, considerations prior to and during transportation should include adequate packaging and handling. This is especially true in hot or cold temperatures.

   Hand delivery—often involves the use of a log to document the receipt of each specimen. In a hospital setting, the blood collection trays or carts are typically arranged to hold numerous specimens awaiting delivery to the laboratory. All specimens should be secured vertically, closures-up, using test tube racks, a holder for microscopic slides, plastic holders, cups, and/or a leak-proof container for ice water. Specimens, such as CSF or bone marrow, that are acquired by invasive procedures, are often delivered by hand.

Pneumatic tube systems—are used to transport specimens, patient records, messages, letters, bills, medications, x-rays, and laboratory test results. The CLSI reports that many studies have documented the validity of laboratory results after specimen transport through a pneumatic tube and suggest that the tests most affected (lactate dehydrogenase, potassium, plasma hemoglobin, and acid phosphatase) are compromised because of the disruption of red cells. Also, if samples must be kept at body temperature (e.g., testing for cryoglobulins and cold agglutinins), they should not be transported in a pneumatic tube system.[4] However, the majority of analytes are not usually affected, so this is an efficient means of specimen transport. It is recommended that blood collection tubes be placed in the pneumatic tube with shock-absorbent inserts padding the sides and with the tubes separated from one another, to prevent spillage or breakage. Clear plastic liners are also commercially available, so that if leaks do occur, they are visible and are contained to prevent contamination of the tube system, the carrier, and the personnel handling the specimens. Gloves should always be worn when loading or unloading specimens from the transport tube container, because they may be contaminated with biohazardous specimen leakage that is not visible to the naked eye.

Transportation by automated vehicles—uses a small motorized and/or computerized container car attached to a network of track that is routed to appropriate sites in the laboratory and nursing stations.

Specimen Storage

Each laboratory should have specific criteria for keeping specimens stable during storage and for determining time and temperature requirements for their testing procedures. Test results may exhibit significant changes caused by time delays. Even though some analytes may be stable for longer periods, CLSI suggests that cells be removed or separated from serum or plasma as soon as possible after collection. The results of some laboratory tests change significantly if the cells remain in contact with the plasma or serum, yet some may remain stable for longer time periods. Manufacturer's guidelines should be followed closely.

Sample Rejection

Because a test result is only as good as the specimen it is performed on, there are occasions when a sample or specimen (e.g., blood or urine) must be rejected. This is an uncomfortable situation because it means that the patient may have to undergo another venipuncture or another trip to the clinic. Box 5-4 ■ indicates important criteria for specimen rejection. One of the most common reasons for sample rejection is that the specimen is hemolyzed. Hemolysis is the red blood cell disruption and lysis that results in the release of hemoglobin from the cells. Hemolysis can interfere with laboratory testing and results. Sometimes it is caused by the patient's condition, however, oftentimes hemolysis is due to a difficult venipuncture and/or improper handling of the blood sample, if the specimen tubes are roughly handled, shaken vigorously, or if supplies are not used correctly during the venipuncture procedure. In the latter case, the problem can be prevented by careful and correct use of phlebotomy equipment and supplies.

When a problem with a blood sample arises, the health care worker who drew the sample and a supervisor should try to solve the problem initially. Errors should be acknowledged and documented with corrective actions. Other personnel may be involved as needed. Honesty and ethical communication are mandatory.

Clinical Alert !

If a blood sample is not acceptable for testing, it should be disposed of properly, a request for a new specimen must be initiated by an authorized individual, the situation should be documented, and the patient's physician should be notified.

Box 5-4	Factors for Sample Rejection

- The test request does not match the labels on the blood sample
- Label is unreadable, or partially missing
- Anticoagulated tube contains blood clots
- Excessive delays in processing the specimen
- Hemolyzed blood specimen (except for tests in which hemolysis does not interfere with the analysis)
- Improper specimen transport temperature or storage
- Improper blood collection tube (the correct additive is a requirement for specific tests)
- Incorrect blood volume (too much or too little) in the collection tube (this can affect the blood to additive ratio and affect the accuracy of test results)
- **Lipemic** blood specimen (cloudy or milky appearance of serum due to ingestion of fatty foods)
- Non-fasting blood specimen (unless appropriately noted)
- Use of outdated supplies to collect the specimen (the expiration date has passed)
- Variation in patient's posture (hormone values change based on whether the patient is sitting or reclining)
- Timed specimens drawn at the wrong time
- Unlabeled, unidentified specimen tubes
- Contaminated urine specimen

Self Study

Study Questions

For the following questions, select the one best answer.

1. Medical records serve what purpose?
   a. coordination of care
   b. maintain technical skills
   c. provide competency statements
   d. certification

2. Bar codes can be used for which type of phlebotomy information?
   a. identification of blood cells
   b. unique patient ID numbers
   c. designation of right from left
   d. inventory of patients' belongings

3. What is the most error-free method for requesting a laboratory test?
   a. handwritten request
   b. electronic request
   c. verbal routine request
   d. verbal STAT request

4. A specimen should be protected from light for which of the following determinations?
   a. bilirubin concentration
   b. hemoglobin level
   c. glucose level
   d. blood cultures

5. A specimen should be chilled for which of the following analyses?
   a. complete blood count (CBC)
   b. bilirubin
   c. ammonia
   d. glucose

6. Normal body temperature (in degrees Centigrade) is:
   a. 25
   b. 37
   c. 98
   d. 100

7. Room temperature (in degrees Centigrade) is:
   a. 25
   b. 37
   c. 98
   d. 100

8. Thermolabile means sensitivity to:
   a. latex
   b. temperature
   c. light
   d. legal liability

9. Photosensitivity means sensitivity to:
   a. latex
   b. temperature
   c. light
   d. seasonal allergies

10. Approximately how long does it take a normal blood specimen (without an anticoagulant or clot activator) to clot?
    a. 1–5 minutes
    b. 6–10 minutes
    c. 30–60 minutes
    d. longer than 120 minutes

Case Study

Blood samples for 12 patients were received via the pneumatic tube system in a large hospital laboratory within 15 minutes of each other. All specimens had been collected by a new phlebotomist. Six of the patients' specimens showed hemolysis and could not be used for laboratory analysis.

Questions

1. What is a likely cause of the hemolysis?
2. What should be done next?

Advocating Patient Safety Case Study

Health care facilities across the country (clinics, hospitals, etc.) are moving toward electronic medical records and automated generation of patient information. This change has implications for phlebotomy practices and laboratory testing.

Questions

1. How would the use of electronic medical records save time over paper-based medical records?
2. Explain how the use of electronically transmitted test requests and blood specimen labels help avoid identification errors.
3. How should errors in laboratory test results be noted in an electronic medical record?

Competency Assessment

Check Yourself: Designing a Test Requisition

Design either a computer version or paper-based **requisition form** that includes all of the appropriate information for a laboratory test. With a peer who has not seen your version, practice giving instructions on how to complete your test request. Practice your communication techniques (from Chapter 1) by double-checking that they completely understand. Ask them specific questions about parts of the requisition that might be hard to remember how to fill out.

Check Yourself: Bar Code Awareness

As you do errands in daily life, become aware of the uses of bar codes. For one week, make a list of everywhere you see a bar code and speculate about how they are used in each place. Describe how bar codes may be useful for phlebotomy practice and laboratory applications.

Competency Checklist: Specimen Transportation

This checklist can be completed as a group or individually.

(1) Completed (2) Needs to improve/Repeat lesson and checklist

_____ 1. List five essential items that should be on laboratory requisitions and specimen labels.

_____ 2. List three methods that are used to transport specimens.

_____ 3. Describe three examples of why a specimen might be unsuitable for laboratory testing.

_____ 4. Describe the three phases of processing and centrifugation of a sample.

_____ 5. Describe three reasons that specimens should be kept covered at all times.

References

1. Frazier, MS, Malone, C, and Moran, C: _Medical Assisting, Foundations and Practices,_ Upper Saddle River, NJ: Pearson, 2010.

2. Clinical and Laboratory Standards Institute (CLSI): Accuracy in Patient and Sample Identification; Approved Guideline, GP33-A, vol. 30, no. 7, Wayne, PA: CLSI: 2010.

3. Clinical and Laboratory Standards Institute (CLSI): Specimen Labels: Content and Location, Fonts, and Label Orientation; Proposed Standard, AUTO12-P, vol. 30, no. 2, Wayne, PA: CLSI: 2010.

4. Clinical and Laboratory Standards Institute (CLSI): _Procedures for the Handling and Processing of Blood Specimens: Approved Guideline,_ 4th edition, vol. 24, no. 38, H18-A4, Wayne, PA: CLSI, 2010.

PEARSON
myhealthprofessionskit™

Go to www.myhealthprofessionskit.com to access the Companion Website created for this textbook. Simply select "Clinical Laboratory Science" from the choice of disciplines. Find this book and log in using your username and password to access interactive learning games, assessment questions, and more.

Chapter 6

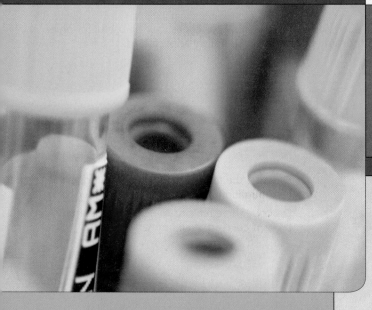

Blood Collection Equipment

CHAPTER OBJECTIVES

Upon completion of Chapter 6, the learner should be able to do the following:

1. Describe the latest phlebotomy safety supplies and equipment.
2. Identify the various supplies that should be carried on a specimen collection tray when a skin puncture specimen must be collected.
3. List the various types of anticoagulants and additives used in blood collection, examples of tests performed on the specimens collected in the tubes containing them, and the color codes for these anticoagulants and additives.
4. Describe the differences between the venipuncture and skin puncture equipment and supplies.
5. Identify the types of safety equipment needed to collect blood by venipuncture and skin puncture.

KEY TERMS

acid citrate dextrose (ACD)
anticoagulants
antiglycolytic agent
butterfly needle
capillary tubes
citrate-phosphate-dextrose (CPD)
citrates
disposable sterile lancet
ethylenediaminetetra-acetic acid (EDTA)
gauge number
glycolytic inhibitor
heparin
holder (adapter)
latex allergic
microcontainers
oxalates
sodium fluoride
sterile gauze pads
vacuum (evacuated) tube
winged infusion set

Introduction to Blood Collection Equipment

Health care workers involved in blood collection use many types of supplies and safety equipment in the collection and transport of blood specimens. Blood collection devices with safety features decrease needlestick injuries. The collection equipment is used for venipuncture (blood collection from a vein), skin puncture (blood collection from a finger and/or an infant's heel), and arterial puncture (blood collection from an artery). Venipuncture equipment includes vacuum tubes (evacuated tubes) and safety-needle collection devices that allow the blood collector to collect a patient's blood, plus a disposable tourniquet to assist in locating a vein, supplies to cleanse the puncture site, labeling supplies, gloves, and special trays for the transport of the blood specimens. Box 6-1 ■ lists the equipment used in routine venipuncture procedures.

Venipuncture Equipment

Venipuncture with a **vacuum (evacuated) tube** (VACUTAINER), as shown in Figure 6-1 ■, is the most direct and efficient method for obtaining a blood specimen. The vacuum tube system requires an evacuated tube, a special needle, and a special safety plastic **holder (adapter)** (Figure 6-2 ■) that covers the needle after blood collection. One end of the double-pointed needle enters the vein, the other end pierces the top of the tube, and the tube's vacuum aspirates the blood. The needle and/or plastic holder that covers the needle after venipuncture has/have safety devices to protect the health care worker from a needlestick injury. State and federal laws require these "safety-engineered devices."

Box 6-1	Equipment for Routine Venipuncture

Antimicrobial hand gel or foam to wash hands

Safety-needle collection device

Needles

Vacuum (evacuated) blood collection tubes

Safety syringes and syringe transfer devices

Safety winged infusion sets (safety butterfly sets)

Needle disposal container

Disposable tourniquets

70% isopropyl alcohol, chlorhexidine and/or iodine pads, or swab sticks

Disposable gloves

Prepackaged gauze pads

Hypoallergenic adhesive bandages and gauze wraps (for more sensitive skin)

Marking pens and labels

Specimen collection tray

Laboratory requisitions or labels

Puncture-resistant disposal container

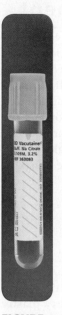

FIGURE ■ 6-1 Vacuum Tube
Source: Courtesy of BD VACUTAINER Systems, Preanalytical Solutions, Franklin Lakes, NJ

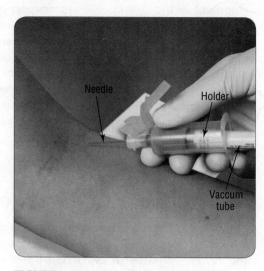

FIGURE ■ 6-2 Vacuum (Evacuated) Tube Holder System and Parts
Source: Courtesy of BD VACUTAINER Systems, Preanalytical Solutions, Franklin Lakes, NJ

Blood Collection Tubes and Additives

Blood collection tubes are available in different sizes, in safety-engineered plastic, to reduce risk of tube breakage and blood spill. Glass collection tubes are not desirable because the risk of exposure to bloodborne pathogens (disease-causing organisms) is increased due to possible breakage. The two criteria used to describe vacuum tube size are: (1) the external tube diameter and length plus (2) the maximum amount of specimen to be collected into the vacuum tube. The smaller sizes (e.g., 2 mL) are useful for pediatric (child or baby) and geriatric (elderly) blood collections and can be purchased with different types of additives (i.e., **anticoagulants**), as well as being chemically clean or sterile. Each vacuum tube top is color-coded according to the additive contained within the tube (see Table 6-1 ■).

Many tubes are designed to be used directly with the chemical, hematological, or microbiological instruments. In these cases, the tube of blood is identified by its bar code and is pierced by the instrument probe, and some blood sample is aspirated (pulled) into the instrument for analyses. In addition, some tubes have plastic tops or screw-on enclosures around the rubber stopper to minimize exposure to blood left on the top of the cap or blood splatters that can occur during cap removal. The expiration dates of tubes should be monitored continuously for quality assurance of accuracy and reliability in blood collection.

Traditionally, in most clinical laboratories, serum and plasma have been used to perform various assays. Heparinized whole blood has become the specimen of choice for several clinical chemical laboratory instruments used in STAT (immediate) situations. Using whole blood as a specimen decreases the time involved in acquiring the test result, because centrifugation is not required before laboratory testing.

Table 6-1	Specimen Type and Collection Vacuum Tubes	
Specimen Type	**Collection Tubes (Top Color/Type)**	**Additive**
Clotted blood/serum	Gray/red or clear	No additive
	Yellow/red	Polymer barrier
	Gold or red/black	Clot activator and polymer barrier
	Red	None or clot activator in plastic tube
	Orange	Thrombin
	Yellow/gray or orange	Thrombin
Whole blood/plasma	Green/gray or light green	Polymer barrier and lithium heparin
	Light blue	Sodium citrate (3.2% or 3.8%)
	Lavender (purple)	K_3 EDTA, K_2 EDTA or Na_2 EDTA
	Gray	Sodium fluoride and potassium oxalate or sodium fluoride and Na_2 EDTA; or sodium fluoride only (SERUM TUBE)
	Green	Lithium heparin
	Green	Sodium heparin or ammonium heparin
	Royal blue	K_2 EDTA sterile tube for toxicology and nutritional studies
	Pink	Blood bank K_2 EDTA
	Tan	K_2 EDTA tube for lead testing
Clotted blood/serum	Royal blue	Clot activator; sterile tube for trace elements, toxicology, and nutritional studies
Whole blood	Lavender (purple)	K_3 EDTA, K_2 EDTA or Na_2 EDTA
	Green	Lithium heparin, sodium heparin, or ammonium heparin
	Black	Sodium citrate for hematology
	Yellow	Sodium polyanethol sulfonate (SPS) or acid citrate dextrose (ACD)

Many coagulation factors are involved in blood clotting, and coagulation can be prevented by the addition of different types of anticoagulants.[1] These anticoagulants often contain preservatives that can extend the metabolism and life span of the red blood cells (RBCs) after blood collection such as **citrate-phosphate-dextrose (CPD)** used in blood donations. Another major use of anticoagulants and preservatives is in the collection of plasma for laboratory analysis. Specific anticoagulants or preservatives must be used depending on the test procedure ordered. Anticoagulants cannot be substituted for one another. Coagulation of blood can be prevented by the addition of anticoagulants such as **oxalates, citrates, ethylenediaminetetraacetic acid (EDTA),** or **heparin.** Oxalates, citrates, and EDTA prevent the coagulation of blood by removing calcium and forming insoluble calcium salts. These three anticoagulants cannot be used in calcium determinations; however, citrates are frequently used in coagulation blood studies. EDTA is used for platelet counts and platelet function tests. Fresh EDTA-anticoagulated blood allows preparation of blood smears for differential (diff) counts because cell sizes are not affected. Heparin is used in assays such as ammonia and plasma hemoglobin, and it prevents blood clotting by inactivating the blood-clotting chemicals thrombin and factor X. Pediatric tubes are available from manufacturers for patient blood collections in which it is anticipated that a "smaller amount of blood" will be collected. These tubes provide accurate laboratory results even though a smaller amount of blood is collected.

Clinical Alert ⚠️

Two important things to remember when using vacuum blood collection tubes:

1. These tubes have been designed for a certain amount of blood to be collected into the tube by vacuum in relation to the amount of prefilled anticoagulant in the tube.

2. If an insufficient amount of blood is collected in the anticoagulated tube, the laboratory test results may be wrong because of the incorrect amount of blood mixed with anticoagulant, and the sample should not be used for testing.

YELLOW-TOPPED TUBES, VACUUM CULTURE VIALS, AND ACD TUBES

Sterile blood specimens are ordered for blood cultures when the patient is suspected of having septicemia (symptoms of sepsis). A major problem with collecting blood for culture is that the patient's sample can become contaminated with microorganisms from the skin. Thus, the blood must be collected in a sterile container (vacuum tube, vial, or syringe) under aseptic conditions. (See Chapter 11 for blood culture collections.) The additive sodium poly-anethol sulfonate (SPS) is in the yellow-topped tubes for blood culture specimen collections in microbiology. The collected blood should be gently inverted in the vacuum tube eight times for complete mixing of SPS with the blood. Also, as shown in Figure 6-3 ■, blood can be collected directly into vacuum vials that contain culture media.

This type of collection minimizes the risk of specimen contamination. The vacuum vials can be purchased with different types of culture media, an unplugged venting unit for aerobic incubation, or a plugged venting unit for anaerobic incubation.

It should be noted that tubes containing **ACD (acid citrate dextrose)** also use the yellow color code. These tubes are mainly used to preserve blood for donation. Also, ACD is used for specialty blood banking, such as human leukocyte antigen (HLA) typing and DNA testing. The yellow-topped tubes need to be gently inverted eight times immediately after blood collection for additive/blood mixing.

LIGHT BLUE-TOPPED TUBES

Many coagulation procedures, such as prothrombin time (PT) and activated partial thrombo-plastin time (APTT), are done on blood collected in light blue–topped vacuum tubes, which contain sodium citrate. Tubes must be filled, or coagulation results will be inaccurate, which could lead to the wrong treatment for the patient. Sodium citrate buffers coagulation factors, making it the best anticoagulant for coagulation testing. The light blue–topped tube should be gently inverted three to four times as soon as the blood is collected.

SERUM SEPARATION TUBES (MOTTLED-TOPPED, SPECKLED-TOPPED, AND GOLD-TOPPED TUBES)

Another tube is the serum separation tube, such as the VACUETTE® serum tube (Figure 6-4 ■) and the BD VACUTAINER plus SST tube. These tubes must be gently inverted after obtaining the blood to ensure mixing of the clot activator. These tubes contain a polymer barrier in the bottom of the tube. The specific gravity (weight compared to water) of this material lies between the blood clot and the serum. After blood is collected in one of these tubes, the tube needs to be gently inverted five to eight times and then allowed to set for 30 minutes prior to centrifugation. During centrifugation, the polymer barrier moves upward to the serum-clot interface, where it forms a stable barrier separating the serum from fibrin and

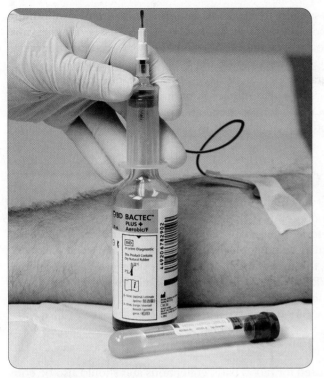

FIGURE ■ 6-3 Collecting Blood for Culture Using the BD BACTEC Culture Vial
Source: Courtesy of BD (Becton-Dickinson and Company), Sparks, MD

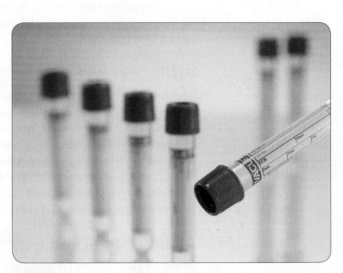

FIGURE ■ 6-4 VACUETTE® Serum Tube
Source: Courtesy of Grenier Bio-One, Kremsmunster, Austria

blood cells. Serum may be aspirated directly from the collection tube, eliminating the need for transfer to another container.

The orange and gray/yellow vacuum topped tubes have the additive thrombin, which completes clotting of the blood in less than five minutes. These tubes are used for STAT (emergency) laboratory procedures requiring serum specimens.

RED-TOPPED SERUM TUBES

The red-topped tubes indicate a tube without an anticoagulant or polymer (gel) barrier and is used for the collection of serum. Thus, the collected blood *will* clot in this tube. After the blood is collected in the tube, the clotting process begins and takes at least 30 minutes for the fibrin clot to form. However, BD VACUTAINER has developed the new red-topped Rapid Serum Tube (RST) that has a five-minute clotting time.

GREEN-TOPPED TUBES

The anticoagulants sodium heparin and lithium heparin are found in green-topped vacuum tubes. These tubes are used in various laboratory assays requiring plasma or whole blood, which are mainly chemical tests.

Lithium heparin tubes are used for many assays, including:

■ glucose;

■ blood urea nitrogen (BUN);

■ ionized calcium;

■ creatinine; or

■ electrolyte studies.

However, this anticoagulant is not suitable for tests involving the measurement of lithium or folate levels.[1] Similarly, sodium heparin tubes should not be used for assays that measure the sodium concentration. Green-topped vacuum tubes should not be used for collections for blood smears. When used for cytogenetic studies, these tubes must be sterile.

Light green–topped or green/gray-topped tubes have a gel to separate the plasma from the red blood cells and are used for assays that require heparinized plasma.

As for other vacuum tubes containing additives and anticoagulants, these tubes should be thoroughly mixed with the blood by eight gentle inversions of the tube immediately after blood collection.

PURPLE (LAVENDER)-TOPPED TUBES

The purple-topped vacuum tubes (containing EDTA) are used for most hematology procedures, such as the complete blood count (CBC), red blood cells (RBCs), white blood cells (WBCs), platelet count, hematocrit, differentials (DIFF), hemoglobin, mean corpuscular hemoglobin (MCH), mean corpuscular hemoglobin concentration (MCHC), and mean cell volume (MCV), among others. Also, this tube is used for molecular diagnostic testing, immunology, and hemoglobin A1c. The EDTA tube needs to be completely inverted 8 to 10 times after blood collection to avoid the possibility of microclots forming in the tube from lack of proper mixing of the EDTA with the blood (Box 6-2 ■).

PINK-TOPPED TUBES

These tubes contain EDTA and are used for blood bank collections and should also be completely inverted 8 to 10 times for complete mixing of the blood with the anticoagulant. This tube has the pink closure and a label that meets the AABB required for blood bank collections.

GRAY-TOPPED TUBES

Gray-topped vacuum tubes usually contain (1) potassium oxalate and sodium fluoride, (2) sodium fluoride and EDTA, or (3) only sodium fluoride (see Box 6-3 ■). This type of collection tube is primarily used for glucose (sugar) tests. The terms **antiglycolytic agent** and **glycolytic inhibitor** are the terms for this tube's additive because it slows the chemical process of glucose breakdown.

ROYAL BLUE-TOPPED AND TAN-TOPPED TUBES

The royal blue–topped tubes are used to collect samples for nutritional studies, therapeutic drug monitoring, and toxicology. The royal blue–topped tube is the trace element tube. The tan-topped tube is used for lead testing and contains EDTA.

BLACK-TOPPED TUBES

From certain manufacturers, a black-topped tube containing sodium citrate is available for blood collections used to determine the erythrocyte sedimentation rate (ESR).

Box 6-2	Purple-Topped Tubes

If a purple-topped tube is underfilled, the patient will have:
- Falsely low blood cell counts
- Falsely low hematocrits
- Staining alterations on blood smears

Box 6-3 | **Contraindications for Gray-Topped Tubes**

Because sodium fluoride destroys many enzymes, the gray-topped tube should *not* be used in blood collections for enzyme determinations that include:

- creatine kinase (CK);
- alanine aminotransferase (ALT);
- aspartate aminotransferase (AST); or
- alkaline phosphatase (ALP).

Likewise, potassium oxalate destroys blood cell features. Thus, gray-topped tubes should not be used for hematological studies because blood cells are identified and counted in these tests.

Also, it should be noted that hemolysis frequently occurs if a gray-topped tube is underfilled with blood.

MOLECULAR DIAGNOSTICS TUBES

Special sterile vacuum tubes for molecular diagnostic studies are available that contain different additives (e.g., sodium citrate and sodium heparin) as required for the different testing procedures. Manufacturers use tops of different color for these tubes.

TUBE ORGANIZER

The TiMO™ Tube Management Organizer (Figure 6-5 ■) is an innovative test tube holder that assists with managing the test tubes during the blood sample collection process. TiMO may be used to collect test tube samples from both patients and blood donors. It holds and organizes test tubes before, during, and after blood sample collection, provides a simple mechanism to keep one patient or blood donor's set of test tubes together, and ensures confident test tube management throughout the entire collection process.

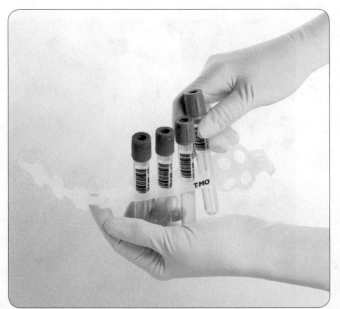

FIGURE ■ 6-5 TiMO Tube Management Organizer
Source: Courtesy of ITL Corp.

Safety Syringes

Some patients' veins are too fragile for blood collection with vacuum tubes, so safety syringes are generally used for the collection process.[2] Syringes are hazardous and pose an increased risk of accidental needlesticks.

Syringes are sometimes used for collecting blood from central venous catheter (CVC) lines. Major parts of the syringe are the needle, safety cover, hub, barrel, and the plunger (Figure 6-6 ■). The barrel and the plunger are made to fit together tightly so that when the plunger is in the barrel and drawn back, a vacuum is created. To fit properly, the needle and syringe must be compatible and are attached at the hub. This vacuum allows blood or other fluids to be aspirated, or sucked, into the barrel as the plunger is pulled back. The barrel of the syringe has graduated measurements in milliliter (mL) or cubic centimeter (cc) increments. For specimen collection purposes, 5- to 20-mL syringes are most often used. The health care worker should ensure that the syringe is the correct size for the amount of blood to be collected.

A safety syringe shielded-transfer device (Figure 6-7 ■) must be used to avoid possible exposure to the patient's blood.[3] The plunger must not be pushed down as the tubes are being filled from the syringe because doing so is extremely hazardous. Also, pushing the plunger may damage cellular components and cause hemolysis because of the forceful expulsion of blood. The syringe needle should be shielded after blood collection, removed, and discarded in a sharps disposal container.[3] The BD blood-transfer device is attached to

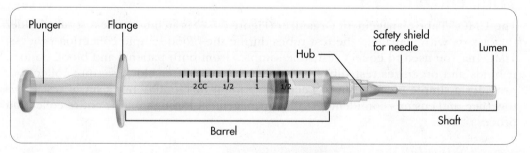

FIGURE ■ 6-6 Example of a Safety Syringe

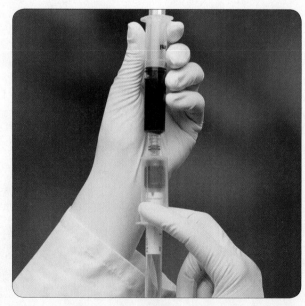

FIGURE ■ 6-7 BD SafetyGlide Needle and BD Blood Transfer Device

Source: Courtesy of BD VACUTAINER Systems, Preanalytical Solutions, Franklin Lakes, NJ

the syringe, and a vacuum tube is inserted into the transfer device. The blood is transferred from the syringe to the tube using the tube's vacuum. Specialized tubes and bottles that fit the adapter are also available for blood culture collection.

Clinical Alert !

- Safety engineering controls (needlestick protection) and safe work practices must be used when collecting blood with a syringe.
- Avoid the use of syringes in blood collection if at all possible.
- Needleless safety blood-transfer devices must be used to transfer the blood from the syringe to the vacuum tube.

Safety Needles/Holders

The gauge and length of a needle used on a syringe or a vacuum tube is selected according to the specific task. The **gauge number** indicates the diameter of the needle; the smaller the gauge number, the larger the needle diameter and the higher the flow rate (Box 6-4 ■).

For example, larger (18-gauge) needles are used for collecting donor units of blood (450 mL or less), whereas smaller (21- and 22-gauge) needles are used for collecting specimens for laboratory assays. When blood is collected from children, a 21- to 23-gauge needle is usually used with a tuberculin, or 3-mL syringe or with a winged infusion set. The length of the needle depends on the depth of the vein to be punctured. Needles are usually available as either 1 or 1½ inch.

Needles are sterilized and packaged by vendors in sealed shields that maintain sterility. These sealed shields are packaged in individual containers that are color coded according to the gauge size of the needles and must be twisted apart before the needles are used in blood collection.

The needle attaches to the safety holder/adapter, or syringe, at its hub. For example, the BD Eclipse safety-shielding blood needle attaches to a holder (Figure 6-8 ■). The BD Eclipse shield is activated immediately after the blood collection tubes are filled and the needle is removed from the vein. When the thumb pushes forward on the shield, as shown in Figure 6-8, an audible click indicates that the safety shield is locked in place. This single-use adapter provides immediate containment of a used needle.

Another protective holder that provides effective, immediate containment of a used needle is the Venipuncture Needle-Pro (Figure 6-9 ■). The safety feature is an integral part of the device and engages with a single-handed technique. The health care worker's hands and fingers remain behind the exposed sharp at all times. Also, the health care worker can easily tell whether the safety feature is activated. The needle is securely locked inside the safety device and remains protected through disposal.

Box 6-4	**Needle Sizes Used for Blood Collection**

- Larger (16- to 18-gauge) needles are used for collecting donor units of blood (e.g., 450 mL).
- Smaller (21- and 22-gauge) needles are used for collecting specimens for laboratory assays.

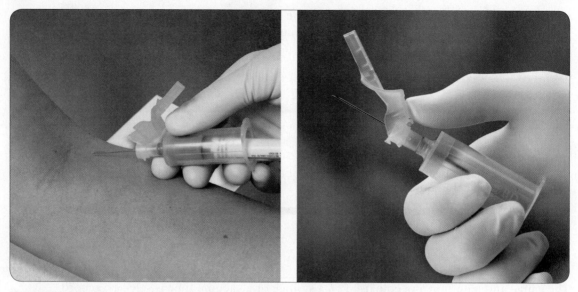

FIGURE ■ **6-8** BD Eclipse Blood Collection Needle Attached to a Holder
Source: Courtesy of BD VACUTAINER Systems, Preanalytical Solutions, Franklin Lakes, NJ

Once engaged, both ends of the needle are covered, protecting the blood collector from an accidental needlestick.

The Vanishpoint blood collection system features a blood collection tube holder and a small tube adapter. The needle is automatically retracted from the patient when the end cap is closed after the last tube has been removed. It virtually eliminates exposure to the contaminated needle and the possibility of needlestick injury (Figure 6-10 ■).

The VACUETTE® QUICKSHIELD Complete PLUS Safety Tube Holder is used to prevent accidental needlestick injuries during venous blood collection (Figure 6-11 ■).

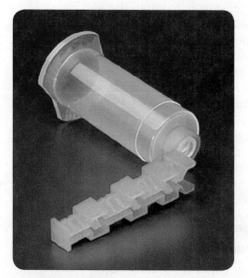

FIGURE ■ **6-9** Venipuncture Needle-Pro Needle Protection Device
Source: Courtesy of Smiths Medical ASD, Inc. Norwell, MA

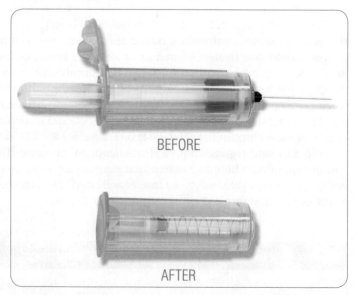

BEFORE

AFTER

FIGURE ■ **6-10** Vanishpoint Blood Collection Tube Holder
Source: Courtesy of Retractable Technologies, Little Elm, TX

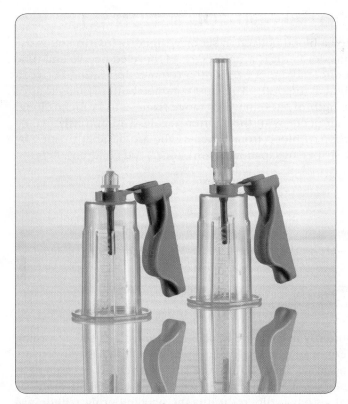

FIGURE ■ 6-11 VACUETTE® QUICKSHIELD Complete PLUS Safety Tube Holder

Source: Courtesy of Greiner Bio-One GmbH, Kremsmünster, Austria

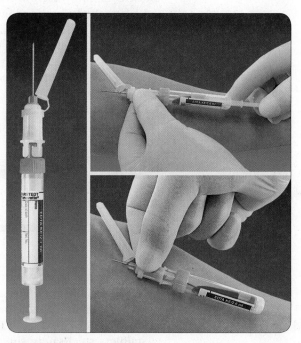

FIGURE ■ 6-12 Sarstedt S-Monovette® Venous Blood Collection System

Source: Courtesy of Sarstedt, Inc., Newton, NC

The safety cap is activated immediately after blood collection using one hand. With the aid of a solid support, the safety cap closes over the needle. A clearly audible "Click" indicates that the safety mechanism has been activated correctly.

Sarstedt, Incorporated, offers the S-Monovette Blood Collection System (Figure 6-12 ■), which is an enclosed multiple-sampling blood collection system that collects blood using either an aspiration or vacuum principle of collection. Using the aspiration procedure replaces syringe draws for patients with difficult veins and can prevent uncomfortable resticks. All tubes are plastic with screw caps, which minimizes the risk of breakage and aerosol formation when caps are removed. Each needle has an integral holder that does not require assembly before use and cannot be disassembled. Thus, it prevents reuse of the holder.

For any of these blood collection needle and tube holder devices, disposing of the tube holder while it is still attached to the needle ensures that the tube-puncturing needle remains protected during and after disposal.[4] This safety method significantly reduces the risks of needlestick injuries and blood exposure because the tube-puncturing needle automatically retracts into it after blood collection.

The tip of each needle should be checked for damage. A blunt or bent tip can be harmful to the patient's vein and may result in failure to collect blood.

It is important to use needles with holders or syringes that are compatible with the needle to avoid the possibility of leaking blood and blood exposure.

THE BUTTERFLY NEEDLE (BLOOD COLLECTION SET)

The **butterfly needle,** also called a blood collection set or **winged infusion set,** is the most commonly used intravenous device. It is a stainless steel, beveled needle and tube with attached plastic wings on one end and a Luer fitting (connection fitting between needle and holder device) attached to the other. The most common butterfly needle sizes are 21- and 23-gauge, and the length of these needles range from ½ to ¾ inches long. The smaller angle of insertion can occur with the shorter needle. The butterfly needle is sometimes used in the collection of blood from patients who are difficult to stick by conventional methods (e.g., elderly persons, patients with cancer, and children). Refer to Chapter 8 for more details.

Clinical Alert !

The safety device *must* be activated on the butterfly needle after venipuncture to avoid needlestick injury.

Numerous types of safety butterfly needles are available and must be used according to OSHA regulations. These safety needles each have a shield that automatically covers the contaminated needle point upon withdrawal from the patient's vein. One example is the MONOJECT ANGEL WING blood collection set (Figures 6-13A ■ and 6-13B ■). It has a stainless steel safety shield that automatically resheaths the needle during withdrawal from the patient.

BD VACUTAINER Systems *Preanalytical Solutions* has the BD VACUTAINER Push Button Blood Collection Set with Pre-Attached Holder (see Figure 6-14 ■), which provides immediate protection against needlestick injury when it is properly activated within the vein and in accordance with the BD directions.

Greiner Bio-One manufactures the VACUETTE® Safety Blood Collection Set (Figure 6-15 ■). It is a winged needle device with a safety shield. Terumo Medical Corporation manufactures

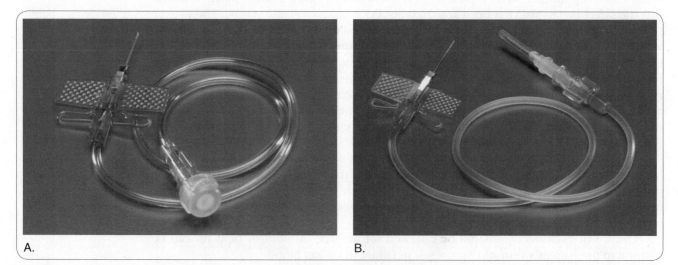

A.   B.

FIGURE ■ 6-13 ANGEL WING Blood Collection Set with (A) Female and (B) Male Luer

Source: ANGEL WING is a trademark of Covidien AG. © Covidien. All rights reserved

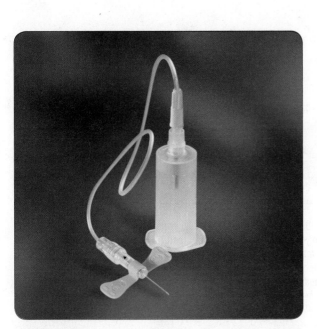

FIGURE ■ 6-14 Blood Collection with BD VACUTAINER Push Button Blood Collection Set

Source: Courtesy of BD VACUTAINER Systems, Preanalytical Solutions, Franklin Lakes, NJ

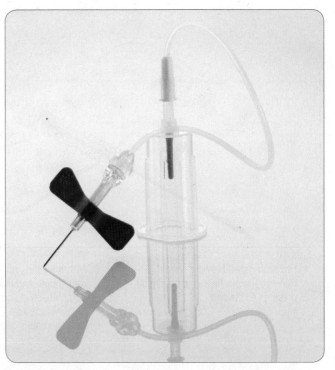

FIGURE ■ 6-15 VACUETTE® Safety Blood Collection Set

Source: Courtesy of Greiner Bio-One GmbH, Kremsmünster, Austria

the Surshield Safety Winged Blood Collection Set (Figure 6-16 ■) a safety-engineered butterfly device for blood collection or IV insertion. No matter what type of safety blood collection set is used, it is important to use a Luer adapter (fitting) from the same manufacturer, to avoid possible blood leakage and exposure.

NEEDLE AND OTHER SHARPS DISPOSAL

Needles, syringes, and lancets (sterile, disposable sharp devices used in skin puncture) must be discarded in rigid, leakproof, plastic containers, reducing the possibility of needlesticks. Each unit is usually orange or red and is disposable as biohazardous waste (Figure 6-17 ■). Several sizes of sharps disposal containers are available for use at the bedside, on the cart, in isolation, and on home health care trays. Before beginning a blood collection procedure, note the location of the nearest sharps container.

Clinical Alert !

Never overfill a biohazard sharps container!

Tourniquets

The tourniquet is a key to successful venipuncture: it provides a barrier to slow down venous flow. Tourniquets are used in specimen collection to apply enough pressure to the arm to slow the return of venous blood to the heart. This slowing of venous return causes pooling of blood in the veins, making the veins more visible and easier to feel and

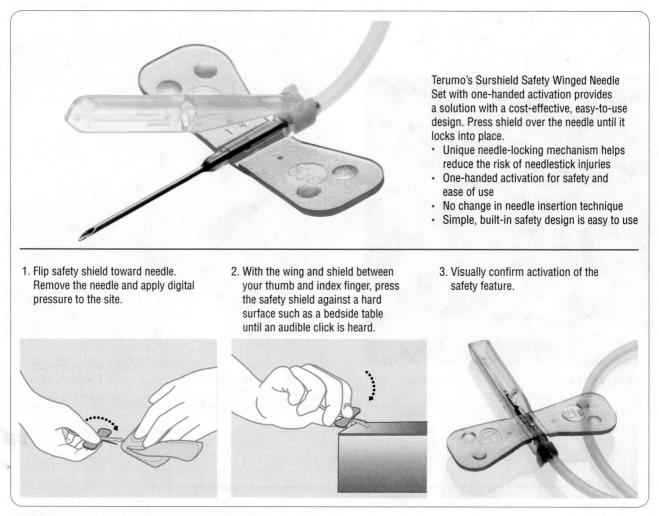

Terumo's Surshield Safety Winged Needle Set with one-handed activation provides a solution with a cost-effective, easy-to-use design. Press shield over the needle until it locks into place.
- Unique needle-locking mechanism helps reduce the risk of needlestick injuries
- One-handed activation for safety and ease of use
- No change in needle insertion technique
- Simple, built-in safety design is easy to use

1. Flip safety shield toward needle. Remove the needle and apply digital pressure to the site.

2. With the wing and shield between your thumb and index finger, press the safety shield against a hard surface such as a bedside table until an audible click is heard.

3. Visually confirm activation of the safety feature.

FIGURE ■ 6-16 Surshield® Safety Winged Blood Collection Set
Source: Courtesy of Terumo Medical Corp., Somerset, NJ

find. A tourniquet should not restrict arterial blood flowing into the arm. Blood should enter the arm at a normal rate and, with the use of a tourniquet, return to the heart at a slower rate. If the tourniquet is too tight, all blood flow will cease, making it difficult to collect.

Tourniquets that are usually used include the pliable strap, the Velcro type, and the blood pressure cuff. The preferred procedure is to use a new tourniquet for each patient or have one new tourniquet assigned to only one patient. This procedure will assist in reducing the spread of nosocomial infection by tourniquets and reduce the risk of cross-contamination between patients and health care workers.[6,7,8]

The blood pressure cuff can be used successfully when veins are difficult to find. However, as for the tourniquet, it is highly recommended to use a single cuff per patient. Another type of tourniquet is the Seraket, which uses a seat-belt design. It allows the health care worker to release the venous pressure partially by using a lever that releases some pressure, but not all. One drawback of this type of tourniquet, however, is the difficulty in cleaning and decontaminating it if it is soiled with blood between each patient use.

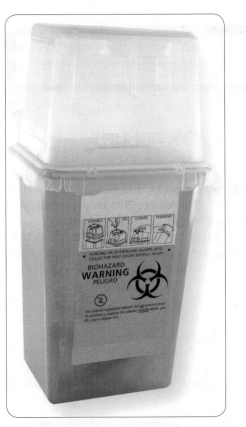

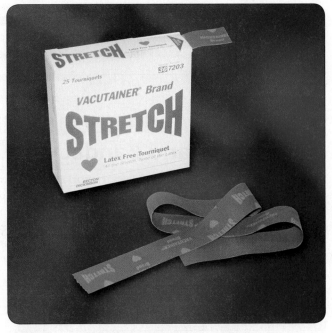

FIGURE ■ **6-18** BD VACUTAINER Latex Free Tourniquet
Source: Courtesy and © Becton, Dickinson and Company

FIGURE ■ **6-17** Sharps Disposal Container
with the Required Biohazard Sign
Source: Steve Carroll/Shutterstock.com

Velcro-type tourniquets are popular because they are easy to apply and comfortable for the patient. Alternatively, because of major concern for infection control in health care institutions, many facilities now use a disposable natural latex tourniquet strap to help prevent cross-contamination. As discussed in Chapter 4, many patients are allergic to latex[5]; thus, other types of tourniquets must be available to use to avoid an allergic reaction. Nonlatex disposable tourniquets are available as a good option for the blood collector and patient (Figure 6-18 ■).

Gloves for Blood Collection

Safety guidelines have been established for health care workers to help them prevent the possibility of acquiring infections, such as hepatitis or those associated with AIDS. These guidelines include the use of gloves during collection of blood from patients (Figure 6-19 ■). It is recommended that health care workers use non latex gloves (see Chapter 4 for **latex allergic** reactions). Also, health care workers should *not* use gloves with powder.

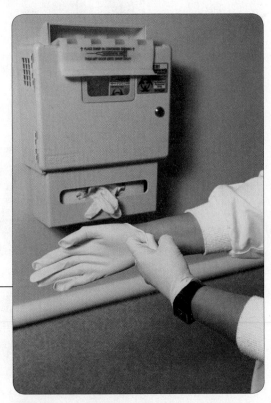

FIGURE ■ **6-19** Use of Gloves

> **Clinical Alert** ⚠️
>
> ■ Use proper hand hygiene and change gloves between each patient's blood collection.
> ■ Do not wash, disinfect, or reuse the gloves.

Antiseptics, Sterile Gauze Pads, and Bandages

The health care worker needs antiseptics, **sterile gauze pads,** and bandages for blood collection by either venipuncture or microcollection. Therefore, 70% isopropyl alcohol preparation and chlorhexidine swab sticks or pads (for blood cultures) are essential items for blood collection. In home health care and other ambulatory health care environments where soap and water may not be available, a waterless antiseptic agent (Figure 6-20 ■) should be carried with other blood collection items and used before and after blood collection.

Microcollection Equipment

Usually, skin puncture blood-collecting techniques are used on adults and infants when small amounts of blood can be used for diagnostic laboratory testing and also if venipuncture is excessively hazardous for a patient. A minimal volume of blood should be collected from adults,

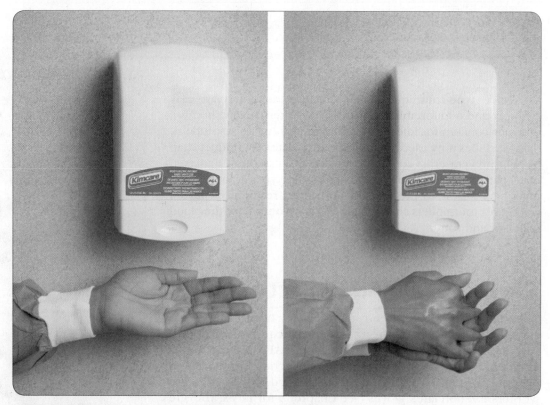

FIGURE ■ 6-20 Waterless Antiseptic Agent
Waterless antiseptic agents can be mounted in wall dispensers or carried with other blood collection supplies in travel-size containers.

neonates (newborns), or older infants to avoid the risk of iatrogenic (induced) anemia caused by large amounts of blood loss due to specimen collection.

LANCETS AND TUBES

For infants, the Clinical Laboratory Standards Institute recommends a penetration depth of less than 2.0 mm on heelsticks to avoid penetrating bone. The BD Quikheel lancet (Figure 6-21 ■) is available for two different incision depths, depending on the needs of the infant. The teal-colored Quikheel Infant lancet has a preset incision depth of 1.0 mm and a width of 2.5 mm. The purple-colored Quikheel Preemie lancet has a preset incision depth of 0.85 mm and a width of 1.75 mm. This lancet blade retracts permanently after activation, to ensure safety to the health care worker.

The BD Microtainer Contact-Activated Lancet (Figure 6-22 ■) is a safety-engineered device that activates only when it is positioned and pressed against the skin, facilitating a consistent puncture depth and providing for the patients' and health care worker's safety.

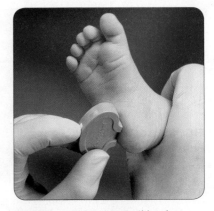

FIGURE ■ 6-21 BD Quikheel Lancet

Source: Courtesy of BD VACUTAINER Systems, Preanalytical Solutions, Franklin Lakes, NJ

Clinical Alert !

■ **Disposable sterile lancets** that are retractable to avoid bloodborne pathogen exposure should be used to puncture the skin for skin puncture collections.

■ Surgical blades should not be used for skin puncture because of the hazard to the patient and health care worker.

The Terumo Capiject[R] lancet (Figure 6-23 ■) is a safety-engineered device for skin puncture blood collection. The Capiject[R] lancet is available in an assortment of puncture widths and depths.

ITC has produced fully automated, single-use, automatically retracting, disposable devices that provide safety both for the neonate and for the health care worker (Figure 6-24 ■). The Tenderlett incises 1.75 mm deep, Tenderlett Jr. incises 1.25 mm deep, and Tenderlett Toddler incises only 0.85 mm deep. The retracting blade of each of these devices eliminates potential injury from an exposed blade contaminated with blood.

Another safety device for microcollection is the MONOJECT Monoletter Safety lancet (Figure 6-25 ■) for fingerstick collections.

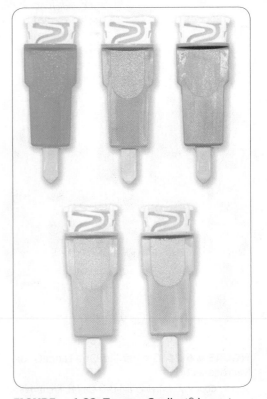

FIGURE ■ 6-23 Terumo Capiject® Lancet

Source: Courtesy of Terumo Medical Corp., Somerset, NJ

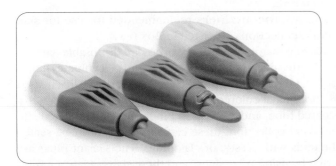

FIGURE ■ 6-22 BD Microtainer Contact-Activated Lancet

Source: Courtesy and © Becton, Dickinson and Company

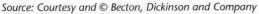

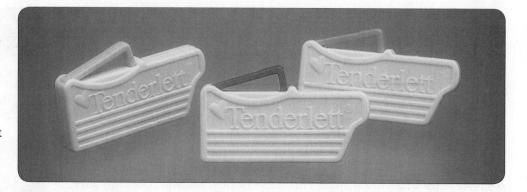

FIGURE ■ 6-24 Tenderlett Automated Skin Incision Device

Source: Courtesy of ITC

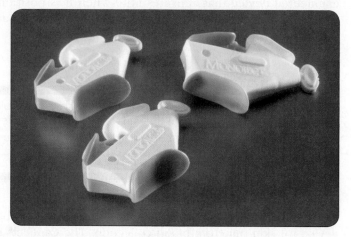

FIGURE ■ 6-25 MONOJECT Monoletter Safety Lancet

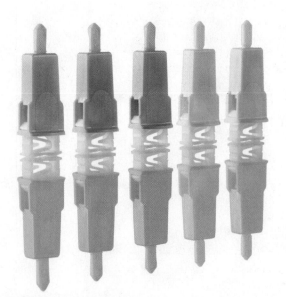

FIGURE ■ 6-26 Greiner Bio-One Lancets for Microcollection

Source: Courtesy of Greiner Bio-One GmbH, Kremsmünster, Austria

The Greiner Bio-One lancet (Figure 6-26 ■) is a safety micro-collection device available for various puncture depths. The Natus Medical NeatNick lancets (Figure 6-27 ■) in both pree-mie and full-term depth controlled sizes has been designed to minimize infant pain through a high-speed nick and pre-cise puncture.

The **microcontainers** recommended for use for skin puncture collections are listed in Box 6-5 ■.

Microhematocrit **capillary tubes** are disposable narrow-bore pipettes that are used for packed red cell volume (hema-tocrit) in microcentrifugation. These plastic or plastic-encased glass tubes have colored bands; a red band indicates a hepa-rin-coated tube, and a blue band indicates no anticoagulant. After blood collection, these capillary tubes must be sealed at the ends with plastic or clay plugs. The sealant plugs are inserted by using "clay slabs" and these slabs create a hazard because they become contaminated with blood and possibly

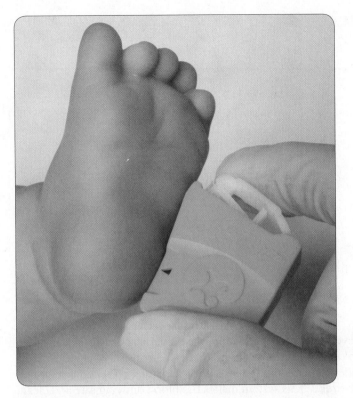

FIGURE ■ 6-27 NeatNick
Preemie Lancet
*Source: Image courtesy of Natus
Medical Incorporated*

glass fragments. These slabs must frequently be discarded in an appropriate sharps container according to the health care facility's safety policies.

Microcollection containers in plastic or glass wrapped, puncture-resistant plastic/film are available for general laboratory collections (e.g., chemistry) and are usually color-coded according to the established protocol for blood collection vacuum tube tops. Thus, purple- or lavender-topped tubes contain EDTA, green-topped tubes contain heparin, red-topped tubes have no additive, and gray-topped tubes have **sodium fluoride** to inhibit blood enzymes that destroy glucose. Some of the manufacturers of microcollection blood tubes produce amber-colored tubes that provides protection for light-sensitive analytes (e.g., bilirubin).

Electrolytes and general chemistry analytes are some of the tests that can be collected in the BD Microtainer tube, which has its own capillary blood collector, self-contained serum separator, and Microgard closure, which is safety engineered to reduce the risk of tube leakage and specimen splatter. Each tube is imprinted with two markings, a minimum 250-microliter line and a maximum 500-microliter line, to assist in collecting appropriate volumes (Figure 6-28 ■).

Alternatively, two or more capillary tubes can be used for electrolyte and general chemistry collection. One advantage of these tubes is that if blood hemolyzes in one capillary tube, another capillary tube containing the patient's sample can be used for the chemical analyses.

Box 6-5	Plastic Microcollection Devices: Various Types Needed

- Serum or plasma separator devices in different color codes (same colors as for vacuum color-topped tubes described earlier according to additives, e.g., purple contains EDTA)
- Disposable plastic calibrated microcollection tubes
- Plastic microhematocrit tubes
- Microdilution systems (e.g., BMP LeukoChek)

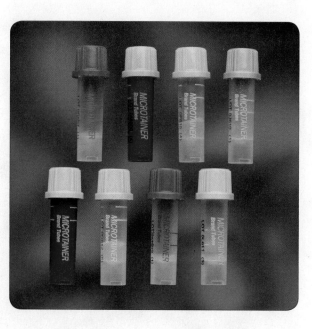

FIGURE ■ 6-28 BD Microtainer Tube
Source: Courtesy of BD VACUTAINER Systems, Preanalytical Solutions, Franklin Lakes, NJ

RAM Scientific, Inc., has developed an unbreakable plastic capillary-receptacle system called the SAFE-T-FILL capillary blood collection system. The device consists of a plastic capillary inserted into a microtube receptacle (Figure 6-29 ■). With the attached receptacle, blood flows directly to the bottom of the tube. This system makes the blood drawing safe and clean. The capillary can then be removed, and the tube is closed with the appropriate color-coded cap.

For most chemical assays using the various types of microcollection devices, lithium and ammonium salts of heparin are the anticoagulants of choice for microcollections. They have rarely been reported to interfere with the determination of electrolytes and most other chemical assays. However, ammonium heparin cannot be used as the additive for the blood collection to test ammonia levels.

Another type of microcollection device is the BMP LeukoChek microdilution system as shown in Figure 6-30 ■. This device serves as a collection and dilution unit for blood samples and, thus, increases the speed and simplicity of leukocyte and platelet counting. These devices are prefilled with buffered ammonium oxalate solution and have been tested to CLIA guidelines.

The BMP Leukocyte Test Kit includes:

1. a disposable, self-filling, diluting pipette consisting of a straight, thin-walled, uniform-bore, plastic capillary tube fitted into a plastic holder, and

2. a plastic reservoir containing a premeasured volume of buffered ammonium oxalate solution.

Specimen Collection Trays

The health care worker collecting blood specimens needs a specimen tray (Figure 6-31 ■) to take on blood-collecting rounds. The tray is usually made of plastic (preferably latex-free) and must be made of a plastic that can be sterilized. The tray should include all necessary collection equipment. For example, when working in a children's hospital, the tray must contain microcollection equipment, such as that described earlier. For home health care providers and reference laboratory couriers, the necessary collection supplies, equipment, and collected blood must be carried in an enclosed container with the biohazard symbol shown on the outside. It should be lockable to protect the contents from tampering or accidental contamination. It also should have a tight seal to reduce the risk of infection from

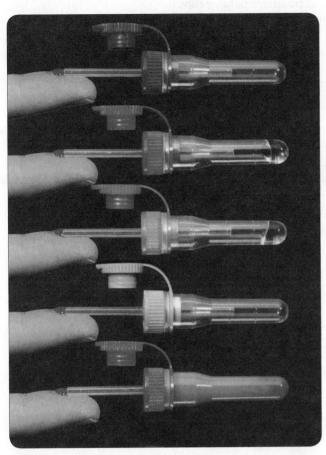

FIGURE ■ 6-29 SAFE-T-FILL® Capillary Blood Collection Tubes
Source: Courtesy of RAM Scientific, Inc., Needham, MA

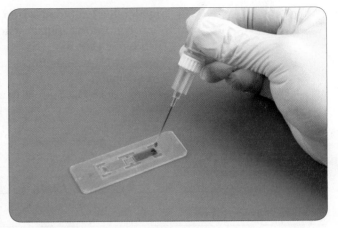

FIGURE ■ 6-30 BMP LeukoChek
Source: Courtesy of Biomedical Polymers, Inc.

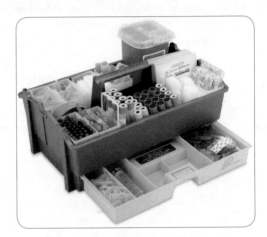

FIGURE ■ 6-31 Specimen Collection Tray
Source: Courtesy of MarketLab www.marketlabinc.com

bloodborne pathogens due to spills or accidents. Refer to Chapter 5 for more information about specimen transportation.

Health care workers who collect blood from adults usually have the following equipment on their trays or in their safety container for travel for home health care:

1. Marking pens or pencils
2. Vacuum tubes containing the anticoagulants designated in the clinical laboratory blood collection manual
3. Safety holders for vacuum tubes
4. Safety needles for vacuum tubes and syringes
5. Safety syringes
6. Disposable tourniquets (nonlatex)
7. Safety blood collection sets (butterfly needle assembly)
8. 70% isopropyl alcohol, iodine, and chlorhexidine pads/swabs
9. Sterile gauze pads
10. Bandages
11. Biohazardous waste containers for used needles, holders, and lancets
12. Safety lancets for skin puncture
13. Microdilution devices for fingerstick blood collection

14. Microcollection blood serum and plasma separator tubes
15. Microcollection capillary whole blood collectors with 0.23 mg of EDTA (200 micro L)
16. Disposable gloves
17. Cloth towel or washcloth
18. Thermometer
19. Antimicrobial hand gel or foam to wash hands without water and soap

Self Study

Study Questions

For the following questions, select the one best answer.

1. The light blue–topped vacuum collection tube has which of the following additives?
   a. lithium heparin
   b. sodium citrate
   c. sodium polyanethol sulfonate (SPS)
   d. EDTA

2. The butterfly blood collection set is frequently used with the needle gauge size of:
   a. 25
   b. 23
   c. 19
   d. 18

3. Which of the following blood analytes is sensitive to light?
   a. cholesterol
   b. glucose
   c. hematocrit
   d. bilirubin

4. Which of the listed needle gauges has the smallest diameter?
   a. 19
   b. 20
   c. 21
   d. 23

5. Which of the following containers is frequently used for the micromeasurement of packed red cell volume?
   a. Microtome
   b. BD Microtainer
   c. RAM SAFE-T-FILL
   d. microhematocrit tube

6. Which of the following is an anticoagulant used in blood donations?
   a. sodium citrate
   b. ACD
   c. EDTA
   d. lithium heparin

7. Specimens for which of the following tests must be collected in gray-topped blood collection tubes?
   a. PT and APTT
   b. glucose
   c. trace elements
   d. ESR

8. Blood collection for toxicology and nutritional procedures can be collected in which of the following tubes?
   a. pink-topped tubes
   b. black-topped tubes
   c. royal blue–topped tubes
   d. light blue–topped tubes

9. A prefilled device used as a collection and dilution unit is the:
   a. MONOJECT tube
   b. BMP LeukoChek
   c. Sarstedt S-Monovette Blood Collection System
   d. RAM SAFE-T-FILL

10. A minimal volume of blood should be collected from a person to avoid the risk of iatrogenic:
    a. leukemia
    b. anemia
    c. lymphoma
    d. polycythemia

Case Study

Ms. Herrara is a diabetic and has come to the health care facility to have her blood glucose (sugar) level checked. In addition, the physician has ordered an APTT and PT to be run on her blood.

Questions
1. Which blood collection tube should be used to obtain the blood for the glucose level?
2. Can the blood from the same tube collected for the glucose be used to obtain a result for the APTT and PT?

Advocating Patient Safety Case Study

Ms. Debbie Halt works for a home health care agency as a phlebotomist. She travels 60 to 100 miles a day to collect blood from home bound patients and returns with the blood specimens to the clinical laboratory for testing. She is faithful in carrying the following blood supplies in her lockable closed container:

1. Marking pens or pencils
2. Vacuum tubes containing the anticoagulants designated in the clinical laboratory blood collection manual
3. Safety holders for vacuum tubes
4. Safety needles for vacuum tubes and syringes
5. Safety syringes
6. A disposable tourniquet (nonlatex)
7. Safety blood collection sets (butterfly needle assembly)
8. 70% isopropyl alcohol, iodine, and chlorhexidine pads/swabs
9. Sterile gauze pads
10. Bandages
11. Biohazardous waste containers for used needles, holders, and lancets
12. Safety lancets for skin puncture
13. Microdilution devices for fingerstick blood collection
14. Microcollection blood serum and plasma separator tubes
15. Microcollection capillary whole blood collectors with 0.23 mg of EDTA (200 micro L)
16. Disposable gloves
17. Cloth towel or washcloth
18. Thermometer
19. Antimicrobial hand gel or foam to wash hands without water and soap

Question
Does she have the appropriate supplies to collect blood from the home bound patients?

Competency Assessment

Check Yourself: Identifying the Proper Equipment for Blood Collection

1. Describe three examples of microcollection lancets. For the microcollection lancets, identify the maximum incision depth that should occur for neonates, children, and adults.

2. Based on your educational readings and/or experience, what do you recommend should be carried on the phlebotomy tray for the type (elderly, healthy adults, children, etc.) of patients from whom you collect blood.

3. Describe the types of blood collection tubes that have been made to collect blood for trace element measurements.

Competency Checklist

This checklist can be completed as a group or individually.

(1) Completed (2) Needs to improve/Repeat lesson and checklist

_____ 1. Correctly identifies blood collection tubes according to additive and color of top.

_____ 2. Identifies safety devices for venipuncture collection.

_____ 3. Lists blood collection equipment necessary for collection from a newborn infant.

References

1. Clinical and Laboratory Standards Institute (CLSI): *Tubes and Additives for Venous and Capillary Blood Specimen Collection; Approved Standard,* 6th ed. (H01-A6). Wayne, PA: CLSI, 2010.

2. Rossen J, Stoker R: *The Compendium of Infection Control Technologies.* Palm City, FL, 2005.

3. Pugliese G, Salahuddin, eds.: *Sharps Injury Prevention Program: A Step-By-Step Guide.* Chicago: American Hospital Association, 1999.

4. Occupational Safety and Health Administration (OSHA), US Dept. of Labor: OSHA Safety and Health Information Bulletin (SHIB): *Re-Use of Blood Tube Holders.* October 15, 2003.

5. Experts address glove-related latex allergies. *Inf Cntrol Today.* http://www.infectioncontroltoday.com/ 10/20/2008 Accessed: 3/22/2011

6. Forseter G, Joline C, Wormser GP. Blood contamination of tourniquets used in routine phlebotomy. *Am J Inf Control* 1990; 18:386–90.

7. Rourke C, Bates C, Read RC. Poor hospital infection control practice in venepuncture and use of tourniquets. *J hosp Inf* 2001; 49:59–61.

8. Golder M, Chan CLH, O'Shea S, Corbett K, Chrystie IL, French G. Potential risk of cross-infection during peripheral-venous access by contamination of tourniquets. *Lancet* 2000; 355:44.

Resources

1. International Sharps Injury Prevention Society. *www.isips.org*

2. Premier Safety Institute. *www.premierinc.com/SAFETY*

3. Kohn LT, Corrigan JM, Donaldson MS, eds: Institute of Medicine. *To Err Is Human: Building A Safer Health System.* Washington, DC: National Academy Press, 2000.

4. Shelton P, Rosenthal K: Sharps injury prevention: select a safer needle. *Nurs Management* 2004:35(6):25–31.

PEARSON
myhealthprofessionskit™

Go to www.myhealthprofessionskit.com to access the Companion Website created for this textbook. Simply select "Clinical Laboratory Science" from the choice of disciplines. Find this book and log in using your username and password to access interactive learning games, assessment questions, and more.

Chapter 7

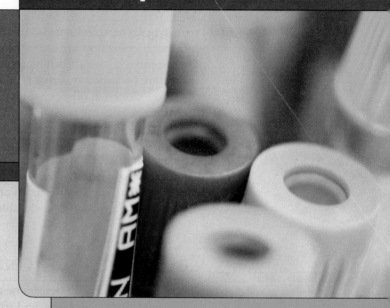

Preexamination/ Preanalytical Complications

KEY TERMS

basal state

edema

fasting

hematoma

hemoconcentration

hemolysis

lipemic

mastectomy

obesity

occluded veins

petechiae

sclerosed veins

syncope

thrombi

turbid

CHAPTER OBJECTIVES

Upon completion of Chapter 7, the learner should be able to do the following:

1. Describe preanalytical (preexamination) complications related to blood collection procedures and affect on patient safety.
2. Explain how to prevent and/or handle complications in blood collection.
3. List at least five factors about a patient's physical disposition (i.e., make-up) that can affect blood collection.
4. List examples of substances that can interfere in clinical testing of blood analytes and describe methods used to prevent these interferences.
5. Describe how allergies, a mastectomy, edema, and thrombosis can affect blood collection.
6. List preanalytical complications that can arise with test requests and identifications.
7. Describe complications associated with tourniquet pressure and fist pumping.
8. Identify how the preanalytical factors of syncope, petechiae, neurological complications, hemoconcentration, hemolysis, and intravenous therapy affect blood collection.
9. Describe methods used to prevent these interferences.

Overview

Preanalytical (preexamination) variables that are important to health care workers involved with blood collection are shown in Box 7-1 ■. The value of laboratory responsibilities to patient-centered care and safety is becoming increasingly apparent, especially as new laboratory testing becomes available (i.e., complex genetic and cancer marker tests).

As mentioned in other chapters, preanalytical variables are particularly critical to health care workers, because most of them can be controlled. Often when a blood collection error occurs it could have been prevented by taking precautions (i.e., proper ID check of patient). Occasionally, however, patient complications during or after the blood collection procedure are unavoidable. If so, the health care worker must be knowledgeable about methods that will decrease the negative impact of the complication to the patient, to the quality of the blood sample, to the health care worker, or to all three. This chapter covers patient complications and the preanalytical variables that are reported most often.

Categories of Preanalytical Variables

Blood specimens used to determine the amount of the patient's glucose, cholesterol, triglycerides, electrolytes, proteins, and so on, should be collected when the patient is in a **basal state**—that is, in the early morning, approximately 12 hours after food intake. The results of laboratory tests on basal state specimens are most constant. However, several factors—including diet, exercise, emotional stress, **obesity,** menstrual cycle, pregnancy, diurnal variations, posture, tourniquet application, and chemical constituents (alcohol or drugs)—can cause changes in the basal state. Health care workers need to have a general understanding of these possible patient changes and their effects on laboratory testing.

DIET

To ensure that the patient is in the basal state, the physician must require the patient to fast overnight. The term **fasting** refers to no food or drinks (except water). The required time period necessary for fasting depends on the test procedures to be performed. Before collecting a specimen, the health care worker should ask the patient whether he or she had anything to eat or drink. The amounts of blood analytes significantly change after meals and, thus, are not correct for many clinical chemistry tests. If the patient has eaten or had anything other than water to drink recently but the physician still needs the test, the word "nonfasting" must be written on the requisition and/or directly on the specimen.

When giving instructions to the patient to fast for blood tests, it is important to gain the patient's cooperation by using professional behavior. Inadequate patient instructions can cause mistakes in specimen collection. Casual instructions are apt to be taken lightly by the patient or even forgotten. If asked to explain fasting restrictions to a patient, the instructions should be thorough and clear, with emphasis on the important points of the procedure.

Box 7-1 Variables Important in Specimen Collection

- Patient assessment and physical disposition
- Test requests
- Specimen collection
- Specimen transport
- Specimen receipt in the laboratory

Some patients assume that the term fasting refers to abstaining from (i.e., avoiding) food and water. Abstaining from water can result in dehydration, which can cause errors in test results. Thus, the health care worker must ensure that the patient understands all the requirements. Written instructions are also helpful, if available.

If a procedure involves some discomfort or inconvenience, the patient should be informed. For example, if blood is to be collected for timed blood glucose levels, cholesterol levels, and/or triglyceride levels, the patient needs to fast for 8 to 12 hours. The health care worker can inform the patient that several specimens will be collected at timed intervals and that he or she may drink water, but that coffee, tea, and chewing gum should be avoided because they may cause an error in the lab results.

OBESITY

More than 60% of adult patients in the United States are overweight.[1] Obese patients generally have veins that are difficult to visualize and/or palpate. (Refer to Chapter 8 to view examples of different arm veins.) If the vein is not entered when first punctured, the health care worker must be careful not to probe (i.e., dig) excessively with the needle, because doing so destroys red blood cells (RBCs) and causes errors in blood test results. Usually the patient him- or herself knows where the "best site" is for venipuncture, so it is helpful to check with the patient before selecting the site. Also, there are longer needles available for collections from obese patients.

DAMAGED, SCLEROSED, OR OBSTRUCTED VEINS

Obstructed, or clogged, veins do not allow blood to flow through them; **sclerosed,** or hardened, veins are a result of inflammation and disease. Patients' veins that have been repeatedly punctured often become scarred and feel hard when the arm is palpated to find a venipuncture site. Because blood is not easily collected from these sites, they should be avoided. Chapter 8 discusses alternative venipuncture sites.

ALLERGIES

Some patients are allergic to iodine, alcohol, or other solutions used to cleanse a puncture site. Check for color-coded armbands or posted signs indicating specific patient allergies. Also, another precaution is to ask the patient if he/she is allergic to a solution or latex. If a patient states that he or she is allergic to a solution, all efforts should be made to use another cleansing agent. (Chlorhexidine has been reportedly used as an alternative to cleanse the skin. After application, it can be wiped off with sterile water.)[2] In addition, some patients are allergic to latex. Latex-free tourniquets, gloves, and bandages must be used for patients who have this allergy. (See Chapter 4 for more information about latex allergy.)

MASTECTOMY

Patients who have undergone a **mastectomy** (i.e., surgical removal of the breast) often have resulting lymphedema (increased lymph fluid) on the side of the surgery. The fluid in the area may make the patient more prone to infections; therefore, the arm and area around the arm on the side of the mastectomy should be protected from cuts, scratches, burns, and blood collection.

EDEMA

Some patients develop **edema** (i.e., an abnormal accumulation of fluid in the tissues) because of reasons other than a mastectomy (e.g., heart failure, renal failure, inflammation, malnutrition, and bacterial toxins). This swelling can be localized or spread out over a larger area of the body. The health care worker should avoid collecting blood from these sites, because veins in these areas are difficult to palpate or locate, and the specimen may become contaminated with fluid. Again, consultation with the physician is sometimes needed to determine whether and where a blood specimen should be taken.

> **Clinical Alert** !
>
> Venipuncture and/or skin puncture should never be performed on the same side as that of a mastectomy (unless *written* approval by the physician is obtained), because the patient is more susceptible to infection, and some analytes in the blood may be altered. Also, the pressure from the tourniquet could lead to injuries in a patient who has had this type of surgery. If the patient has had a double mastectomy, fingersticks are better sites for blood collection. However, the physician should provide written permission for this blood collection to occur.

THROMBOSIS

Thrombi are solid masses derived from blood constituents that reside in the blood vessels. A thrombus may partially or fully occlude (close) a vein or artery, and such occlusion will make venipuncture more difficult.

> **Clinical Alert** !
>
> **Burned, Scarred, or Tattooed Areas**
>
> Areas that have been burned, scarred, or tattooed should be avoided during phlebotomy. Burned areas are very sensitive and susceptible to infection, and veins under scarred areas are difficult to palpate. Collecting specimens from these sites can be very painful. Tattoos contain dyes that may interfere with laboratory tests. Also, tattooed areas are susceptible to infections and impaired circulation.

VOMITING

Sometimes the thought or sight of blood before or during blood collection leads to nausea and possibly vomiting. If this reaction occurs, have the patient take deep breaths and use a cold compress on his or her head. Follow the health care facility's protocol. Also, contact the phlebotomy supervisor and patient's physician about this complication.

Complications Associated with Test Requests and Identification

IDENTIFICATION DISCREPANCIES

Improper identification is the most dangerous and costly error a health care worker can make, because it can be life-threatening. Identification should include a match between the patient's identification, his or her verbal confirmation, and the test requisition. At least two patient identifiers are necessary to avoid an identification error. Bed labels, water pitchers, or door charts should not be used as a patient identifier. Even armbands are not completely reliable. (Refer to Chapter 8 for more details on identification procedures.)[3] Sometimes a phlebotomist is the first to detect a discrepancy between a name on the requisition and the name that the patient states or the name on the armband. In these cases, the discrepancy should be reported to a supervisor and/or nurse and may result in the prevention of other errors related to that patient. These discrepancies must be resolved before the collection of any samples.[4]

TIME OF COLLECTION

Timing factors can affect test results. In some cases, such as testing drug levels, the timing of the collection must coincide with when the dosage was given. Early morning specimens are most commonly requested in hospital settings, because a fasting specimen is preferred (given that reference ranges are based on fasting specimens). If a health care worker is running late, the specimen might be collected after an inpatient has eaten breakfast and would require a special notation about his or her "nonfasting" condition.

REQUISITIONS

Checking the requisition to match the laboratory tests requested with the appropriate type of collection tube is essential to minimize the amount of blood collected from each patient. Too much blood loss because of excessive specimen removal can result in anemia.

Complications Associated with the Specimen Collection Procedure

TOURNIQUET PRESSURE AND FIST PUMPING

Laboratory test results can be falsely elevated or decreased if the tourniquet pressure is too tight or is maintained for too long. The pressure from the tourniquet causes biological analytes to leak from the tissue cells into the blood, or vice versa. For example, plasma, cholesterol, iron, lipid, protein, and potassium levels will be falsely elevated if the tourniquet pressure is too tight or prolonged. These falsely elevated results may be seen with as short as a 3-minute application of the tourniquet (the recommended time for tourniquet application is no longer than 1 minute at a time).[5] In addition, some enzyme levels can be falsely elevated or decreased because of tourniquet pressure that is too tight or prolonged. Also, pumping of the fist before venipuncture should be avoided, because it leads to an increase in the plasma, potassium, lactate, and phosphate concentrations.

REDUCING RECOLLECTIONS FOR BLOOD

Several factors may cause the health care worker to "miss the vein." These factors include not inserting the needle deep enough, inserting the needle all the way through the vein, holding the needle bevel against the vein wall, or losing the vacuum in the tube (as demonstrated in Figure 7-1 ■). During needle insertion, the gloved index finger can be used to help locate the vein. The needle may need to be moved or withdrawn somewhat and redirected. The only acceptable redirections are backward and forward in a relatively straight line. In an elderly (geriatric) patient, the vein may be "tough" during needle entry, and it may roll; such rolling can cause the needle to slip to the side of the vein instead of properly puncturing it. Thus, the health care worker must securely anchor the vein before blood collection, to prevent rolling. If the vein rolls, it is the fault of the blood collector, because the anchoring technique used on the vein was not sufficient. Do not blame the patient.

On occasion, a blood collection vacuum tube will have lost some of its vacuum and the blood slowly trickles into the collection tube or the tube may have no vacuum because of a manufacturer's error, the age of the tube, or tube leakage after a puncture. Therefore, an extra set of tubes should be readily available to change to another tube in case this should happen during venipuncture. Also, needles for evacuated tube systems have been known

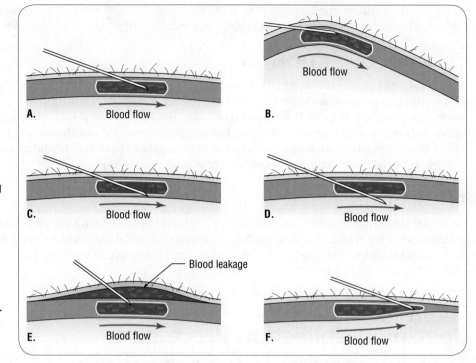

FIGURE ■ 7-1 Needle Positioning and Failure to Draw Blood

A. Correct insertion technique; blood flows freely into needle.
B. Bevel on the vein upper wall does not allow blood to flow.
C. Bevel inserted into the vein's lower wall does not allow blood to flow. D. Needle inserted too far.
E. Needle partially inserted, which causes blood leakage into tissue.
F. Collapsed vein.

to unscrew from the barrel during venipuncture. If this happens, the tourniquet should be released immediately and the needle removed from the arm as the safety device is activated over the needle, to avoid a needlestick to the blood collector.

FAINTING (SYNCOPE)

Syncope is the sudden loss of consciousness caused by a lack of oxygen to the brain that results in an inability to stay in an upright position. Patients usually recover their orientation quickly, but injuries (e.g., abrasions and cuts) often result from falling to the ground. Syncope may be caused by a variety of things, including low blood glucose levels, heart ailments, rapid breathing, mental conditions, or medications. Many patients become dizzy and faint ("get weak in the knees") at the thought or sight of blood. Also, patients who have donated blood recently and/or fasting patients frequently become faint. Therefore, the health care worker should be aware of the patient's condition throughout the collection procedure. This can be done by asking ambulatory patients whether they tend to faint or have ever previously fainted during blood collections. Also, look for signs of fainting such as sweating, paleness in the face, anxiety, hyperventilation, and nausea. If so, they should be moved from a seated position to a lying position. Even for an ambulatory patient without a history of fainting, it is still extremely important to use a blood collection chair with a "locked" armrest to avoid the possibility of a fall if he or she faints. If you are a home health care provider, you need to have the patient seated in a chair with arm supports or have him/her lie down. A recliner chair with arm rests is also a good safe place for the blood collection. If a seated patient feels faint, the needle should be removed, the patient's head should be lowered between the legs, and the patient should breathe deeply. If possible, the health care worker should ask for help and move the patient to a lying position. Talking to patients can often reassure them and distract their attention from the blood collection procedure. Bed-bound patients may also faint during blood collection, although rarely. In any case, the health care worker should stay with the patient for at least 15 minutes until he or she recovers or until a nurse or physician takes over. A wet towel gently applied to the forehead or a glass of juice or water may help the patient feel better.

Clinical Alert !

If a patient faints during or after the procedure, the health care worker should try to end the venipuncture procedure immediately and make sure that the patient does not fall or become injured. Sometimes controlling the situation is difficult because of the patient's physical size; however, the health care worker should use common sense about the safest position for a patient. If a patient has fainted and is in a secure position, the health care worker should quickly request assistance from the nursing staff or a physician. A patient who has fainted should recover fully before being allowed to leave and should be instructed not to drive a vehicle for at least 30 minutes. Patients often think too soon that they have recovered, but when they try to stand up, they collapse again, risking injury. An incident report must be filed with the health care facility regarding the fainting incident and any injuries resulting from the fall, the immediate precautions taken, and what instructions were provided to the patient to prevent the possibility of long-term complications (e.g., a car accident after the fainting incident).

HEMATOMAS

When the area around the puncture site starts to swell, usually blood is leaking into the tissues and causes a **hematoma.** A hematoma can occur when the needle has gone completely through the vein, the bevel opening is partially in the vein, or not enough pressure is applied to the site after puncture. This swelling results in a large bruise after several days (Figure 7-2 ■). If a hematoma begins to form, the tourniquet and the needle should be removed immediately, and pressure should be applied to the area for approximately 2 minutes. If the bleeding continues, a nurse should be notified.

PETECHIAE

Petechiae, small red spots appearing on a patient's skin, indicate that minute amounts of blood have escaped into outer skin layers (Figure 7-3 ■). This complication may be a result of a blood clotting abnormality such as thrombocytopenia—that is, a low platelet count—and should be a warning that the patient's puncture site may bleed excessively. Petechiae also occur during illnesses with fever.

EXCESSIVE BLEEDING

Most patients stop bleeding at the venipuncture site within a few minutes. Patients receiving anticoagulant therapy and/or high dosages of arthritis medication or other medication, however, may bleed for a longer period. Often, elderly patients are receiving these medications and must be watched carefully for excessive bleeding. Also, coagulation abnormalities can cause excessive bleeding. Thus, anytime a venipuncture is performed, pressure must be applied to the venipuncture site until the bleeding stops.

Clinical Alert !

The health care worker must not leave the patient until the bleeding stops or a nurse takes over to assess the patient's situation. In rare instances, the health care worker may accidentally puncture an artery instead of a vein. An artery has pulsating pressure that causes the blood to squirt out in pulses. These cases require that pressure be applied as quickly as possible to stop the bleeding and that a nurse and/or supervisor be notified as soon as possible.

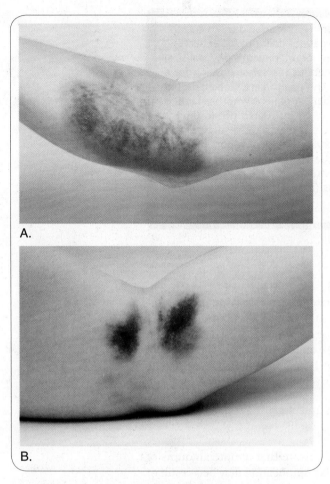

A.

B.

FIGURE ■ 7-2 Patient's Hematoma after Venipunctures
Source: A. © Powered by Light/Alan Spencer/Alamy
B. © Julie Thompson/Alamy

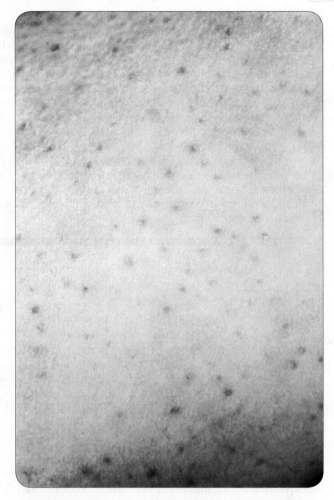

FIGURE ■ 7-3 Petechiae of the Skin in a Patient
Source: CDC Public Image Library

NEUROLOGICAL COMPLICATIONS

If the health care worker accidentally inserts the needle all the way through the vein, he or she may hit the nerve below the vein. If this happens, the patient will most likely have a sharp, electric tingling (and painful) sensation that radiates down the nerve. The tourniquet should be released immediately, the needle removed, and pressure held over the blood collection site. An incident report on the occurrence should be completed and given to the supervisor.

Clinical Alert !

A rare but serious complication that may occur during blood collection is a seizure (a sudden attack or convulsion). Try to keep the patient from hitting things. If a patient begins to have a seizure, the health care worker should immediately release the tourniquet, remove the needle, move the patient to a lying position if they have not fallen already, attempt to hold pressure over the blood collection site, and call for help from the nursing station. No attempt should be made to place anything in the patient's mouth unless the health care worker is experienced and authorized to do so.

HEMOCONCENTRATION

Hemoconcentration, the increase in red blood cells, and other cells and solids in the blood is caused from loss of fluid in the surrounding tissues around the venipuncture site. These may be due to several factors, including prolonged (i.e., longer than 1 minute) tourniquet application; massaging, squeezing, or probing a site; long-term intravenous (IV) therapy; and sclerosed or **occluded veins.** All of these practices and/or sites for venipuncture should be carefully avoided.

INTRAVENOUS THERAPY

Every time a catheter (IV) is used, vein damage occurs. Circulatory blood is rerouted to branching veins and can result in hemoconcentration. As a consequence, patients on IV therapy for extended periods often have veins that are palpable and visible but damaged or occluded (blocked). An arm with the IV line should not be used for venipuncture, because the specimen will be diluted with IV fluid. Instead, the other arm or another site should be considered. Alternatively, sometimes the nurse or the physician can disconnect the IV fluid and collect blood from the line that is already inserted. In this situation, the first few milliliters of the specimen should be discarded to remove the IV fluid, and a note should be made on the laboratory requisition that this step was performed.

Also, blood collections through an IV device increase the risk of hemolysis since the IV cannula (IV tubing) is not designed for blood collection.[6]

HEMOLYSIS

Hemolysis results when RBCs are lysed (i.e., destroyed), hemoglobin is released, and serum or plasma, which is normally straw colored, becomes tinged with pink or red. If a specimen is grossly hemolyzed, the serum or plasma appears very dark red. Hemolysis can be caused by improper phlebotomy techniques, such as using a needle that is too small (i.e., 25-gauge), expelling the blood vigorously into a tube, shaking or mixing tubes vigorously, performing blood collection before the alcohol has dried at the collection site, or pulling a syringe plunger back too fast (although syringes are not recommended for routine use). Hemolysis may also be the result of physiological abnormalities (e.g., sickle cell diseases, exposure to drugs or toxins, artificial heart valves, some infections).[7] Hemolysis due to poor technique or sample handling causes falsely increased results for many analytes, including potassium, magnesium, iron, lactate dehydrogenase, phosphorus, ammonia, and total protein. Hemolysis also shows falsely decreased RBC counts, hemoglobin, and hematocrit. These problems can easily be prevented with appropriate handling. The health care worker should document the fact if he or she notices that a specimen is hemolyzed.

COLLAPSED VEINS

Veins collapse when blood is withdrawn too quickly or forcefully during venipuncture, especially when blood is being collected from smaller veins (see Figure 7-1F) and/or the veins of geriatric patients. Thus, the health care worker should use a smaller blood collection tube and/or a smaller needle size (i.e., 23-gauge) during the collection process for patients with smaller veins and/or geriatric patients. A collapsed vein should not be probed with the needle. The health care worker will notice that the tube is filling properly, but then the blood entering the tube starts to slow and stops flowing. A smaller tube size should be used for the remainder of the blood collections. If the problem is not resolved, then the patient's blood should be recollected using a syringe because the health care worker can control the force of vacuum exerted on the vein.

TURBID OR LIPEMIC SERUM

After the cells have settled or have been separated from the serum or plasma, it is normally clear, light yellow, or straw colored. **Turbid** serum or plasma appears cloudy or "milky" and can be a result of bacterial contamination or high lipid levels in the blood. Turbidity is primarily caused by ingestion of fatty substances, such as meat, butter, cream, and cheese. If a patient has recently eaten fatty substances, he or she may have a temporarily elevated lipid level, and the serum will appear **lipemic,** or cloudy. Because lipemic serum or plasma does not represent a basal state and may indicate some chemical abnormalities, documentation about the appearance of the serum or plasma may be useful to the physician.

IMPROPER COLLECTION TUBE

Learn which common laboratory tests require which collection tubes. However, there are so many possible laboratory tests and tubes available that you should also be familiar with how and where to seek information (electronically, via laboratory reference manual, etc.) about test and tube requirements that you are unfamiliar with. An example of a blood specimen collected in the wrong tube would be as follows: green-topped tubes containing lithium heparin are not suitable for a patient's lithium studies because laboratory values will be falsely high, suggesting that the patient has a toxic level of lithium when he or she really does not.

Self Study

Study Questions

The following questions may have more than one answer.

1. What does the term "preexamination" refer to in phlebotomy practice?
   a. variables that affect the blood specimen during testing
   b. equipment malfunction during analysis
   c. variables that affect the specimen prior to laboratory testing
   d. when a test result is reported incorrectly

2. What is the ideal time for blood specimens to be collected?
   a. at midnight
   b. 6 hours after the last ingestion of food
   c. 12 hours after the last ingestion of food
   d. 24 hours after the last ingestion of food

3. If blood is to be collected for a timed blood glucose level determination, the patient must fast for how long?
   a. 4–6 hours
   b. 6–8 hours
   c. 8–12 hours
   d. 14–16 hours

4. If a patient is overweight and the phlebotomist cannot access the vein when the needle is first inserted, what should the phlebotomist do?
   a. probe around with the needle until the vein is found
   b. repalpate and adjust/move the needle very slightly forwards or backwards
   c. push the needle all the way in because the vein is probably under layers of fat
   d. push to the left and right with the needle to see if the vein is there

5. If the tourniquet is applied for longer than 3 minutes, which of the following analytes will most likely become falsely elevated?
   a. glucose
   b. bilirubin
   c. cholesterol
   d. lithium

6. To ensure that the patient is in the basal state for laboratory testing,
   a. the patient must sleep for at least 8 hours
   b. the physician must require the patient to fast overnight for 8 to 12 hours
   c. the physician must require the patient to fast and not drink water overnight
   d. the patient must rest for at least 13 hours and not drink water or eat any food

7. Which of the following should stop the health care worker from collecting blood from a patient's arm vein?

   a. heart attack that occurred the previous day

   b. cardiac bypass surgery two days ago

   c. high blood pressure

   d. mastectomy

8. The appearance of small red spots on a patient's skin due to a blood clotting abnormality is referred to as:

   a. hemoconcentration

   b. petechiae

   c. hemolysis

   d. syncope

9. What is the effect on a patient if a phlebotomist punctures a nerve with the blood collection needle?

   a. It should not have an effect on the patient or blood specimen.

   b. The patient will feel a sharp radiating pain and the procedure should be discontinued.

   c. The blood specimen may be contaminated with interstitial fluid.

   d. The patient's arm may tingle slightly but it should not interfere with the rest of the procedure.

10. A hemolyzed specimen can lead to falsely increased results for:

    a. RBC count

    b. hematocrit

    c. hemoglobin

    d. potassium

Case Study

Mary, a new health care worker at the Northlake Ambulatory Clinic, had a requisition to collect a fasting blood specimen from Mr. Martinez, who had come to the laboratory area at 9 a.m. for the specimen collection. Mary followed through with the necessary protocol to check Mr. Martinez's identification and to prepare for the blood collection. During her preparation for blood collection, she asked Mr. Martinez whether he had eaten anything since the night before. Mr. Martinez stated that he had not had any food since 7 p.m. the night before. As she looked at both arms to assess the best venipuncture site, she discovered that both arms were totally covered from the wrist to the shoulder with tattoos.

Question
How should Mary proceed with the fasting blood specimen for the blood glucose test?

Advocating Patient Safety Case Study

After the phlebotomist, Ms. Shilling, had prepared the venipuncture site on the young teenage patient, Ms. Howard, she inserted the needle into the antecubital venipuncture site. As she did, Ms. Howard immediately jerked forward and vomited.

Question
What should Ms. Shilling do?

Competency Assessment

Check Yourself: Ready to Give Patient Instructions for Fasting Blood Specimens

1. Write out the instructions you would give to a patient who needs to fast before a blood collection procedure. Try to think of all the most usual and unusual questions that the patient might ask about eating or drinking.

2. Practice giving the instructions to a friend or coworker. Practice your communication techniques by double checking that they completely understand; ask them specific questions about their comprehension of the fasting process; and ask them to give a friendly and constructive critique of your instructions.

Competency Checklist: Preanalytical Complications in Blood Collection

This checklist can be completed as a group or individually.

(1) Completed (2) Needs to improve/Repeat lesson and checklist

_____ 1. List five factors about a patient's physical disposition that can affect blood collection.

_____ 2. List three examples of substances that can interfere in clinical testing of blood analytes.

References

1. Organization for Economic Co-operation and Development. Obesity and the Economics of Prevention: Fit Not Fat. September 23, 2010.

2. Ernst, D: Iodine disinfectant for infants, tips from the clinical experts. *Med Lab Obs* July 2003:54, www.mlo-online.com.

3. Kahn, S: Specimen mislabeling: A significant and costly cause of potentially serious medical errors. http://www.bloodgas.org. April, 2005. Last accessed on 06/27/06.

4. Clinical and Laboratory Standards Institute (CLSI): Accuracy in Patient and Sample Identification: Approved Guideline GP33-A. Wayne, PA:CLSI, 2010.

5. Saleem S, Mani V, Chadwick MA, Creanor S, Ayling RM: A prospective study of causes of haemolysis during venepuncture: Tourniquet time should be kept to a minimum. *Ann Clin Biochem* 2009;46(Pt 3): 244–246.

6. Lowe G, Stike R, Pollack M, Bosley J, O'Brien P, et al.: Nursing blood specimen collection techniques and hemolysis rates in an emergency department: Analysis of venipuncture versus intravenous catheter collection techniques. *J Emerg Nurs.* 2008;34(1):26–32.

7. Arzoumanium L: BD Tech Talk. *What Is Hemolysis: What Are the Causes.* Vol. 2, No 2: 10/2003.

Resources

1. Weight Watchers: Welcome brochure. Woodbury, NY: Weight Watchers. Available at: *www.weightwatchers.com.* Accessed January 13, 2011.

2. Guder, WG, Narayanan, S, Wisser, H, et al.: *Samples: From the Patient to the Laboratory.* Munich, Germany: Git Verlag Publishers, 1996.

3. McGlasson, DL: Laboratory variables that may affect test results in prothrombin times (PT)/international normalized ratios (INR). *Lab Med* 2003;34(2):124–9.

4. Clinical and Laboratory Standards Institute (CLSI). *Procedures for the Collection of Diagnostic Blood Specimens by Venipuncture.* Approved Standard 6th ed. (H3-A6). Wayne, PA: CLSI, 2007.

PEARSON
myhealthprofessionskit™

Go to www.myhealthprofessionskit.com to access the Companion Website created for this textbook. Simply select "Clinical Laboratory Science" from the choice of disciplines. Find this book and log in using your username and password to access interactive learning games, assessment questions, and more.

Chapter 8

Venipuncture Procedures

KEY TERMS

butterfly system

Clinical and Laboratory
  Standards Institute
  (CLSI)

decontaminate

evacuated tube system

hand hygiene

physician–patient
  relationship

specimen rejection

STAT

syringe method

therapeutic drug
  monitoring (TDM)

timed specimen

tourniquet

winged infusion
  system

CHAPTER OBJECTIVES

Upon completion of Chapter 8, the learner
should be able to do the following:

1. Describe the patient identification
   process.
2. Explain the use of venipuncture supplies
   in a typical venipuncture procedure.
3. Describe when hand hygiene and gloving
   procedures should be used.
4. Identify the most appropriate sites for
   venipuncture.
5. Describe how to apply a tourniquet to
   a patient's arm and its effects on the
   venipuncture process.
6. Describe the decontamination process
   for a venipuncture site.
7. Describe the detailed steps of a
   venipuncture procedure.
8. Describe the "order of draw" for collection
   tubes.
9. Describe the importance of timed, fasting,
   and STAT specimens.
10. Explain at least three potential
    errors related to the incorrect use of
    venipuncture supplies.

Blood Collection Process

There are essential steps that are part of every successful blood collection procedure. Figure 8-1 ■ is a flow chart that demonstrates the basic venipuncture process. Many health care facilities have their own very specific procedures to follow for this process. Employees must be trained to abide by each facility's protocols. In some cases, steps may occur simultaneously (e.g., checking the patient's physical condition while confirming the identification); in others, a problem may arise that prevents the health care worker from going further in the procedure (e.g., the verbal identity of the individual does not match the written documentation or the supplies needed for the venipuncture have expired). Each step of the patient encounter must be evaluated carefully in a detailed manner, with care taken not to omit any of the essential components.[1,2] However, the most basic and essential elements of all venipuncture procedures involve the following steps:

1. Prepare yourself by cleansing hands and reviewing laboratory test orders.
2. Approach, identify, and position the patient comfortably and safely.
3. Assess the patient's physical disposition, including diet and/or whether the patient is sensitive to latex or skin cleansing products.
4. Select and prepare equipment and supplies.
5. Find a suitable puncture site.
6. Prepare/decontaminate the puncture site.
7. Choose a venipuncture method.
8. Collect the samples in the appropriate tubes and in the correct order.
9. Discard contaminated supplies in designated containers.
10. Label the samples.
11. Assess the patient to ensure bleeding has stopped.
12. Decontaminate hands.
13. Manage and document any special circumstances that occurred during the phlebotomy procedure.

Using Standard Precautions

Precautionary measures such as **hand hygiene** and the use of gloves should be considered routine procedures and are covered in detail in Chapter 4: Safety and Infection Control. These procedures are vital to the well-being of the patient and the health care worker and must be practiced continuously. Hand hygiene and gloving procedures are most commonly done as soon as the health care worker is in visual contact with each patient, *before* beginning the actual procedure. This gives the patient a visual assurance of cleanliness and reinforces a safety-conscious gesture for both the patient and the health care worker. Glove removal and hand hygiene should be performed again *after* each patient encounter. Refer back to Procedures 4-1, 4-2, and 4-3 for hand hygiene and gown, mask, and gloving techniques. These procedures should be mastered and practiced diligently by every health care worker who has contact with patients. Adherence to hand hygiene techniques (handwashing or use of alcohol-based hand rubs) has been shown to significantly reduce outbreaks of infections, including antimicrobial-resistant infections (e.g., methicillin-resistant *Staphylococcus aureus,* MRSA).[3,4]

In addition, a clean, pressed uniform or "scrubs" with a laboratory coat is comfortable attire and instills a sense of professionalism and hygiene, which is gratifying to patients and promotes a safer work environment (see Procedure 8-1 ■). Each facility will have guidelines about when and where protective clothing is needed so health care workers must follow their employers' protocols.

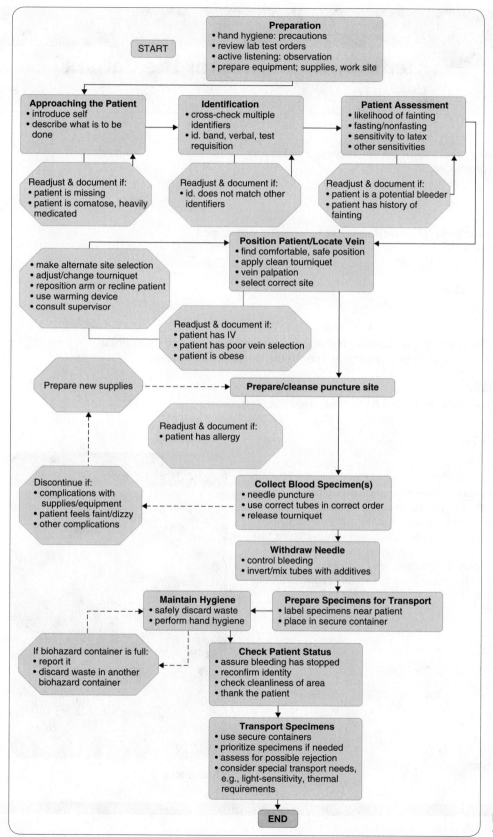

FIGURE ■ 8-1 Flow Chart of the Venipuncture Process

Procedure 8-1

Mentally Preparing for the Patient Encounter

RATIONALE

To help the health care worker mentally focus on the importance of the individual patient and prepare for that specific venipuncture procedure.

EQUIPMENT

- Phlebotomy supplies
- Personal protective equipment (PPE) (gloves, clean uniform, laboratory coat, etc.)
- Test requisitions
- Writing pen
- Bar code reader/scanner (if applicable)

PREPARATION

1 Prepare and assemble PPE, phlebotomy supplies, test requisitions, writing pen, and appropriate patient information before the patient encounter and prior to the venipuncture process.

2 Identify the patient properly.

3 Wash or sanitize your hands with an alcohol hand rinse, then put on gloves.

PROCEDURE

4 The health care worker needs a positive, professional appearance (neat and clean) and temperament (optimistic and open-minded) before beginning the patient encounter. Take a deep, cleansing breath before beginning (Figure 8-2 ■). As you do this, focus on the individual patient and the requests for that particular patient. Use the cleansing breath to center your attention on the upcoming venipuncture task as you temporarily remove yourself from other distracting factors in the workplace (e.g., TV noise, telephones, and other conversations). Use your keen observations to determine any special circumstances or needs that the patient may have.

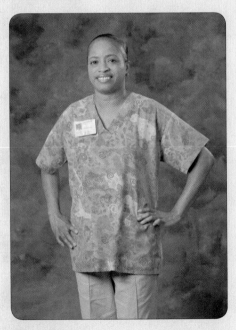

Figure ■ 8-2

(**5**) Arrange and check phlebotomy supplies, test requisitions, writing pen, and appropriate patient information before beginning the patient encounter and venipuncture process (Figure 8-3 ■).

(**6**) If the patient information is incomplete on test requisitions, the health care worker may not be able to identify the patient correctly, or he or she may not know in which tubes to collect the blood. In such cases, obtain assistance from a laboratory supervisor or a nurse before collecting the sample.

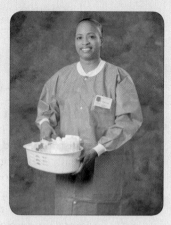

Figure ■ 8-3

Clinical Alert !

Remember that the use of gloves does not eliminate the need for hand hygiene, nor does good hand hygiene eliminate the need for gloves. Hands should be cleaned or **decontaminated** before and immediately after specimen collection procedures, and new gloves should be used for each patient. These are requirements for proper technique and for reducing the risk of transmitting microorganisms from one person to another.

Be familiar with policies regarding precautions for handling blood and body fluids. *All specimens should be treated as if they are hazardous and infectious*, according to the standard precautions described in detail in Chapter 4.

Assessing, Identifying, and Approaching the Patient

TEST REQUISITIONS

Laboratory test requests are usually transmitted electronically or as a paper requisition. Electronic (computer-generated) requests contain the same required information as paper requisitions. And, in some cases, the medical record may be used as verification for a test requisition; however, each facility should have specific instructions for health care workers and their level of authority in making decisions about laboratory requests. Whatever the circumstances, the health care worker should be familiar with procedures used in his or her facility.

Clinical Alert !

If the health care worker does not understand the test ordered, a supervisor, laboratory technologist, or nurse should be consulted *before* the procedure. Knowing which tests are requested helps the health care worker to prepare the patient appropriately and collect the specimen in the appropriate tubes and in the correct order. Failure to do so results in preanalytical errors, misleading test results, and repeated venipunctures.

Patient Identification Process

Positive patient identification is one of the most crucial responsibilities for which a health care worker is held accountable (see Procedure 8-2 ■). In hospital settings, it begins with registration and admission when the patient is typically issued an identification (ID) band, usually worn on the wrist. Some hospitals use color-coded ID bands to denote specific patient conditions such as red for allergy alerts, yellow for patients who are at risk of falling, and purple for patients with a "do not resuscitate (DNR)" order.[5]

Whenever taking blood samples or administering medications or blood products, the Joint Commission recommends using "at least two ways to identify patients."[6] The identifiers can include name, date of birth, government-issued ID with photograph, etc. However, it is *not acceptable* to use the following items as patient identifiers: hospital room numbers, bed tags, charts in holders near a patient or on a table, or tags on IV equipment because these items may not change as patients are moved or discharged so they are not consistently reliable identifiers. Patient identification errors can occur at any time during the laboratory workflow process, including at the time of phlebotomy (for example, placing the wrong label on the specimen) or as the specimen is being prepared for testing (for example, after centrifugation when the specimen is divided into aliquots). The process of identifying patients varies slightly on the basis of the patient's location (inpatient, outpatient, or emergency room), the type of patient (pediatric or adult), whether the patient is conscious or unconscious, and the available information at the time (armband or picture identification). CLSI recommends that extra care is needed when identification occurs in certain *high-risk* situations:[5]

- a patient does not understand the language. In this case, all efforts to find an interpreter must be made;
- siblings or twins are being cared for at the same time;
- patients with similar sounding names are being treated;
- patients have common names (for example, Rodriguez, Smith, Jones,);
- patients have similarly spelled names (for example, Cho, Chou, Chow, Chiu, Chung, Chu, etc.).

Clinical Alert !

If there is a discrepancy in the identification process, the specimen should *not* be obtained until identity can be verified. Discrepancies should be reported immediately. Identification errors can be life-threatening for the patient and pose significant liability to both the health care worker who makes the error and the health care facility that employs him or her. Never base identity on records or charts placed on the patient's bed or equipment. Identity errors occur because of inaccurate requisitions, mixed-up paperwork, or failure to follow identification procedures. All discrepancies should be reported to a supervisor.

Procedure 8-2

The Basics of Patient Identification

RATIONALE

To use appropriate patient identifiers whenever taking blood samples.

EQUIPMENT

Not applicable

PROCEDURE

Patient identification involves *at least 3 steps*

1. After introducing oneself, and greeting a conscious patient (Figure 8-4 ■), *ask the patient to state his or her full name, spell the last name, and state his or her birth date.* (You may also request the patient's hospital identification number and/or home address.) For example: "Sir, could you please confirm your full name and date of birth? Could you please spell your last name for me?" (Do not ask the patient "yes or no" questions; ask open-ended questions as in the example above for a more reliable way to confirm identity.)

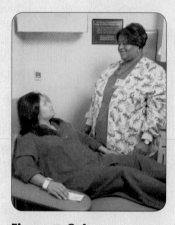

Figure ■ 8-4

2. *Compare the information stated with the information on the patient's ID band* (Figure 8-5 ■). (If the patient does not have an ID wristband, other forms of reliable, verifiable, person-specific identification may be used such as a government-issued photo ID card, a nurse, or a parent. If the patient does not have an ID wristband, document the source of identification.)

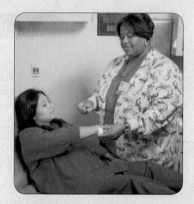

Figure ■ 8-5

3. Confirm the information (from steps 1 and 2) with the sample labels and/or requisitions (Figure 8-6 ■).

If *all three steps* indicate the same identity, proceed with the rest of the specimen collection procedure.

Refer to Chapter 5 for more information about requisitions.

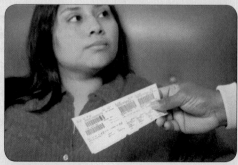

Figure ■ 8-6

> **Box 8-1** Advances in Identification Systems
>
> As mentioned in Chapter 5, bar codes are quick, accurate, cost-effective, and widely used for patient and specimen identification and tracking. Wireless technology, such as radio frequency identification (RFID) which uses radio waves to transmit data, is also being used for patient identification and tracking specimens. Electronic identification systems have been shown to reduce identification errors. Some hospitals have also incorporated a small picture of the patient into his or her armband as an additional visual verification step. In addition, biometric technology (fingerprints, voice recognition, iris or retinal patterns, and digitized signatures) are emerging in the health care market for use as identification tools.

INPATIENT IDENTIFICATION

Hospitalized patients (except those just entering an emergency room) must wear an ID wristband indicating the first and last names and a designated hospital number (sometimes called a unit number). Hospital identification numbers provide a unique number for each patient and help hospital personnel to distinguish between patients with the same first and/ or last names (see Box 8-1 ■).

Information on the identification bracelet may also include the patient's room number, bed assignment, and physician's name. As mentioned in Procedure 8-2, a three-way match should be made with the patient's statement and spelling of his or her name, birthday, or address, the ID wristband, and the test requisition.

> **Clinical Alert** !
>
> In some hospitals, there are special cases that involve patients with severe burns or in isolation, in which the identification is attached to the patient's bed rather than the arm. These are the only circumstances in which a health care worker may use a bed-labeled identification tag to confirm identity. This step should be followed up by a nurse's confirmation and appropriate documentation.

IDENTIFICATION OF PATIENTS WHO ARE SLEEPING

A patient who is sleeping should be awakened and have the patient identity verified before blood is collected. Verbal information should be compared with the information on the identification bracelet, and the requisition/labels.[5]

> **Clinical Alert** !
>
> The health care worker should *not* ask, "Are you Ms. Doe?" because an ill patient on medication may mistakenly utter anything, nod, or answer yes. Therefore, remember that the best tactic is to ask an open-ended question, "What is your name?" or "Please state your name and birthday," and let the patient reply. The patient must be correctly identified by his or her identification bracelet. If the patient does not have an identification bracelet, the nurse responsible for the patient must be asked to make the identification. The name of the nurse should be noted.
>
> Also, patients who are semiconscious, comatose, cognitively impaired, or sleeping may jerk unexpectedly during the blood collection process, particularly as the needle is inserted into the arm. If the patient cannot be awakened, be prepared by seeking assistance from an authorized health care worker during the procedure to help secure the patient's arm.

IDENTIFICATION OF PATIENTS WHO ARE UNCONSCIOUS, COGNITIVELY IMPAIRED, TOO YOUNG TO IDENTIFY THEMSELVES, DO NOT SPEAK THE LANGUAGE, OR HAVE SENSORY IMPAIRMENTS

There are also special cases in which health care workers must deviate from the standard ID procedure. A nurse, relative, or friend may identify patients in the listed circumstances:[5]

- unconscious or comatose (Figure 8-7 ■)
- cognitively impaired
- too young to identify themselves; i.e., pediatric patients
- cannot speak the health care worker's language
- have sensory impairments such as deafness

The nurse or relative should be asked to identify the patient by name, address, and ID number, and/or birth date. The name of the person identifying the patient and his or her relationship to the patient (nurse, spouse, brother, etc.) must be recorded. Again, this information should be compared with the information on the patient's ID wristband if he or she is an inpatient, and with the test requisition and/or labels to confirm identity. Any discrepancy should be reported to a supervisor.

In the case of language barriers or sensory impairments such as deafness, attempts should be made to find an interpreter (for non-English languages or sign language) if possible. However the same ID procedure mentioned above may be used when an interpreter is not available. Refer to Chapter 1 for additional strategies to care for these patients.

EMERGENCY ROOM PATIENT IDENTIFICATION

Patients often come to the emergency room (ER) unconscious and/or unidentified. Most ER departments have similar identification methods but all health care workers should be knowledgeable of the specific procedures at their own facility. Typically, a temporary master identification number (e.g., unique hospital number attached to the patient's body by wristband or other suitable device) may be provided until a positive identification can be made. When in the ER, the phlebotomist must often complete a requisition or sample labels, either electronically or handwritten, and it is imperative that all requisitions and sample labels can be cross-referenced to the ER patient's master ID number.[5] This will link the specific laboratory test results back to the patient, even if he or she does not have a confirmed ID by name.

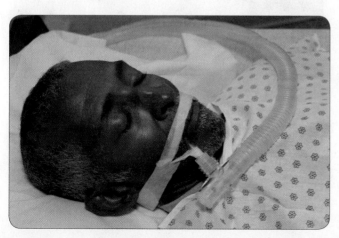

FIGURE ■ 8-7 Sleeping Patient

Later, when the name, birthdate, address, etc., are confirmed, the patient's name is usually electronically entered and linked to the master ID number, and from then on, the name and other pertinent information is available.

Health care workers in ERs must take extra care in the ID procedure because each situation has the potential to be hectic and stressful. Many critically ill patients may be cared for simultaneously and sometimes multiple unconscious, unidentified patients will need to have laboratory tests performed at the same time. Blood samples from the ER are usually considered as priority specimens or for STAT processing, testing, and results reporting (Figure 8-8 ■).

IDENTIFICATION OF NEONATES AND BABIES

In a hospital pediatric setting, neonates and babies under the age of 2 may have an ID band placed on the lower leg or ankle rather than on the wrist, or on *both* the ankle and the wrist. Whatever the case, CLSI recommends that a nurse, guardian, family member or relative state the baby's name and date of birth so that it may be compared with the ID band AND with the requisition. All the following elements should be confirmed:[5]

- Name of baby if designated
- Date of birth
- Baby's gender
- Medical record number or unique identifier
- Mother's last name, or the last name used at registration

The name of the person who identified the baby and his or her relationship to the patient must be documented. Keep in mind that neonates do not always have a given name when they are first born so their ID bands are typically linked to the birth mother (Figure 8-9 ■). If the mother had twins, she may wear her own ID band plus ID bands that reference each of her babies. In some circumstances, the baby may have a different last name that was provided

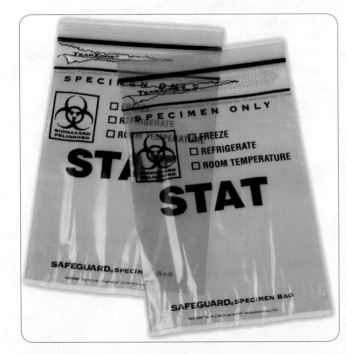

FIGURE ■ 8-8 A STAT Blood Sample Transportation Bag

Source: Courtesy of MarketLab: www.marketlabinc.com

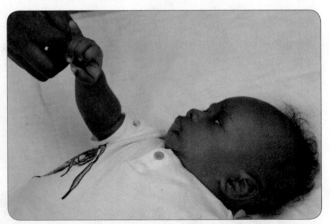

FIGURE ■ 8-9 Infant Holding his Mother's Finger

upon registration. Whatever the case, all the criteria must match before proceeding with blood sample collection. Also, as mentioned previously, in the case of multiple births, extra care and sometimes, additional procedures must be taken not to confuse the identity of siblings.

OUTPATIENT/AMBULATORY PATIENT IDENTIFICATION

Ambulatory patients may be seen in hospital clinics or physicians' offices, and/or may be receiving services such as diagnostic radiology and/or laboratory testing and they require positive ID but do not require armbanding. Ambulatory patient ID is handled in much the same way as previously discussed, except that as there is not a wristband to cross-reference, other identifiers are used. Typically, an ambulatory patient is called by his or her name or a waiting room number into a private or semi-private blood collection area from a waiting room. Thus, ambulatory patient identification takes more time, because the patient first has to walk into the specimen collection area, and be seated in a comfortable, safe phlebotomy chair or recliner. It is preferable for the identification process to take place in a private location since personal information is being revealed.

For a positive ID, the ambulatory patient must be asked to state his or her first and last name, and birthdate, and spell the last name while the health care worker cross checks this information with the test requisitions, then he or she should be asked to show some form of identification (e.g., health care ID card, driver's license, or government-issued ID).[5] If the patient has an ID card available, positive identification using a 3-way match (verbal, ID, and requisition) can occur in the same manner as with hospitalized patients. If there are discrepancies or problems with ID, a supervisor should be consulted prior to collecting blood samples.

Patients who are undergoing outpatient surgery, or receiving sedation or blood products must have an ID wristband (or if the armband is not possible, an ankle band). This is issued at registration. At minimum, it should include the patient's full name and medical record number.[5] Thus, for these patients, positive ID is essentially the same as for inpatients.

PHYSICAL CLUES FOR ASSESSMENT OF THE PATIENT

As mentioned previously, factors related to the physical or emotional disposition or age (pediatric versus geriatric) of the patient may affect the blood collection process. The health care worker can get clues about the patient's disposition by being observant and alert and by listening carefully—for example, if there is an empty food tray by the patient's bedside, it is likely that the patient has eaten recently, and documentation about the nonfasting condition should be made after confirming the observation with the patient. The following statement might confirm it with the patient, "Mr. Jones, it looks like you might have finished your breakfast recently, could you tell me when you last ate or drank anything?" A clue about something unusual may come after talking to the patient or after the identification process has taken place. In the case of ambulatory patients, it is important to know if they have fainted during prior venipunctures. A simple question may evoke more information, for example, "Mr. Jones, have you ever fainted during or after a blood-collection procedure?" If the answer is yes, the health care worker might move the patient to a recliner prior to beginning the venipuncture procedure. This assures a safer and more comfortable position in case he feels faint.

APPROACHING THE PATIENT

Several professional and courteous behaviors and phrases can help make the patient–health care worker encounter a smooth interaction (Box 8-2 ■). The first of these is a polite knock (no banging) on the patient's door before entering the patient's room. The health care worker should introduce him- or herself and state which department he or she is from—e.g., the laboratory—and that he or she has come to collect a blood sample. Sometimes, the health care worker may need to explain to the patient that the physician ordered the laboratory

Box 8-2   Typical Health Care Worker–Patient Interaction

The following scenario is one example of a health care worker and patient interaction just before the blood collection. It begins when the health care worker politely knocks on the patient's door and slowly enters the room.

Health care worker: Good morning. I am Ms. Smith from the laboratory, and I have come to collect a blood sample.

(Use a normal voice, not loud or sudden. Pause to give the patient an opportunity to speak or ask a question. If the lights are off or dimmed, explain that you need to turn the lights on. Doing so gives the patient a moment to wake up and adjust to the idea of bright lights if he or she has been asleep.)

Health care worker: Could you please state your name and your birthday while I check your armband? Please spell your last name.

Patient: My name is John Jones. J-O-N-E-S. My birthday is June 25, 1985.

Health care worker: Thanks, I'll double check this information with the laboratory requests.

(Cross check the armband, the verbal ID, and the laboratory requisitions. If all three match, proceed.)

Health care worker: This will take only a few minutes.

Patient: Will it hurt?

Health care worker: It will hurt a little, but it will be over soon. Please allow me to look at your arm veins. I am going to palpate the area to feel for a vein. Is that okay with you?

Patient: No problem, it's okay.

(Proceed with the remainder of the procedure, maintaining a highly professional atmosphere and a respectful attitude. Ascertain whether the patient has been fasting.)

Health care worker: Mr. Jones, when was the last time you ate or drank anything?

(Do not use the term fast *because some patients may not understand it completely.)*

Patient: Last night when I had dinner.

(As supplies are being readied, the health care worker could demonstrate that she is opening a new needle. She should also inquire about any allergy sensitivities such as latex if using latex products, e.g., gloves or a tourniquet.)

Health care worker: Mr. Jones, naturally I'll be using a new tourniquet and needle to collect your blood sample. Have you ever fainted during or after a blood collection procedure?

Patient: No, never.

Health care worker: Are you allergic to any products like latex or skin cleansing products?

Patient: No, I'm not allergic to anything.

Health care worker: Okay then, please hold still while I check your arm for a vein, and then I'll collect the blood sample. You will feel a needle prick.

After the blood samples are collected and labeled, as a confirmatory step, ask the following:

Health care worker: Mr. Jones, could you confirm that these blood sample labels have your name on them?

(The health care worker can hold the sample tubes out for the patient to see and confirm the labels.)

Patient: Yep, they do.

At the end of the procedure, say the following:

Health care worker: Let me check your arm one more time to make sure the bleeding has stopped. Thank you, Mr. Jones.

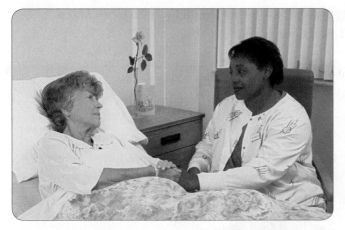

FIGURE ■ 8-10 On occasion, a health care worker may need to actually sit down near the patient to spend extra time explaining the procedure or to answer questions. This health care worker is actively listening to the patient's concerns in a compassionate manner.

test or tests. The health care worker may also need to explain the procedure as supplies are being set up or as gloves are put on (Figure 8-10 ■).

Also during setup, standard precautions, hand hygiene, gloving, and other infection control procedures that were discussed in Chapter 4 should be carefully followed. For example, the phlebotomy supply tray should not be placed on the patient's eating table or bed, because the bed is not a stable surface, and because of the risk of contamination. Avoiding the transmission of microorganisms is a key factor in preventing hospital acquired infections. As supplies are being readied and the vein is being palpated, the health care worker may try to alleviate some of the patient's fears. It may be reassuring to purposefully show the patient that the supplies are "new" and "unused."

Clinical Alert !

If a physician, clergy, or nurse is consulting with the patient, the specimen collection procedure should be delayed until the consultation is completed. The **physician–patient relationship** has priority over a phlebotomy procedure unless the request is for a timed or STAT specimen. If either of these is the case, ask for permission to proceed.

When friends or relatives are in the room, politely explain to the patient that a blood sample is needed and ask whether the guests would mind leaving the room temporarily. The patient may also give permission for the guests to stay during the venipuncture procedure.

Equipment Selection and Preparation

SUPPLIES FOR VENIPUNCTURE

Being prepared means having all supplies readily available. As discussed in more detail in Chapter 6, supplies for venipuncture differ according to the method used (i.e., **evacuated tube system** or winged infusion **butterfly system** or **syringe method**) and the tests that have been ordered. Supplies common to most methods of blood collection are the following:

- Written, printed, or electronic laboratory requisitions and/or labels
- Marking pens
- Gloves
- Nonlatex tourniquets
- Alcohol pads/skin disinfectants
- Disinfectant swab sticks for blood culture skin preparation

- Safety needles with single-use, evacuated tube holders and winged infusion sets
- Safety syringes and syringe transfer devices
- Blood collection tubes
- Plastic capillary tubes with tube sealer
- Nonlatex bandages and sterile gauze pads
- Glass microscope slides
- Puncture-proof sharps container

Supplies should be readily available and selected just prior to the procedure (Figure 8-11 ■).

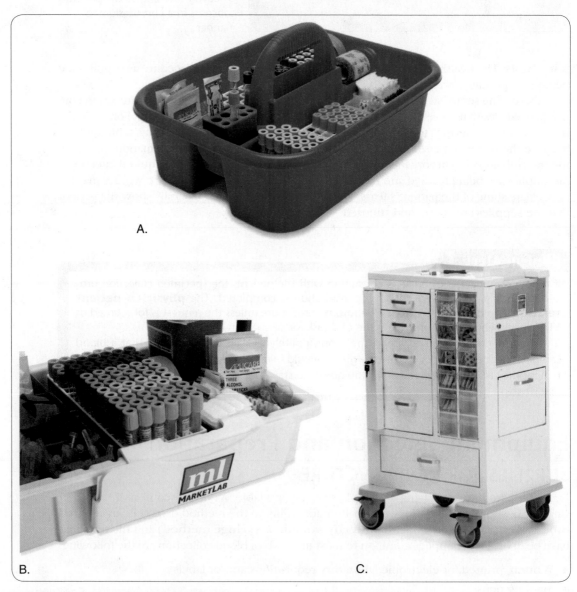

A.

B.

C.

FIGURE ■ 8-11 There are several ways to transport phlebotomy supplies
A-D demonstrate several commercially available carts and trays ranging from basic trays to
the use of mobile phlebotomy carts.
Source: Courtesy of MarketLab: www.marketlabinc.com

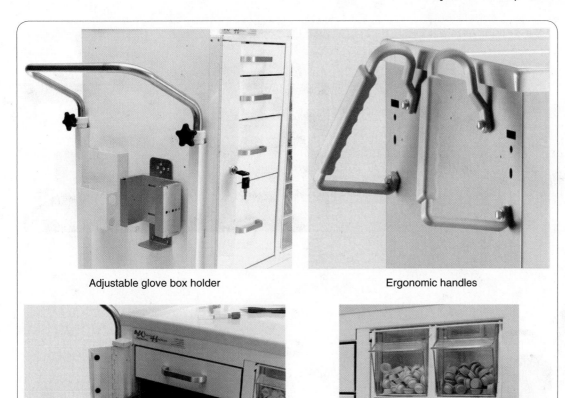

Adjustable glove box holder

Ergonomic handles

3" and 4" drawers are removable
trays with dividers

Clear tilt bins for easy access and
monitoring of supply levels

D.

FIGURE ■ **8-11** Continued

POSITIONING OF THE PATIENT

It is important to make the patient comfortable and safe and to choose the least hazardous site for blood collection by skin puncture or venipuncture. Health care workers should know about useful devices and the positions and locations of veins (Figures 8-12 ■ and 8-13 ■).

VENIPUNCTURE SITE SELECTION

The most common sites for venipuncture are in the antecubital area of the arm just below the bend of the elbow, because this is where the median cubital, cephalic, and basilic veins lie close to the surface of the skin and are most prominent. The least hazardous site for venipuncture should be selected when possible.

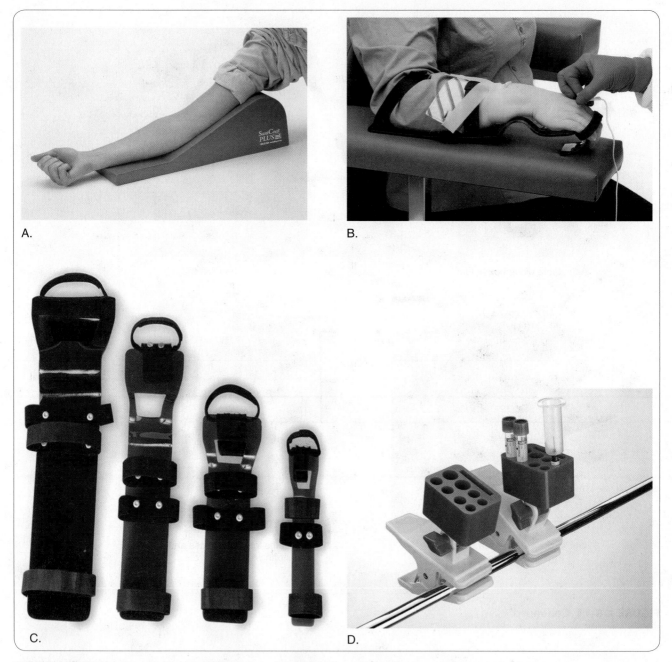

A.

B.

C.

D.

FIGURE ■ 8-12 Devices to Assist in Positioning of the Patient and Supplies

A. A phlebotomy wedge is available to help stabilize the patient's arm. It has an anti-microbial protective vinyl coating that does not absorb liquids and can be wiped clean after each use. B. A hand immobilizer can be useful when hard-to-get hand veins are utilized for phlebotomy. C. The plastic devices come in various sizes, have adjustable straps, and can be disassembled for cleaning. D. Clamps for holding supplies close to the patient during the venipuncture procedure can be attached to bed rails, chair arms, wheelchairs, or countertops.

Source: Courtesy of MarketLab: www.marketlabinc.com

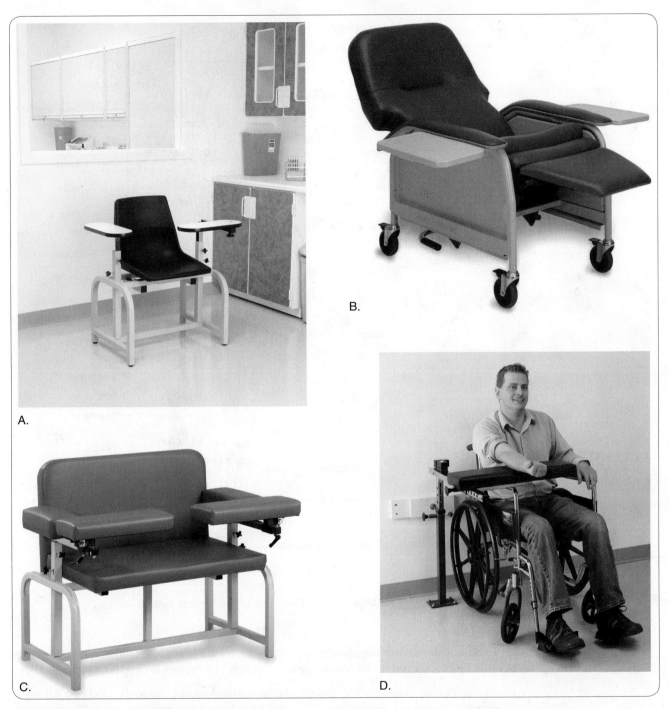

FIGURE ■ 8-13 Blood Collection Chairs

A. A typical phlebotomy chair with adjustable arms B. Recliner style chairs with adjustable arms and/or shelves are available in a variety of styles, often with electronic height adjustments to facilitate comfort and safety for the patient and health care worker. C. Extra wide chairs for large and obese patients D. Some facilities have a mounted wheelchair draw station. It is an adjustable phlebotomy "arm" that enables wheelchair-bound patients to stay comfortable and secure in their wheelchair during the procedure. E. Extra tall chairs are more comfortable for the health care worker because they eliminate back strain. They should be used with patients who have the greatest mobility and are not likely to lose their balance or have trouble getting in/out of the chair. Some chairs have electronic height adjustments so that the health care worker can allow the patient to sit comfortably, then raise the height of the chair to a comfortable level during the procedure and then lower it after the procedure.

Source: Courtesy of MarketLab: www.marketlabinc.com

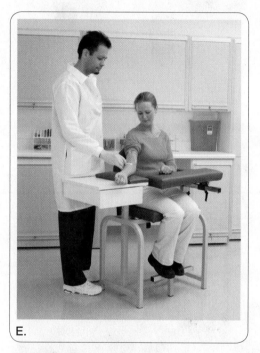

FIGURE ■ 8-13 Continued

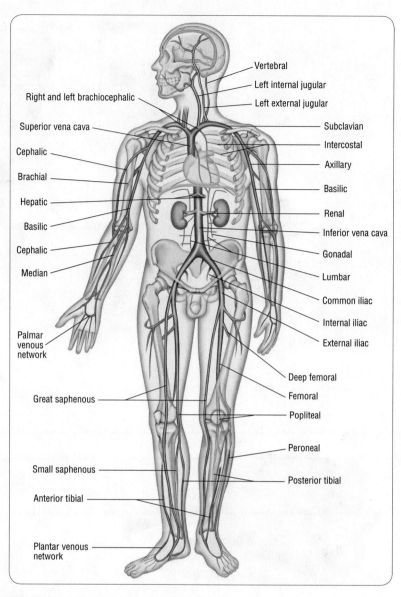

FIGURE ■ 8-14 Overview of the Venous System

To reduce the risks of puncturing an artery or injuring a nerve, CLSI recommends that vein selection be considered in the following order:[1] (Refer to Figures 8-14 ■, 8-15 ■, and 8-16 ■.)

1. Median cubital (sometimes called the median vein)—most commonly used vein for venipuncture because it is the easiest to obtain blood from, has been reported to be less painful, and is less prone to injury if the needle is not placed precisely in the vein. It is best to check both arms for a suitable median cubital vein prior to using the other choices.
2. Cephalic vein—on the outer edge (thumb side) of the arm.
3. Basilic vein—on the inside edge of the antecubital fossa area (the side of the pinkie finger); it is in close proximity to the median nerve and the brachial artery so the other choices are preferable. Sometimes the phlebotomist has to check both arms to choose the least hazardous site. Only use the basilic vein if the other veins on both arms are not prominent.[1,7]

Palpating the entire antecubital area enables the health care worker to get an idea of the size, angle, and depth of the vein. The patient can assist in the process by holding his or her

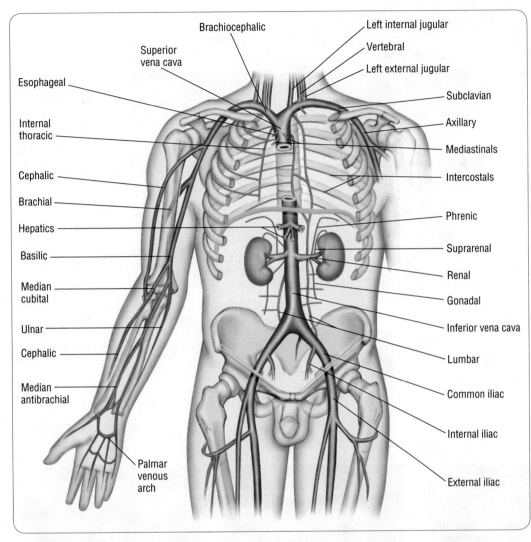

FIGURE ■ 8-15 Venous Circulation of the Abdomen and Chest

arm straight or slightly bent at the elbow. It is *not* recommended that the patient "make a fist" and/or "pump up the vein" because opening and closing the fist multiple times can lead to hemoconcentration. However, in some cases, making a fist once and keeping it closed for a short period of time (*not* pumping the fist) can facilitate the venipuncture until blood flows into the tube. Also, some patients prefer to make a fist as a means to remain steady or still during the needle puncture. If so, ask the patient not to "pump" their fist and remind them to open it as soon as the needle puncture occurs or blood begins to flow.

Because selected veins may also be used for blood product transfusion, infusion, and therapeutic agents, sometimes physicians request that veins have restricted use (or are "reserved") for those purposes only. Health care facilities and educational programs may vary their specific procedures so health care workers should follow the procedures at their respective sites.

ALTERNATIVE PUNCTURE SITES

Alternative sites for blood collection when the antecubital area cannot be used are hand veins and, in some cases with proper training and physician approval, foot veins. In addition, Chapter 9 discusses the alternative of capillary or fingerstick specimens.

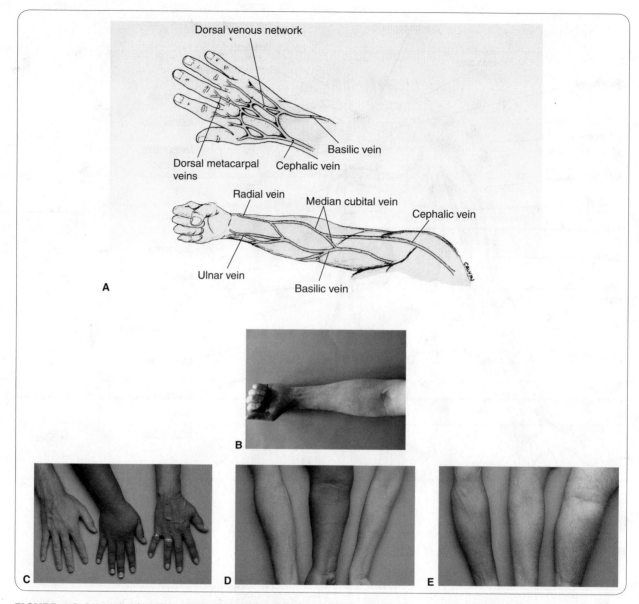

FIGURE ■ 8-16 Individual Vein Variations in the Hand and Arm

Vein patterns are dramatically different among individuals. Learn to *feel* the veins prior to venipuncture, not just simply see them. A. A typical human hand and arm labeled with prominent veins. B. An arm of an adult, white male. C. Dorsal hand veins show up in different locations and in varying degrees of visibility in the three hands. The first is a young, adult, white male; the other two are African American females, one young adult, and one middle-aged. Note the variations in skin tone and elasticity or tightness. D. These arms are all adults of different ages with varying skin tones, muscle mass, fatty tissue, and bone structure. E. Note that in the arms with more muscle mass and fatty tissue, the veins are hardly visible at all. Always rely on feeling the vein rather than simply visualizing it.

Hands

Veins on the dorsal side of the hands or wrists (i.e., the back side) are acceptable venipuncture sites if the median cubital, cephalic, or basilic veins are inaccessible on both arms. Veins in the wrist (and ankle) tend to move, or roll aside, as the needle is inserted; therefore, it may be helpful to have the patient extend the hand (or foot) into a position that helps hold the

Clinical Alert !

- Serious patient injury can occur due to excessive probing, poor site selection, deep needle penetration all the way to a nerve, or if the patient suddenly moves or jerks his arm during the venipuncture procedure. If the patient complains of severe pain during the procedure, the needle must be removed *immediately* and the procedure discontinued. Assistance should be sought from a nurse or supervisor. Only a physician can evaluate whether or not nerve damage has occurred. Nevertheless, the incident should be documented. Figure 8-17 ■ depicts the proximity of nerves in relation to the veins.

- Arteries do not feel like veins and should not be confused. Arteries pulsate, are more elastic, and have a thick wall. Accidental arterial puncture can result in excessive bleeding and hematoma (bruising caused by localized bleeding) formation. If an artery is punctured, the needle should be removed immediately, and direct pressure should be applied to the site for at least 5 minutes or until bleeding has stopped.[1] A supervisor or nurse should be notified.

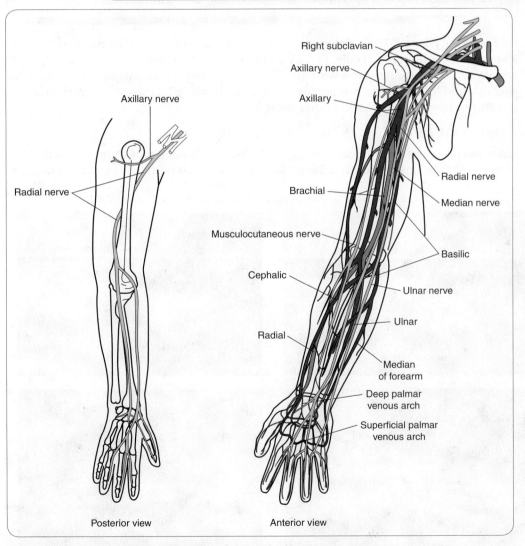

Posterior view   Anterior view

FIGURE ■ 8-17 Arm Veins (blue), Arteries (red), and Nerves (yellow)

Note that several important nerves and arteries pass very close to, or through, the antecubital area where most venipunctures occur. In particular, note the position of the brachial artery and median nerve as they pass through the antecubital area, both are close to the basilic vein. This is why the basilic vein is not a first choice for a venipuncture site.

> ## Clinical Alert ❗
>
> The patient's arm veins CANNOT be used for venipuncture in the following circumstances:
>
> - Intravenous (IV) lines in both arms (If the IV is on one side only, the unaffected arm may be used.)
> - Burned or scarred areas
> - Areas with a hematoma
> - Cast(s) on arm(s)
> - Thrombosed veins (thrombosed veins lack resilience, feel much like a rope cord, and roll easily)
> - Edematous arms (swollen area because of excessive amounts of tissue fluids)
> - Mastectomy on one side only (use of the arm on the unaffected side is acceptable for venipuncture)
> - Mastectomy on both sides (Unless approved by a physician, neither arm should be used because of fluid accumulation. Sometimes, if *no other puncture sites are available,* the doctor may allow blood to be collected; and the situation should be documented.)

vein taut (see Figure 8-18 ∎). Venipuncture in small veins is facilitated by the use of a 21- to 23-gauge safety butterfly needle, by careful placement of the hand/wrist in a comfortable and stable position (sometimes with the use of a clean towel underneath to raise the wrist slightly), and by anchoring/positioning the vein with one hand (holding it taut) while the needle insertion occurs with the other hand.

Ankles or Feet

Ankle and foot veins (on the dorsal, or upper, side) should be used *only* if arm veins have been determined to be unsuitable and if the health care worker has been trained and authorized to

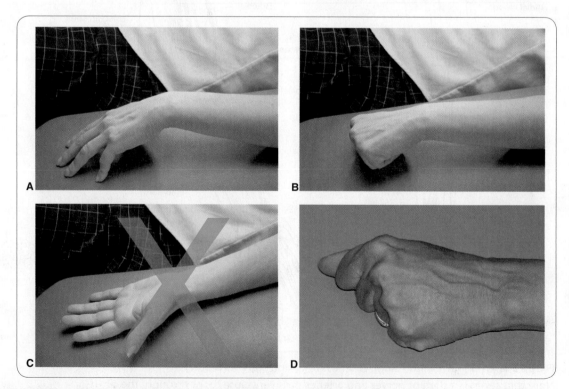

FIGURE ∎ 8-18 Dorsal or Back Side of the Hand
A. Dorsal or back side of the hand. B. Veins are lightly visible and palpable. C. Do not use the underside of the wrist for venipuncture. D. Dorsal hand veins are more prominent if the hand is held taut.

do so. Arm veins are sites preferred over foot or ankle veins, because coagulation and vascular complications tend to be more troublesome in the lower extremities. Thus, foot and ankle veins should not be used for cardiac or diabetic patients. Some hospitals do not allow the use of the lower extremities (foot and ankle) for blood-sampling sites. Other hospitals allow sampling from these sites only after permission has been granted by the patient's physician and after the health care worker has been properly trained. If allowed, a smaller needle is again recommended.

It can take time to find a suitable puncture site in some patients. However, performing a venipuncture on a nontraditional site simply because the "vein looks good" is hazardous, increases the risk of injury to the patient, and will likely result in legal liability to the phlebotomist and health care facility.

HARD-TO-FIND VEINS

Sometimes it is very difficult to feel a suitable vein. Warming the puncture site helps facilitate phlebotomy by increasing arterial blood flow to the area. Several warming devices are available commercially that are quick and easy to activate and provide localized heat to the potential venipuncture area. Another method is to use a clean towel or a washcloth heated to about 42°C. When the warm towel is wrapped around the site for 3 to 5 minutes, the skin temperature can increase several degrees. The wrap can be encased in a plastic bag to help retain heat and/or keep the patient's bed dry. The health care worker may leave the warm wrap on the patient while he or she collects specimens from other patients, and then return to the original patient after several minutes.

Another method to improve vein location if one cannot be felt initially is to have the patient dangle his or her arm by their side in a downward position for 1–2 minutes. This allows the blood to fill the arm veins to capacity, then the tourniquet may be reapplied and the area repalpated.

Clinical Alert !

For hand vein punctures, the posterior, or dorsal side (the back of the hand; i.e., the side that shows off a wedding ring), should be used. Do *not* use the anterior side or the palmar venous network in the wrist, because nerves are easily injured by needle probing in this area (Figure 8-18).

TOURNIQUET APPLICATION AND CLEANSING THE PUNCTURE SITE

A **tourniquet** (preferably single-use, latex-free) makes veins more prominent and easier to puncture by causing venous filling.[1] The tourniquet slows down blood flow toward the heart so that it pools or gathers in the veins. A soft rubber tourniquet about 1 inch (2.5 cm) wide and about 15 to 18 inches (45 cm) long is most comfortable for patients, affordable, and easy to use, and it comes in a variety of colors. Brightly colored tourniquets are preferred to skin-tone tourniquets because they are more noticeable and thus, less likely to be left on or near a patient accidentally. Practices differ slightly on the use of a tourniquet. Experienced health care workers are often able to find a puncture site by palpating the antecubital area without a tourniquet, then applying the tourniquet just before the needle puncture. However, less experienced health care workers are encouraged to take their time in finding a suitable puncture site, so it may be necessary to apply the tourniquet while palpating the antecubital area, then release the tourniquet for a short period of time while the supplies are readied, then reapply it before the needle puncture. A tourniquet should not be left on for more than one minute. Procedure 8-3 ■ provides basic steps for applying a tourniquet, but again, health care workers should follow the procedures at their facilities.

Procedure 8-3

Use of a Tourniquet

RATIONALE

Tourniquet application causes veins to fill with blood, thereby assisting in location of a suitable venipuncture site and enabling easier blood flow once the needle has been inserted.

EQUIPMENT/SUPPLIES

- Latex-free clean tourniquet, preferably for single-use
- Gloves
- Alcohol-based hand disinfectants

PREPARATION

1 Identify the patient properly.

2 Wash or sanitize your hands using appropriate agents, dry them, and then put on gloves.

PROCEDURE

3 Use a clean, latex-free tourniquet (Figure 8-19 ■). It is preferable to use a "single-use" tourniquet for each patient.

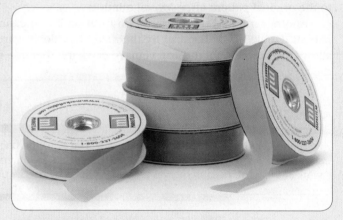

Figure ■ 8-19

Source: Courtesy of MarketLab: www.marketlabinc.com

4 Ask the patient to extend his arm fully. Stretch the ends of the tourniquet around the patient's arm about 3–4 inches (7.6 cm–10 cm) above the venipuncture area (antecubital area). Hold both ends of the tourniquet in one hand while the other hand tucks in a section next to the skin and makes a partial loop with the tourniquet (Figure 8-20 ■).

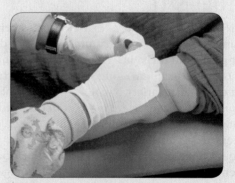

Figure ■ 8-20

(5) The tourniquet should be tight but not painful to the patient. Do *not* leave it on for more than 1 minute. Do *not* place it over sores or burned skin; however, depending on the policies of each health care facility, it may be placed over a hospital gown sleeve.

Palpate the antecubital area to locate the safest vein. (Remember that some health care workers palpate the area prior to placing the tourniquet on the patient, others place the tourniquet on first before palpating.)

Once a vein is selected, cleanse the area as indicated in Procedure 8-4 ■.

(6) Release the tourniquet *after* the needle puncture, when blood has begun to flow into the collection tubes. Release the tourniquet with one hand, because the other hand will be holding the needle and tubes. The partial loop should allow for easy release by the health care worker.

(7) Once released, it can remain loosely on the arm or surface of the work area (e.g., bed or blood collection chair) until the procedure is completed and the health care worker is cleaning up (Figure 8-21 ■).

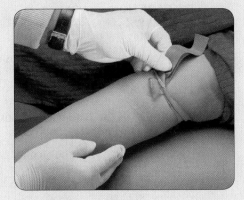

Figure ■ 8-21

Clinical Alert !

A tourniquet should not be left on for more than 1 minute because it becomes uncomfortable and causes hemoconcentration, e.g., increased blood concentration of large molecules (proteins, cells, coagulation factors).

Also, the health care worker should never stick a vein unless it can be felt. If no vein becomes apparent, or "pops up" after tourniquet application, efforts should be made to increase blood flow to the area (warming or lowering arm), then repalpate the area to feel again. It is better to defer the patient to someone else who can search for a palpable vein than to take a blind chance.

Clinical Alert !

Once the patient's skin has been cleansed, it should never be touched with any nonsterile object. The alcohol should be allowed to dry (for approximately 30–60 seconds), or it should be wiped off with sterile gauze after the site is prepared; otherwise, the puncture site will sting, and the alcohol may cause hemolysis and/or interfere with test results, such as blood alcohol levels. Blowing on the site to hasten the drying process is not advised, because doing so may re-contaminate the site.

Procedure 8-4

Cleansing the Puncture Site

RATIONALE

To provide a clean, decontaminated area of the skin in which to make the needle puncture.

EQUIPMENT/SUPPLIES

- Gloves
- 70% isopropanol (isopropyl alcohol) gauze pad (commercially available) or chlorhexidine pads

PREPARATION

(1) Identify the patient properly.

(2) Wash or sanitize your hands using appropriate agents, dry them, then put on gloves.

PROCEDURE

(3) Once the site is selected, cleanse it with a 70% isopropanol (isopropyl alcohol) pad.

(4) Rub the site with the alcohol pad, working in concentric circles from the inside out. If the skin is particularly dirty, repeat the process with a new alcohol pad (Figure 8-22 ■).

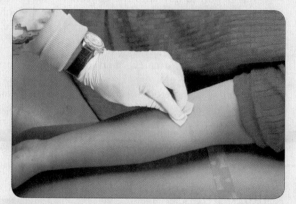

Figure ■ 8-22

(5) If you intend to palpate or touch the site again for any reason, repeat the cleansing again with a new alcohol pad. Air-dry the site or dry it with sterile gauze (Figure 8-23 ■).

(Commercially-available preparation kits/packs are used for drawing blood samples for blood gas analysis and blood cultures. The site must be sterilized prior to venipuncture. Follow the manufacturer's directions for appropriate results.)

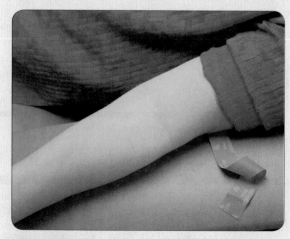

Figure ■ 8-23

Venipuncture Methods

EVACUATED TUBE SYSTEM AND WINGED INFUSION SYSTEM, OR BUTTERFLY METHOD

CLSI recommends that venipuncture specimens be collected with a system that enables blood to flow directly into the tubes.[1] Evacuated tube systems and **winged infusion systems (butterfly)** are widely available, equipped with safety devices, come with needles of varying sizes, and comply with this recommendation. Procedure 8-5 ■ demonstrates a *basic* venipuncture technique. However, some health care facilities and/or educational programs may vary their venipuncture procedures slightly. Health care workers should follow those procedures accordingly.

Procedure 8-5

Performing a Venipuncture

RATIONALE

To provide a safe, effective, and efficient method to obtain a blood specimen.

EQUIPMENT

- Personal protective equipment (PPE) (gloves, clean uniform, laboratory coat, etc.)
- Written or electronic laboratory requisitions/labels
- Marking pens
- Non-latex tourniquet
- Alcohol pads/skin disinfectants
- Chlorhexidine gluconate prep kits for blood cultures
- Safety syringes and syringe transfer devices
- Safety needles with single-use, evacuated tube holders and winged infusion sets
- Blood collection tubes
- Plastic capillary tubes with tube sealer
- Non-latex bandages or sterile gauze pads
- Glass microscope slides
- Puncture-proof sharps container
- Bar code reader/scanner (if applicable)

PREPARATION

Preparation phases prior to venipuncture are described in Procedures 8-1 through 8-4.

1. After greeting and identifying the patient, cleanse hands and don gloves.
2. Check the antecubital area for a suitable vein.

(continued)

Procedure 8-5

Performing a Venipuncture *(continued)*

3 Assemble equipment in the presence of the patient. Double check the expiration dates and integrity of the blood collection tubes. Offer to answer any questions for the patient (Figure 8-24 ■).

4 Position the patient's arm in a straight (or slightly bent) downward manner that is comfortable.

5 Prepare equipment according to the manufacturer's instructions, including attaching a needle onto the appropriate holder, and checking the supplies for defects and expiration dates. For an evacuated tube system, the most commonly used, the safety needle is attached securely and directly onto the tube holder. (For a safety winged-infusion or butterfly apparatus, the smaller needle [1/2–3/4 inch in length and 21–23-gauge in diameter] comes attached to a thin tubing with a Luer adapter that, in turn, must be attached to a tube holder. It *must* be attached, either prefabricated by the manufacturer or by the health care worker, *prior* to the puncture.)

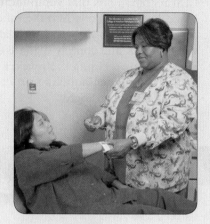

Figure ■ 8-24

6 Select the site, apply the tourniquet in the correct location. Remember to feel for the median cubital vein first on both arms before searching for other options because it is usually bigger and anchored better, then search for the cephalic vein (depending on its size) which is the second choice because it does not roll and bruise as easily as the basilic, and then search for the basilic vein (the last choice). If a suitable vein is not felt, remove the tourniquet. Remember, do not leave the tourniquet on for more than 1 minute at a time on either arm. Choose a vein that feels the fullest. If necessary, warm the site or lower the arm further in a downward position to pool venous blood (Figure 8-25 ■).

7 Cleanse the patient's skin with an alcohol pad in a circular motion from inside to outside (Figure 8-26 ■). Allow it to air dry, and do not blow on it. (The tourniquet can be removed during this step and reapplied when the site is dry.) Do not allow the patient to vigorously clench their hand or "pump" their fist because it may affect some laboratory values. (It is acceptable however, for a patient to make a fist temporarily by holding a ball or other item until the puncture has

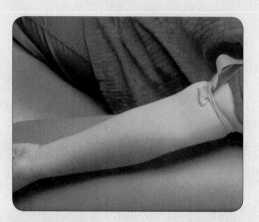

Figure ■ 8-25

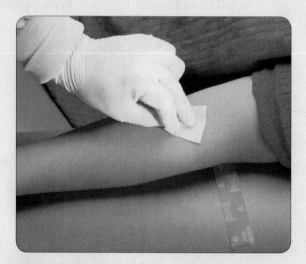

Figure ■ 8-26

happened and blood begins to flow.) Never say that "this will not hurt"; simply mention to the patient that he or she will "feel a stick" or say, "Please remain still while I begin the procedure, you will feel a slight prick." Be mindful that from this step forward a patient may feel faint and/or lose consciousness.

PROCEDURE

Venipuncture can be done by either an evacuated tube system or a winged-infusion/butterfly needle system. The steps listed here are the same for both systems. However, special considerations for the winged-infusion method are listed at the end of the procedure.

⑧ Remove the needle cap carefully so as not to touch anything that would contaminate it. Check the needle tip for defects. If the needle has nicks or burrs, or if the needle touches any surface that is not sterile, replace it with a new needle assembly and discard the old one. Hold the needle assembly in one hand while anchoring the vein with the other hand 1 to 2 inches below the puncture site. (Some health care workers use the thumb and forefinger of the "free hand" to temporarily anchor the vein. Others place the last three fingers of the "free hand" under the elbow to steady the arm even more.) Position the needle so that it is parallel or running in the same direction as the vein. Insert the needle quickly, with the bevel side up, and at a 30-degree angle (or less) with the skin. (If the angle of insertion is too steep, greater than 30 degrees, there is a higher risk of going completely through the vein, and/or hitting a nerve, artery, or tendon.) A slight "pop" should be felt as the needle enters the vein (Figure 8-27 ■).

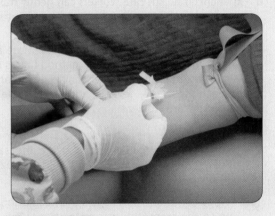

Figure ■ 8-27

⑨ While keeping the needle assembly stable in the vein, place the first collection tube in the holder and *gently* press the tube onto the sheathed needle inside the tube holder. Blood should begin to flow into the tube. If blood does not flow, palpate gently above the puncture to feel for the vein and possibly reorient the needle *slightly.* Do not probe! Use *very small* movements to reorient the needle and not cause damage.

⑩ As the blood begins to flow, release the tourniquet. (The tourniquet can be left on until after the tubes have filled if it appears that blood flow is slow and *if* it has not been more than a minute; however, *always* remove it before withdrawing the needle.) If the patient has made a fist, ask them to relax their fist. If more collection tubes are needed, carefully remove the first tube from the holder with a *gentle* twist-and-pull motion and again, *gently* push the second evacuated tube into the holder so that the tube closure is punctured by the inside needle and blood can enter. Try to orient the tube in a downward position (Figure 8-28 ■).

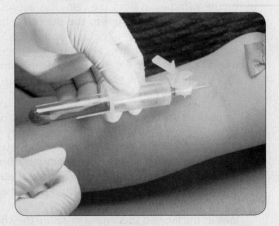

Figure ■ 8-28

⑪ Allow the blood to flow into the tube until it stops so that the proper dilution of blood to additive can occur. Watch carefully to see when the blood flow ceases.

(continued)

Procedure 8-5

Performing a Venipuncture *(continued)*

During tube transfer, be mindful of these key issues:

- Hold the needle apparatus firmly and motionlessly so that the needle remains comfortable and in the vein during tube changes.
- Follow the correct order of draw.
- Remember that blood stops flowing between tube changes because of the inner needle design, which allows a sleeve to block flow if it is not in use.
- Always remove the last tube from the holder's inner needle before removing the needle from the patient's arm.
- Experienced health care workers can gently mix/invert a full tube in one hand while holding the needle apparatus and waiting for another tube to fill.
- Some health care workers switch hands to use a dominant hand during tube exchange. Use the method that is recommended by your health facility, supervisors, or instructors, and/or find the approach that is safe, reliable, and comfortable for both patient and health care worker.

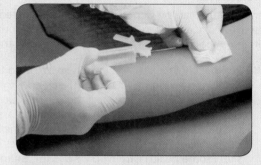

Figure ■ 8-29

12 When all tubes have been filled and removed from the holder, withdraw the needle and activate the safety device, move it away from the patient, and hold a gauze pad over the site (Figure 8-29 ■).

13 The safety device that covers the needle should be used according to the manufacturer's instructions. This involves activating/resheathing/ or somehow covering the needle once it has been withdrawn or manipulating a device that renders the needle blunt before withdrawal from the vein. It is acceptable to instruct the patient to apply pressure to the site using the gauze as long as the health care worker checks it until bleeding stops. (If necessary, continue gentle inversion of the specimen tubes for complete mixing of additives with the blood. Remember: do not shake the tubes.) Dispose of the entire needle apparatus. Do *not* disassemble it prior to disposal.

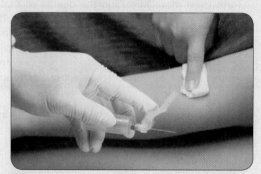

Figure ■ 8-30

14 Assure that the bleeding has stopped or keep pressure applied until it does (Figure 8-30 ■). Additional gauze may be needed. Properly dispose of contaminated gauze. Keep an eye on the patient for signs of syncope. Label the blood samples appropriately (patient's first and last name, identification number, date, time of collection, and health care worker's initials) and place them in an appropriate container. For another identity check, the patient can be asked to look at the labeled specimens to assure they have his or her name on them (Figure 8-31 ■).

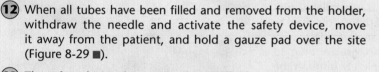

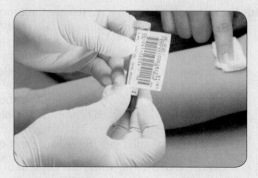

Figure ■ 8-31

AFTER THE PROCEDURE

(15) Dispose of contaminated supplies and equipment in the correct containers.

(16) Double-check to make sure that the bleeding has stopped and apply a bandage, if appropriate.

(17) Wash or sanitize hands.

(18) Thank the patient for cooperating and depart with *all* blood samples and *all* remaining supplies. Do not leave anything at the patient's bedside.

(19) Deliver the samples to the appropriate locations for laboratory testing.

Special Considerations for the Winged Infusion/Butterfly Method

A safety winged infusion system, butterfly needle assembly, or scalp needle set can be used for certain patient populations or for particularly difficult venipunctures. This type of method may be useful in the following circumstances:

- Patients with small veins
- Pediatric or geriatric patients
- Patients having numerous needlesticks (e.g., cancer patients)
- Patients in restrictive positions (e.g., traction and severe arthritis)
- Patients who are severely burned
- Patients with fragile skin and veins
- Patients who specifically request it because they feel it is less painful
- Short-term infusion therapy

Special Notes:

- Use of winged infusion or butterfly systems requires training and practice because of the small tubing involved, but they are widely used because patients report that they are less painful than other methods.
- While the procedural steps are the same as for the evacuated tube system, there is a difference when tubes are filled. Because the tubing from the winged-infusion system contains some air, the first tube will under-fill with blood by 0.5 mL, thus affecting the additive-to-tube ratio in collection tubes that contain anticoagulants or other additives. Therefore, a nonadditive tube should be filled first, then, the order of draw can follow the usual order recommended. Follow the procedures in each health care facility for the use of this system. This is especially important for coagulation testing when only one tube is required. In this circumstance, many hospitals require a discard tube to remove the air displacement prior to collecting the sample tube for coagulation studies.

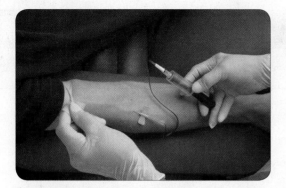

■ Health care workers should be extra cautious as the butterfly needle apparatus is removed from the patient, because it tends to hang loose on the end of the tubing and may sometimes recoil unexpectedly. Therefore, the safety device that covers the needle should be activated immediately. Failure to activate the safety devices correctly as described by the manufacturers may result in a higher incidence of needlestick injuries (Figure 8-32 ■).

FIGURE ■ 8-32

Procedure 8-6

Syringe Method

RATIONALE

Syringes are *not* routinely used for venipuncture because of many safety concerns, issues of accidental cross-contamination of anticoagulants if the blood specimen is injected into multiple evacuated tubes using the same needle and syringe, excessive or forceful withdrawal such that the sample is adversely affected, and potential clotting in the syringe. However, use of a blood transfer device can minimize these problems. There are also circumstances when a syringe is helpful, such as for veins that collapse easily. Syringes are helpful in this case because the pressure withdrawing the blood can be more easily and gently controlled.

EQUIPMENT

■ Same as for other venipuncture procedures
■ Safety needles
■ Syringe and transfer devices

PREPARATION

(1) After greeting, assessing, and identifying the patient, cleanse hands and don gloves.

(2) Assemble supplies in the presence of the patient. Double check the expiration dates and integrity of the collection tubes. Offer to answer any questions for the patient.

PROCEDURE

(3) Prepare equipment according to the manufacturer's instructions. Use a syringe needle with a safety device. Check the needle tip for defects. Remember that a syringe can also be attached to a winged infusion set.

(4) Before the needle is inserted, move the syringe plunger back and forth to allow for free movement and to expel all air.

(5) Use the same approach to needle insertion (holding skin taut, bevel orientation, and insertion angle) as that used for the evacuated tube method. Try to orient the syringe so that the graduated markings are visible. Ask the patient to "please remain still, you will feel a slight prick."

(6) Once the needle is in the vein, draw back the syringe plunger slowly until the required amount of blood is drawn.

> **Clinical Alert** !
>
> Do not panic if blood does not flow immediately after the puncture is made. The following suggestions may help:[1]
>
> ■ Recheck the needle placement and vein by palpating gently above the needle insertion site.
> ■ Change the needle position *slightly, but do not probe;* that is, pull *gently* outward or push *gently* forward or rotate slightly so that the bevel is positioned correctly in the vein. These should be small movements so as to minimize the risk of complications.
> ■ If no blood flows, attempt the collection from one other site. Do not make more than two attempts.

(7) Take care not to accidentally withdraw the needle while pulling back on the plunger, and do not pull too hard because it can cause hemolysis (i.e., rupture of the cells) or collapse of the vein. Release the tourniquet as soon as possible after the blood begins to flow.

(8) After releasing the tourniquet and collecting the appropriate amount of blood, withdraw the entire needle assembly quickly and activate the safety device immediately. Depending on the manufacturer's specifications, the safety device may be activated at a different time, some require activation prior to needle removal. Whatever the case, follow the correct procedure carefully. Ask the patient to apply pressure to the site with a clean gauze pad.

(9) Remove the needle apparatus or winged-infusion set and discard it appropriately.

(10) Immediately apply the syringe transfer device and fill the evacuated tubes for testing. Follow the manufacturer's instructions for filling tubes. It usually involves holding the transfer device vertically and allowing the tubes to fill until the flow stops (Figure 8-33 ■).

(11) Fill the tubes until flow stops; there is no need to push the plunger to expel blood.

(12) Fill the tubes in the same order as that for the evacuated tube method. Mix the additive tubes according to the manufacturer's instructions.

AFTER THE PROCEDURE: BANDAGE THE PUNCTURE SITE

(13) Apply a dry, sterile gauze pad with pressure to the puncture site for several minutes or until bleeding has ceased. If the patient has a free hand, ask them to apply the pressure. Keep the patient's arm straight or slightly bent at the elbow. Always make sure the bleeding has stopped completely before leaving the patient. Observe for hematoma formation or for signs that bleeding has not stopped completely (oozing, leakage, incomplete clot formation, or excessive bleeding). If the patient continues to bleed, apply pressure yourself until the bleeding stops. Then apply a bandage. If the patient continues to bleed, notify a nurse and/or supervisor. Remember that excessive bleeding may be a rare event but can lead to serious complications including anemia, blood transfusions, and others.

(continued)

Procedure 8-6

Syringe Method *(continued)*

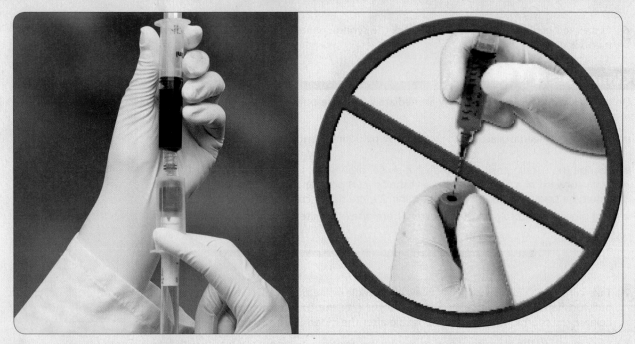

Figure ■ 8-33 Blood Transfer Device

A. This image shows the health care worker inserting a tube into the blood transfer device after the needle (with safety device activated) was removed from the syringe and disposed of properly. B. This image is the incorrect way to transfer blood from a syringe into a collection tube. Note that the needle might have easily punctured the health care worker's index finger or thumb accidentally while holding the tube.

Source: © Becton, Dickinson and Company

14. Label the tubes appropriately. Double check the identity on the labels or ask the patient to double check that the labels match his or her identity.

15. Discard all disposable or contaminated equipment into appropriate containers.

16. Cleanse your hands.

17. Thank the patient for cooperating and depart with *all* blood samples and *all* remaining supplies.

18. Transport the samples to the laboratory.

Clinical Alert !

Use Once and Discard Immediately

Needles, lancets, syringes, and other bloodletting devices—collectively called *sharps*—that are capable of transmitting infection from one person to another should be used only *once,* then immediately discarded. Sharps must be discarded in puncture-resistant containers that are easily accessible, located in areas where they are commonly used, and have proper warning labels. Blood tube holders should be used only once because of the potential needlestick hazards associated with the double-ended needle at and after disposal. Shearing or breaking of contaminated sharps is illegal and strictly prohibited. Bending, recapping, or removing contaminated needles is not acceptable practice.

Other contaminated supplies such as gauze, alcohol wipes, etc., should be discarded in designated biohazard containers, depending on the workplace setting and the health facility's procedures.

ORDER OF DRAW FOR BLOOD COLLECTION TUBES

Because multiple blood tests are usually ordered simultaneously for a patient, it is common for multiple tubes to be collected. Many tubes contain various additives, therefore collecting blood sample tubes in the correct order reduces the chances of erroneous laboratory test results due to additive carry-over from one tube to the next. Additive carry-over may cause erroneous laboratory test results. During the actual venipuncture process of filling tubes with blood, tube manufacturers and the **Clinical and Laboratory Standards Institute (CLSI)** recommends the following specific order (order of draw) (Figure 8-34 ■) when collecting blood in multiple tubes (either glass or plastic) via the evacuated method or the syringe transfer method (Box 8-3 ■):[1]

1. Blood culture tubes (yellow closure) or blood culture vials. Blood cultures are always drawn first after special skin decontamination procedures, to decrease the possibility of bacterial contamination. (Blood cultures are discussed in more detail in Chapter 11.)
2. Coagulation tube (sodium citrate) (light blue closure).
3. Serum tube, with or without clot activator, with or without gel (red or speckled closure). (Glass, nonadditive serum tubes can be filled before the coagulation tube. However, plastic serum tubes containing a clot activator may interfere with coagulation tests.)
4. Heparin tube (green closure) with or without gel plasma separator.*
5. EDTA tube (purple/lavender closure) used for routine hematology tests.
6. Glycolytic inhibition tube (potassium oxalate/sodium fluoride or lithium iodoacetate/heparin) (gray closure).

* A Tip Worth Remembering: If laboratory test requests require blood cultures (yellow), serum tubes (red), and heparin tubes (green), remember this phrase related to traffic lights: "yellow light, red light, green light, go." Even though it does not account for all tubes, it helps with the order of draw in these cases.

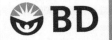

Helping all people
live healthy lives

BD Vacutainer® Order of Draw for Multiple Tube Collections

Designed for Your Safety

Reflects change in CLSI recommended
Order of Draw (H3-A5, Vol 23, No 32, 8.10.2)

* When using a winged blood collection set for venipuncture and a coagulation (citrate) tube is the first specimen tube to be drawn, a discard tube should be drawn first. The discard tube must be used to fill the blood collection set tubing's "dead space" with blood but the discard tube does not need to be completely filled. This important step will ensure proper blood-to-additive ratio. The discard tube should be a nonadditive or coagulation tube.

Closure Color	Collection Tube	Mix by Inverting
BD Vacutainer® Blood Collection Tubes *(glass or plastic)*		
	• Blood Cultures - SPS	8 to 10 times
	• Citrate Tube*	3 to 4 times
or	• BD Vacutainer® SST™ Gel Separator Tube	5 times
	• Serum Tube *(glass or plastic)*	5 times (plastic) none (glass)
	• BD Vacutainer® Rapid Serum Tube (RST)	5 to 6 times
or	• BD Vacutainer® PST™ Gel Separator Tube With Heparin	8 to 10 times
	• Heparin Tube	8 to 10 times
or	• EDTA Tube	8 to 10 times
	• BD Vacutainer® PPT™ Separator Tube K₂EDTA with Gel	8 to 10 times
	• Fluoride (glucose) Tube	8 to 10 times

Note: Always follow your facility's protocol for order of draw

Handle all biologic samples and blood collection "sharps" (lancets, needles, luer adapters and blood collection sets) according to the policies and procedures of your facility. Obtain appropriate medical attention in the event of any exposure to biologic samples (for example, through a puncture injury) since they may transmit viral hepatitis, HIV (AIDS), or other infectious diseases. Utilize any built-in used needle protector if the blood collection device provides one. BD does not recommend reshielding used needles, but the policies and procedures of your facility may differ and must always be followed. Discard any blood collection "sharps" in biohazard containers approved for their disposal.

= 1 inversion

BD Technical Services
1.800.631.0174
BD Customer Service
1.888.237.2762
www.bd.com/vacutainer

1 Becton Drive
Franklin Lakes, NJ 07417
www.bd.com/vacutainer

BD, BD Logo and all other trademarks are property of Becton, Dickinson and Company. © 2010 BD
Franklin Lakes, NJ, 07417   1/10   VS5729-6

FIGURE ■ 8-34 Order of Draw and Mixing Requirements for Multiple Tube Collections
Source: Courtesy and © Becton, Dickinson and Company

Box 8-3	Other Issues Related to Filling the Blood Collection Tubes

- During the venipuncture procedure, care should be taken that the additive or anticoagulant present in one tube does not come into contact with the multisample needle as the tubes are changed. To minimize the transfer of anticoagulants from tube to tube, holding the tube horizontally or slightly downward during blood collection is recommended. If an anticoagulant is inadvertently carried into the next tube, it may cause erroneous test results.

- Be attentive to the "fill" rate and volume in each tube. Evacuated tubes with anticoagulants must be filled for the proper mix of blood with the anticoagulant: i.e., the blood-to-additive ratio.

- Although the use of a syringe should be restricted to special cases, occasionally a large volume (more than 15 mL) of blood needs to be drawn using a syringe. Sometimes more than one syringe of blood is needed. In this case, it is best to use a winged-infusion set and ask for assistance in transferring the blood to tubes, while a second syringe is being collected. Thus one health care worker is collecting the sample while the other is transferring the blood from the first syringe into the tubes. This reduces the risk of blood clotting in the syringe.

- Also, closures/stoppers on the sample tubes should not be removed to inject blood from the syringe; rather, a transfer device should be used to transfer the blood into the tubes.

Clinical Alert !

Special Considerations for Coagulation Testing[1]

- Each health care worker should use the procedure adopted by his or her own facility. However, if coagulation studies are the *only* tests ordered, and a *winged infusion (butterfly) system* is to be used for collection, a "discard" tube should be collected before drawing the citrate tube. This is the only way to rid the specimen of the air in the winged infusion tubing. If this air in the "dead space" enters the citrate tube, it causes an inaccurate blood-to-citrate ratio, and false test results.

- When a syringe method is used to collect a large volume of blood, usually two syringes are used, so blood from the *second* syringe should be used for the coagulation tube as it is less likely to have begun clotting.

- Because coagulation tests require a specific plasma concentration of sodium citrate, "overfilling" the tube may cause artificial results or falsely short clotting times.

- If a tube is "underfilled," the opposite occurs, and artificial results indicate falsely prolonged clotting times.

- Immediately after collection, coagulation tubes should be mixed gently to prevent clotting in the tube. However, over-mixing by an excessive number of inversions or vigorous mixing can lead to platelet activation and shortening of clotting times when tested.

SPECIMEN IDENTIFICATION AND LABELING

Completed labels should be firmly attached to the patient's specimens in the presence of the patient.[4] Labels must accompany all blood specimens (Box 8-4 ■). The health care worker may write directly on the container label if necessary. Commercial collection tubes may have affixed blank labels for this purpose. Similarly, hospitals often use computer-generated labels for collection tubes; however, capillary tubes, microcollection tubes and vials, or other containers without labels must be identified, either by labeling them directly

---

Box 8-4 Labels for Blood Specimens

Specimens should be labeled (usually bar-coded labels) immediately *at the patient's bedside* or ambulatory setting, *before leaving the patient.* Laboratory procedure manuals should contain explicit instructions about labeling requirements and reconfirmation that the samples and patient have the same identity. Supervisors should spend ample time not only training new employees in correct identification and labeling practices but also observing as they perform the steps. Sometimes labels need to be placed in specified locations on a tube due to automated processing and analytical requirements.

Remember, tubes should *never* be pre-labeled because they may be erroneously picked-up and used for another patient which could cause significant errors. Also, a different health care worker may complete the venipuncture if the initial health care worker is unsuccessful. In that case, the prelabeled tubes may display the initials of the first health care worker and, therefore, be inaccurate. In addition, if the prelabeled tubes are not used, tearing off the old or unused label may be difficult because of the adhesive; thus, either a new label (from a different patient) would have to be placed on the tube with a partially torn label or the unused tube would have to be discarded. Either option is unsatisfactory, messy, and wasteful.

---

with a permanent felt-tipped pen, wrapping an adhesive label around them, or placing them into a larger labeled test tube for transport. In some cases, small electronically-generated adhesive labels with printed information are available with, and detachable from, the requisition form.

Whatever the type of label may be (handwritten or electronically generated) blood sample labels should consistently include the following information:[1,2]

1. Patient's full name
2. Patient's identification number
3. Date of collection
4. Time of collection
5. Identification of the person who collected the sample
6. Patient's room number, bed assignment, or outpatient status (optional)

Clinical Alert !

Before leaving the patient, be cognizant of the following issues.

■ The health care worker should always make sure the bleeding has stopped; the sample tubes are correctly labeled, identified, and placed in a secure location for transport; supplies are safely disposed of or stored; hands are cleaned; that the patient does not feel faint, and has been thanked for their cooperation. This must occur before leaving to draw blood from another patient.

■ The date and time are necessary information because physicians need to know exactly when the specimen was drawn so that they may correlate results with any medications given or with changes in the patient's condition. Requisition forms only indicate the date and time when a laboratory test was *ordered,* whereas the label indicates the date and time when it was *collected.*

■ The health care worker's initials are necessary to help clarify questions about the specimen or patient if any arise during laboratory processing or testing.

■ All supplies and equipment must be removed from the patient's bedside (see Procedure 8-7 ■).

Procedure 8-7

Leaving the Patient

RATIONALE

To assure that the patient is no longer bleeding, does not feel faint, and has no further complications related to the venipuncture procedure.

EQUIPMENT

- Nonlatex bandages
- Pen
- Alcohol-based hand rub or soap/water
- Biohazard containers
- Bar-code scanner (if applicable)

PREPARATION

(1) Visually scan all surfaces near the patient for extraneous supplies.

(2) Before leaving the room, wash or sanitize your hands.

PROCEDURE

Before leaving the patient's side, perform the following steps:

(3) Check the puncture site to observe for hematoma formation, blood leakage, or excessive bleeding. Continue to apply pressure until bleeding has stopped or call for a nurse or supervisor if bleeding complications appear serious. Assure that the bleeding stopped and check that the patient does not feel faint if they are ambulatory.

(4) Apply an adhesive bandage if the patient is agreeable.

(5) Ensure that all tubes are appropriately labeled. Ask the patient to double check that the sample labels indicate his or her name.

AFTER THE PROCEDURE

(6) Cleanse hands again.

(7) Remove all items that were brought in or appropriately discard used supplies.

(8) Prepare the specimens for transportation.

(9) Thank the patient.

Clinical Alert !

Excessive bleeding after a venipuncture procedure may be due to an inadvertent or accidental arterial puncture. Although this is a rare occurence, it can lead to serious complications for the patient so the health care worker should call for assistance from a nurse or supervisor to assure that the bleeding is adequately contained.

Also, bandages are not recommended for infants or very young children because of possible irritation and the potential of swallowing or aspirating the bandage if it comes off.

Prioritizing Patients

During the course of a day's work at a busy hospital or clinic, a health care worker may have to make decisions about the order in which blood work is obtained. Priorities must be set and adhered to, whether they concern the order in which certain blood tests are drawn on a particular patient or which patients are to be drawn first from among a group. If these distinctions are not made properly, test results can be affected, and interpretation of the results may be difficult (see Box 8-5 ■: Ideas for Improving Venipuncture Practices).

Timed specimens—If a test is ordered for blood sample collection at a particular time, the health care worker is responsible for drawing the blood as near to the requested time as possible. Timed samples are important for various reasons such as the timing of administering medications (e.g., digoxin), therapeutic drug monitoring to establish drug dosing (e.g., chemotherapy agents), fasting restrictions (e.g., glucose), or circadian rhythms (e.g., cortisol.) Physicians will make medical decisions based on the laboratory values at the specified times. Timed specimens are crucial for TDM because the laboratory results taken from blood samples for TDM are used in establishing a patient's drug dose.

STAT, or emergency, specimens—STAT blood samples must be collected and delivered to the laboratory for testing as quickly as possible. These terms are used because the patient has a medical condition, possibly life-threatening, that must be treated or responded to as a medical emergency. Some health care facilities utilize other terms that indicate a priority status (as soon as possible or ASAP, etc.) but not a critical emergency status. Familiarity with each facility's terms related to order of priority is essential.

Box 8-5	**Ideas for Improving Venipuncture Practices**

All members of the health care team should strive to improve phlebotomy practices. Sometimes this involves coordination across departments and hospital units. A few suggestions for improving efficiency and quality include:

- Coordination of laboratory requests among *all* staff physicians and nurses working with the patient, to reduce duplicate and triplicate laboratory orders.
- Possible modifications to the laboratory test panel menu and better education of physicians to be aware of all the tests on each laboratory panel.
- The laboratory could be notified when multiple timed tests are ordered. For example, if a patient needs a hemoglobin test at 2:00 P.M. and a glucose test at 3:00 P.M., coordinating the times and drawing both specimens during one venipuncture may be possible. Common analyses that are time-dependent are glucose tolerance tests and drug levels so coordination of other venipunctures should be carefully considered.
- Reassessment of STAT test orders to make sure that they are clinically necessary.
- **Therapeutic drug monitoring (TDM)** (i.e., timed laboratory analysis of serum drug levels to determine adequate therapeutic dosing) should be coordinated among laboratory, nursing, and pharmacy personnel.
- The laboratory should be aware of patient transfers.
- The number of times that a patient can be punctured should be monitored. (Generally, a health care worker should not puncture a patient more than twice before calling for a second opinion.)
- The number of times that a patient can be punctured in one day should be coordinated and minimized.
- The total volume of blood that can be drawn daily from a patient, especially for infants and children (Appendix 4), and critically ill patients must be monitored.
- When conversing with the patient, health care workers should restrict discussion about a patient's clinical information to very basic facts about the tests that have been ordered. It should be emphasized that the patient's physician ordered the tests and can answer questions about them in more detail.
- Procedures for documenting a patient's refusal to have blood collected should be established. All patients have a right to refuse treatment. Explain to the patient that laboratory results are used to help the physician make an accurate diagnosis, establish proper treatment, and monitor the patient's health status and that the patient's cooperation would be greatly appreciated. If the patient continues to refuse, remain professional and acknowledge his or her right to refuse. Documentation of the refusal should be made and the patient's physician notified.

continued

Box 8-5	Ideas for Improving Venipuncture Practices *(cont.)*

- Guidelines for **specimen rejection** (i.e., criteria that relate to the suitability of a specimen for testing or when it may not be used) should be periodically reviewed. These policies generally include circumstances related to inaccurate identity, collection in the wrong tube, inadequate volume of blood in the tube, hemolyzed or clotted specimens when they are not supposed to be, improper transportation or storage, use of outdated/expired supplies, contaminated samples, patient did not comply with diet restrictions, or a timed sample that was collected at the wrong time. In all these situations, the health care worker should learn how to proceed with corrective actions and error documentation based on SOPs for each facility.
- Communication, honesty, and ethical, professional behavior are the keys to an efficient and reliable health care environment. Refer to Chapter 7 for further discussion about Preexamination/Preanalytical Complications.

Self Study

Study Questions

The following questions may have more than one answer.

1. An unconscious emergency patient may be identified by which of the following means?
   a. a name on the patient's bed
   b. temporary identification label
   c. patient's backpack
   d. ER clerk

2. Identification procedures for outpatients may include asking for which of the following?
   a. photo identification
   b. birth date
   c. address
   d. identification by a family member

3. The most common sites for venipuncture are in which of the following areas?
   a. the dorsal side of the wrist
   b. the antecubital area of the arm
   c. the middle finger
   d. the earlobe

4. Applying a tourniquet is useful for:
   a. providing an indication of the size of the vein
   b. distracting the patient from the discomfort of the procedure
   c. providing an indication of the depth of the vein
   d. allowing blood to pool in the veins

5. What effect does warming the arm have on venipuncture?
   a. prevents veins from rolling
   b. makes veins stand out
   c. causes hemoconcentration
   d. increases localized blood flow

6. How long should the tourniquet be placed around the patient's arm?
   a. approximately 4 minutes
   b. until the needle is removed
   c. until the entire venipuncture is completed
   d. no more than 1 minute

7. How many times should one patient be punctured during a procedure?
   a. only once
   b. no more than twice
   c. three times
   d. four times

8. Which of the following blood sample tubes should always be drawn first?
   a. blood culture
   b. lavender-topped tube
   c. light blue-topped tube
   d. red-topped tube

9. When should the needle safety device be activated during a venipuncture procedure?
   a. before beginning the procedure
   b. just before sticking the patient so that no one will get hurt
   c. immediately after withdrawal from the vein unless the manufacturer recommends otherwise
   d. just before putting it in the waste container

10. During a venipuncture procedure using evacuated tubes when should the tourniquet be released?
    a. before the blood flows into the tube
    b. after the blood flows into the tube
    c. before the needle is inserted
    d. after the needle has been withdrawn

Case Study

A health care worker was assigned to collect blood samples from a hospitalized, comatose patient. The health care worker entered the hospital room to begin the identification process. The sign on the patient's bed indicated that the patient was Annie Bentsen; however, the laboratory requisitions were for Ann Beaumont. As the health care worker approached the patient to check for identification, she noticed that the patient had an IV in one arm and appeared to be asleep.

Question
What should the health care worker do to confirm the identification of the patient and to collect the blood sample?

Case Study

The following laboratory tests were ordered for a patient who had recently had a mastectomy on her left side: PT and PTT, blood cultures, hemoglobin and hematocrit, electrolytes, and cell counts (WBC and RBC).

Questions
1. What site would be most appropriate for the venipuncture?
2. What would be the correct order of drawing the evacuated tubes during the venipuncture?

Advocating Patient Safety Case Study

Many health care workers feel that when they perform a venipuncture procedure their work is done once they collect a patient's blood sample. He or she may feel that the "hard part is over" once they have the blood tubes in their hands. If the workload is heavy that day, it is possible that they may want to stick the tubes in the pocket of their uniform and continue on with the next assignment. However, the health care worker is ultimately responsible for several important steps after the actual venipuncture procedure.

Question
List and describe at least three key patient safety issues that are the phlebotomist's responsibility after the blood sample tubes are collected.

Competency Assessment

Check Yourself: Patient Identification and Name Clarification

1. Patients frequently have the same or similar last name. Common ones are Smith, Jones, and Johnson. As a self-assessment exercise or with a partner, pretend you are tired and at the end of a busy work shift. Practice saying the names listed below and describe what you would do if any of these patients appeared for venipuncture at the same time:

   Betsy Johnson and Betty Johnston
   P. Garcia and J. C. Garza
   Jan Cheung and Jen Chang
   John Riley and Jon Reilly

2. Consider how important each step of the identification process is in these (and all) situations. Next, come up with a list of names that you are familiar with. "Tune-in" your eyes and ears to notice different spellings and verbal pronunciations of these names. Practice using phrases to request the exact spelling of a patient's name. Remember that language differences and/or accents may cause one name to sound like another, therefore resulting in misunderstandings. However, if the identification process is followed carefully and thoroughly, mistakes can be prevented. Remember to notice precautionary labels that indicate an alert for name likenesses. All discrepancies in the identification process should be reported to a supervisor.

Competency Checklist: Patient Identification

This checklist can be completed as a group or individually.

(1) Completed (2) Needs to improve/Repeat lesson and checklist

_____ 1. List three ways to confirm a patient's identity.

_____ 2. List three methods _that would not be reliable_ for confirming a patient's identity.

Competency Checklist: Preparing for the Patient Encounter

This exercise can be done during an actual patient encounter or as a mock encounter. If possible, record a video of the encounter to aid in the assessment critique.

(1) Completed (2) Needs to improve/Repeat lesson and checklist

_____ 1. The health care worker demonstrates a positive, professional appearance and introduces him or herself with name, department where he or she works, and purpose of the encounter.

_____ 2. The health care worker demonstrates positive body language, including a pleasant facial expression and good posture before beginning the patient encounter.

_____ 3. The health care worker has protective equipment, phlebotomy supplies, test requisitions, writing pen, and appropriate patient information before beginning the venipuncture process.

_____ 4. The health care worker can describe what to do if he or she cannot identify the patient correctly or if information is incomplete.

_____ 5. The health care worker uses the correct hand hygiene and gloving techniques.

Competency Checklist: Use of a Tourniquet and Site Selection

Practice on a partner several times before practicing on a patient.

(1) Completed (2) Needs to improve/Repeat lesson and checklist

_____ 1. A clean, latex-free tourniquet is used by stretching the ends of the tourniquet around the patient's arm about 3 inches (7.6 cm) above the venipuncture area (antecubital area). The tourniquet is applied tightly but it should not be painful to the patient. It is not left on more than 1 minute.

_____ 2. The antecubital area is palpated appropriately. (Not too hard, not too softly.)

_____ 3. Veins are located and identified appropriately. One or more options can easily be identified in the antecubital area.

_____ 4. When it is time to release the tourniquet, the partial loop should allow for easy release by the health care worker using only one hand, because the other hand will be holding the needle and tubes.

_____ 5. Next, practice applying the tourniquet on the lower arm to identify dorsal hand veins.

_____ 6. Palpate and identify the best option for venipuncture on the dorsal side of the hand.

_____ 7. Release the tourniquet during the appropriate time frame.

Competency Checklist: Decontamination of the Puncture Site

Choose a partner to work with. Your partner or supervisor can evaluate the extent to which the site is adequately decontaminated.

(1) Completed (2) Needs to improve/Repeat lesson and checklist

_____ 1. Once the site is selected, it is cleansed with an alcohol-soaked gauze or a commercially packaged alcohol pad.

_____ 2. The site is rubbed with moderate pressure applied to the alcohol pad, working in concentric circles from the inside out.

_____ 3. Adequate time is allotted for the site to dry.

Competency Checklist: Performing a Venipuncture

The steps listed below are typical for either venipuncture system. They should be completed individually and preferably in a practice setting using a mannequin or a real person.

(1) Completed (2) Needs to improve/Repeat lesson and checklist

_____ 1. After greeting and identifying the patient, performing hand-hygiene, donning gloves, and preparing equipment in the presence of the patient, the health care worker offers to answer any questions for the patient.

_____ 2. The health care worker checks and prepares equipment according to the manufacturer's instructions, including attaching a needle onto the appropriate holder.

_____ 3. The patient's arm is positioned properly.

_____ 4. A clean tourniquet is applied and potential sites are checked by palpating the vein.

_____ 5. If a suitable vein is not felt, the tourniquet is removed and applied to the other arm.

_____ 6. Practice warming the site or lower the arm further in a downward position to pool venous blood.

_____ 7. An appropriate site is selected and cleansed with an alcohol pad in a circular motion from inside to outside. It is allowed to air dry.

_____ 8. The patient is asked to "please hold your arm straight and still."

_____ 9. The patient is told that he or she will "feel a stick" or "please remain still while I begin the procedure, you will feel a slight prick."

_____ 10. The patient's arm is held below the site, gently pulling the skin taut.

_____ 11. The needle assembly and arm are held appropriately.

_____ 12. The needle is parallel to the vein and at the appropriate angle.

_____ 13. After blood begins to flow, the tourniquet is released.

_____ 14. Evacuated tubes are gently pushed into the holder in an appropriate manner.

_____ 15. Evacuated tubes are filled in the correct order and until the blood flow stops in each tube.

_____ 16. Each tube is removed from the holder with a gentle twist-and-pull motion and replaced with the next tube.

_____ 17. Tubes are gently mixed in one hand while holding the needle apparatus and waiting for another tube to fill.

_____ 18. When all tubes have been filled, the needle is withdrawn in an appropriate manner.

_____ 19. Bleeding is adequately controlled by applying a sterile gauze.

_____ 20. The safety device is activated according to the manufacturer's instructions.

_____ 21. The patient is asked to apply pressure to the site using the gauze.

Competency Checklist: Order of Draw

The following cases indicate tests requested for laboratory evaluation. Practice numbering the tubes in the correct order of collection for a venipuncture.

(1) Completed (2) Needs to improve/Repeat lesson and checklist

_____ 1. ___ Lavender closure used for hematology tests (CBC), ___ yellow closure used for blood cultures, ___ serum closure used for many chemistry tests

_____ 2. ___ Heparin (green), ___ serum electrolytes (red speckled), ___ coagulation (light blue)

_____ 3. ___ Blood cultures, ___ coagulation, ___ hematology

_____ 4. ___ Coagulation, ___ serum protein

_____ 5. ___ Heparin, ___ EDTA, ___ serum cholesterol, ___ coagulation

_____ 6. Using a butterfly method: ___ coagulation, ___ hematology

Competency Checklist: Leaving the Patient

This checklist can be completed as a group or individually.

(1) Completed (2) Needs to improve/Repeat lesson and checklist

_____ 1. The health care worker rechecks the puncture site to see if the bleeding has stopped, to observe for hematoma formation, and to ask if the patient wants a bandage.

_____ 2. The health care worker asks whether the patient is feeling faint.

_____ 3. The health care worker labels all samples appropriately and asks the patient to double check that the labels are correct.

_____ 4. Used supplies are discarded appropriately.

_____ 5. Specimens are readied for transport in a safe, secure fashion.

_____ 6. Gloves are removed and discarded appropriately. Hands are cleaned again after the procedure.

_____ 7. The health care worker thanks the patient before leaving the room

Competency Checklist: Putting all the Elements Together

This checklist is a basic summary and combination of the procedures listed above and should be completed individually after all the separate procedures have been mastered. This checklist can be completed, first, in a mock patient situation and if it is successful, again, in a real situation under supervision. It is suggested that multiple tubes be used to assess the correct order of draw. (Keep in mind that some organizations may slightly modify the sequence of steps and sometimes steps can be combined or performed simultaneously.)

(1) Completed (2) Needs to Improve/Repeat lesson and checklist

_____ 1. The health care worker demonstrates a positive, professional appearance and introduces him or herself and states the department where he or she works, and purpose of the encounter.

_____ 2. The health care worker demonstrates positive body language, including a pleasant facial expression and good posture before beginning the patient encounter.

_____ 3. The health care worker has protective equipment, phlebotomy supplies, test requisitions, writing pen, and appropriate patient information before beginning the venipuncture process. Supplies are checked for expiration dates and/or defects.

_____ 4. The health care worker uses three ways to confirm a patient's identity.

_____ 5. The health care worker uses the correct hand hygiene and gloving techniques and has supplies ready for the procedure.

_____ 6. A clean, latex-free tourniquet is correctly applied.

_____ 7. The antecubital area is palpated appropriately. (Not too hard, not too softly.)

_____ 8. Veins are located and identified appropriately. The best option is identified in the antecubital area.

_____ 9. The site is appropriately cleansed using an alcohol pad and working in concentric circles from the inside out.

_____ 10. Adequate time is allotted for the site to dry.

_____ 11. The patient's arm is held below the site, gently pulling the skin taut.

_____ 12. The needle assembly and arm are held appropriately.

_____ 13. The needle is parallel to the vein and at the appropriate angle.

_____ 14. The puncture takes place in a smooth and gentle manner. As blood begins to flow, the tourniquet is released.

_____ 15. Evacuated tubes are gently pushed into the holder in an appropriate manner.

_____ 16. Evacuated tubes are filled in the correct order and until the blood flow stops in each tube.

_____ 17. Each tube is removed from the holder with a gentle twist-and-pull motion and replaced with the next tube.

_____ 18. Tubes may be gently mixed in one hand while holding the needle apparatus and waiting for another tube to fill.

_____ 19. When all tubes have been filled, the needle is withdrawn in an appropriate manner.

_____ 20. Bleeding is adequately controlled using a sterile gauze.

_____ 21. The safety device is activated according to the manufacturer's instructions.

_____ 22. The patient is asked to apply pressure to the site using the gauze.

_____ 23. The health care worker labels all samples appropriately and asks the patient to double check that the labels are correct.

_____ 24. Used supplies are discarded appropriately.

_____ 25. The health care worker rechecks the puncture site to see if the bleeding has stopped, to observe for hematoma formation, to ask if the patient wants a bandage, and to assure that the patient is not feeling faint.

_____ 26. Specimens are readied for transport in a safe, secure fashion.

_____ 27. Gloves are removed and discarded appropriately. Hands are cleaned again after the procedure.

_____ 28. The health care worker thanks the patient before leaving the room.

References

1. Clinical and Laboratory Standards Institute (CLSI), formerly the National Committee for Clinical Laboratory Standards (NCCLS): *Procedures for the Collection of Diagnostic Blood Specimens by Venipuncture,* Approved Standard, 6th Ed., document H3-A6. Wayne, PA: CLSI, 2007.

2. Clinical and Laboratory Standards Institute (CLSI): *Procedures and Devices for the Collection of Diagnostic Capillary Blood Specimens,* Approved Standard, CLSI document H04-A6. Wayne, PA: CLSI, 2008.

3. Centers for Disease Control and Prevention: Hand Hygiene in Healthcare Settings, www.cdc.gov/handhygiene/, accessed 1-17-2012.

4. World Health Organization (WHO), World Alliance for Patient Safety: WHO guidelines on hand hygiene in health care, 2009, http://www.who.int/gpsc/5may/tools/9789241597906/en/# accessed 1-17-2012.

5. Clinical and Laboratory Standards Institute (CLSI): Accuracy in Patient and Sample Identification; Approved Guideline, GP33-A, CLSI, 940 West Valley Road, Suite 1400, Wayne PA 19087, 2010, www.clsi.org.

6. Joint Commission on Accreditation of Healthcare Organizations: 2012 National Patient Safety Goals, www.jointcommission.org, 2011. accessed 1-17-2012.

7. Kirven, DR: A Painless Truth, Maintaining good phlebotomy practices today can save time, money and injury tomorrow. Advance for Medical Laboratory Professionals, http://laboratorian.advanceweb.com, posted on Jan 31, 2011, accessed 1-17-2012.

Resources

1. American Society for Clinical Pathology: ASCP LABQ-P, continuing educational exercises for phlebotomy. *http://www.ascp.org/*

2. Clinical and Laboratory Standards Institute (CLSI): Consensus standards for all phases of specimen collection that assist with regulatory and accreditation requirements, and quality improvements. *www.clsi.org.*

3. The Joint Commission: *www.jointcommission.org.*

4. Phlebotomy Today, e-newsletter, *www.phlebotomy.com*

PEARSON
myhealthprofessionskit

Go to www.myhealthprofessionskit.com to access the Companion Website created for this textbook. Simply select "Clinical Laboratory Science" from the choice of disciplines. Find this book and log in using your username and password to access interactive learning games, assessment questions, and more.

Chapter 9

Capillary Blood Specimens

KEY TERMS

capillary action

capillary blood

cyanotic

dehydrated

differentials

feathered edge

interstitial (tissue) fluid

osteochondritis

osteomyelitis

peripheral circulation

CHAPTER OBJECTIVES

Upon completion of Chapter 9, the learner should be able to do the following:

1. Describe reasons for acquiring capillary blood specimens.
2. Identify the proper sites for performing a skin puncture procedure.
3. Explain reasons for controlling the depth of the incision.
4. Describe the procedure for making a blood smear.

Indications for Skin Puncture

Skin punctures are particularly useful for both adult and pediatric patients when small amounts of blood can be used for laboratory testing (Box 9-1 ■). For pediatric patients it is crucial to withdraw *only the smallest amounts of blood needed* for laboratory testing to reduce the effects of blood-volume reduction. Thus, for neonates and infants, use of capillary blood samples is the preferred method of collection. In contrast, a 10-mL blood sample taken using a venipuncture method, which could be tolerated by most adults, would represent 5% to 10% of the *total* blood volume in a neonate's body.[1]

If small amounts of blood are acceptable for laboratory tests, skin punctures or "finger-stick" procedures are used when the following conditions occur in adult patients:[1,2]

- Fragile veins (e.g., in geriatric patients) or difficult-to-access veins
- When veins are being "saved" for therapy (e.g., for cancer patients)
- Patient has already had multiple unsuccessful venipunctures and tests require small amounts of blood
- Home testing (e.g., blood glucose monitoring)
- Point-of-care testing (POCT)
- Severe burns or scarring on the common venipuncture sites
- Obese patients
- Thrombotic tendencies
- Patient is receiving IV therapy in both arms
- Patient is fearful/anxious about venipunctures
- Patient may need only one blood test that could be done on a small sample volume

Fingerstick procedures are *not recommended* if the following circumstances are present:[1,2]

- Laboratory testing requires large amounts of blood (such as blood cultures, and erythrocyte sedimentation rates [ESR])
- The patient has swollen fingers. If a fingerstick is performed, the interstitial fluids may dilute the blood sample
- The patient is **dehydrated** (lacking/loss of water from the body)
- A patient may have poor **peripheral circulation** (near the outer surfaces of the body)
- Coagulation studies (because of a dilution effect with interstitial fluid)

Box 9-1 Laboratory Tests Commonly Performed Using Capillary Blood Samples[2]
Blood smears for a white blood cell differential (manual blood smears on microscope slides)
Complete Blood Count (CBC), hemoglobin and hematocrit (H&H)
Electrolytes
Neonatal blood gases
Neonatal bilirubin
Neonatal screening (using filter paper or blood spot testing)
Point-of-care testing (POCT) and/or home testing (blood glucose monitoring, etc.)

> **Clinical Alert** !
>
> Venipuncture in children, especially infants, should be avoided when possible because of the risk of complications due to taking too much blood (iatrogenic hazards) or difficulties with the puncture site. These complications may include anemia, cardiac arrest, hemorrhage, venous thrombosis, damage to surrounding tissues or organs, infections, and injuries from restraining the child during the procedure.[1]

Composition of Capillary Blood

Capillary blood acquired by skin puncture is different from that of venous or arterial blood samples acquired by other methods. Capillary blood is more of a mixture, composed of blood from:

- arterioles
- venules
- capillaries
- intracellular and **interstitial (tissue) fluids** (fluids that form within tissue layers and gaps)

Generally speaking, capillary blood has slightly more arterial blood than venous blood because the arterial pressure in the capillaries is stronger than the venous pressure. Thus, there are slight differences in laboratory values of glucose, potassium, total protein, and calcium when serum or plasma have been compared with capillary blood. In all cases, except glucose, the values are lower in skin puncture blood.[1]

Collecting Diagnostic Capillary Blood Specimens

The first steps used for the venipuncture procedure also apply to skin puncture procedure (preparing oneself and supplies, identifying the patient, asking about latex allergies and fainting, performing hand hygiene, and cleansing the puncture site). However, subsequent steps are slightly different (Figure 9-1 ■).

Supplies for Skin Puncture

Supplies for skin puncture are available from many manufacturers (see Chapter 6) and, depending on the actual tests that are ordered, the supplies may differ, but the basic list includes the following (Figure 9-2 ■):

- Disposable gloves
- Commercially available warming pack, heating pad, towels, etc., for warming the site
- Sterile, disposable, single-use puncture device with a permanently retractable blade or needle. (There are many types of puncture devices available based on style, size, and depth. Use the appropriate device for each patient situation based on the manufacturers' instructions and the procedures at each facility.)

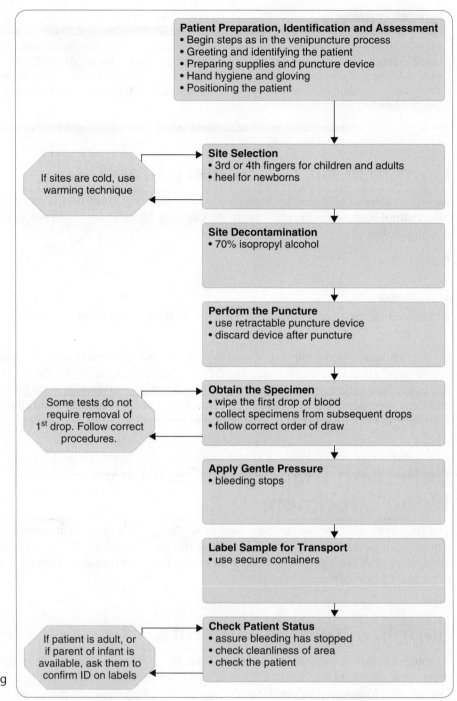

Patient Preparation, Identification and Assessment
• Begin steps as in the venipuncture process
• Greeting and identifying the patient
• Preparing supplies and puncture device
• Hand hygiene and gloving
• Positioning the patient

If sites are cold, use warming technique

Site Selection
• 3rd or 4th fingers for children and adults
• heel for newborns

Site Decontamination
• 70% isopropyl alcohol

Perform the Puncture
• use retractable puncture device
• discard device after puncture

Some tests do not require removal of 1st drop. Follow correct procedures.

Obtain the Specimen
• wipe the first drop of blood
• collect specimens from subsequent drops
• follow correct order of draw

Apply Gentle Pressure
• bleeding stops

Label Sample for Transport
• use secure containers

If patient is adult, or if parent of infant is available, ask them to confirm ID on labels

Check Patient Status
• assure bleeding has stopped
• check cleanliness of area
• check the patient

FIGURE ■ 9-1 Flow Chart: Collecting Capillary Blood Samples

■ Disinfectant pads (70% isopropanol)
■ Sterile, nonlatex bandages and gauze pads
■ Glass microscope slides (if needed for manual WBC differentials)
■ Diluting fluids as required by manufacturers
■ Plastic microcollection tubes
■ Plastic-coated capillary tubes

- Capillary tube sealers or closures
- Laboratory request slips or labels
- A marking pen
- A puncture-proof biohazard discard container

Clinical Alert !

Glass capillary tubes should *not* be used because they break easily and can cause injury. Use plastic capillary tubes instead. Refer to Chapter 6 for more information.

SKIN PUNCTURE SITES

Skin puncture in adults and older children most often involves one of the fingers. The fleshy, central palmar surface of the distal phalanx (fingertip section) of the third (middle) finger or fourth (ring) finger of the nondominant hand is the preferred site for puncture. The non-dominant hand is often less callused so the puncture is more effective. The puncture should be made at the thickest part of the finger, just off-center (not the sides or extreme tip where the tissue is not as thick)[1] (Figures 9-3 ■ and 9-4). The site should be warm and free of calluses, burns, cuts, scars, bruises, or rashes. The finger should not be cyanotic (bluish color due to lack of oxygen), edematous or infected.

For infants less than 1 year old, or neonates, the recommended site for skin puncture is the lateral or medial plantar surface of the heel.[1] The heelstick procedure is covered in detail in Chapter 10.

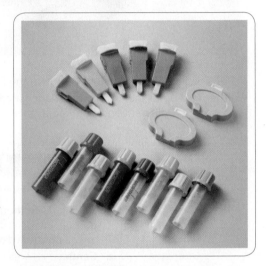

FIGURE ■ **9-2** Capillary Blood Collection Devices and Tubes

Source: Courtesy and © Becton, Dickinson and Company

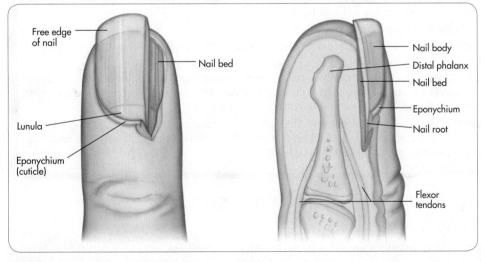

FIGURE ■ **9-3** Structures of the Finger and Nail

Note the positioning of the distal finger bone (called the distal phalanx) and how close it is to the actual end of the fingertip. Also remember that the bone is located in the central part of the finger so the best site to puncture the skin is slightly off-center, but still in the thickest part of the finger and away from the very tip of the finger.

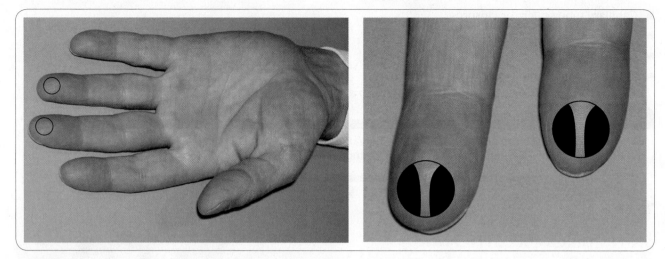

FIGURE ■ 9-4 Sites for Skin Puncture on the Fingers
On the close-up of the fingers, the shaded areas of the circle represent the most suitable puncture sites. However, each patient is different and slight adjustments may be required.

Clinical Alert !

The following sites are *not generally recommended* for routine skin punctures:[1]

■ Earlobe (Even though the earlobe is still used by some, it is not a preferred site because of possible interference with pierced earrings; also, because of the site's close proximity to the eyes, a puncture device may cause undue anxiety to a patient resulting in a jerking of the head.)

■ Central arch area of an infant's heel and posterior curve of the heel (because of the risk of injuring nerves, tendons, cartilage, and bone)

■ Fingers of a newborn or infant less than 1 year old (because of the risk of hitting the bone and causing infections)

■ The fifth (pinky) finger (because the tissue of this finger is considerably thinner than that of the others and there is a risk of hitting the bone)

■ The thumb (because it has a pulse)

■ The index (pointer) finger (because it may be more sensitive and/or it is more likely to be callused)

■ Swollen, infected, callused, burned, cut, scared, bruised, have a rash, or previously punctured sites (because accumulated fluid may contaminate the specimen and the site may be bruised, thus causing more pain if it is punctured again)

■ Fingers on the side of a mastectomy (because the removal of lymph nodes during surgery may result in excessive lymph fluid on the side of the surgery; consult with the ordering physician in the case of a bilateral mastectomy)

WARMING THE SKIN PUNCTURE SITE OR LOWERING THE ARM

Although clinical practices are variable in health care facilities, warming the skin puncture site helps facilitate phlebotomy by significantly increasing arterial blood flow to the area, thus "arterializing" the site. Several easy-to-use methods of warming are commercially available, or the site can be warmed with a heated surgical towel or a washcloth heated with warm water to 42°C, which will not burn the skin. Some facilities ask the patient to wash their hands in warm water to take advantage of the warming effects.

In addition, sometimes it helps to simply lower the patient's arm for a few minutes by pointing the fingers downward towards the floor. This allows gravity to fill the capillary beds of the fingertips.

CLEANSING THE SKIN PUNCTURE SITE

The skin puncture site should be cleaned with a 70% aqueous solution of isopropyl alcohol and allowed to thoroughly dry before being punctured. If alcohol drips or pools at the site, it can cause hemolysis and contaminate testing for glucose determinations. Also, alcohol present during the puncture will sting the patient and prevent the formation of well-rounded drops of blood, which are best for making blood smears on microscopic slides.[1]

Skin Puncture Procedure

Because skin punctures require different procedures when performed on infants, refer to Chapter 10 for information about skin puncture collections on newborn babies, blood spot testing for newborn screening, heel puncture procedures, and specimens for pediatric blood gases. However, there are some precautions that are applicable to both adult and infant skin punctures (Procedure 9-1 ■). Skin puncture devices should be sterile, disposable, for a single-use, and have a permanently retractable safety blade or needle. Some lancets have a needle-type puncture device and others are designed with an incision-type device. Health care workers should understand and follow the manufacturers' directions for the use of each device. Puncture devices are made to control for variable depth and length, depending on the patient's age and weight. The average depth of a skin puncture should be 2 to 2.5 mm for adults and less than 2.0 mm for small children and infants, to avoid injuring the bone. Laser devices are also available as skin puncture alternatives. They provide a smaller hole (about 250 μm wide and 1–2 mm deep).

Procedure 9-1

Basic Skin Puncture for Capillary Blood Collection

RATIONALE

To obtain blood samples in smaller amounts and in a less invasive manner than venipuncture procedures. Remember to follow the procedures adopted by your health care facility and the manufacturers' instructions.

EQUIPMENT

- Disposable gloves
- Sterile, disposable, single-use puncture devices with a permanently retractable blade or needle
- Disinfectant pads (70% isopropyl alcohol)
- Sterile bandages
- Prepackaged gauze pads (2 × 2 or 3 × 3 inches)

(continued)

Procedure 9-1

Basic Skin Puncture for Capillary Blood Collection *(continued)*

- Glass microscope slides (as needed)
- Diluting fluids for specified tests
- Plastic microcollection tubes or plastic-coated capillary tubes
- Capillary tube sealers or closures
- Laboratory request slips or labels
- A marking pen
- A puncture-proof biohazard discard container

PREPARATION

(1) Be emotionally prepared and greet the patient to put him or her at ease.

(2) Ensure proper patient identification and review the test requisitions.

(3) Prepare supplies and choose the correct puncture device(s). Remember to use the correct puncture device for each patient. If the wrong size is used, it may result in prolonged collection, excessive squeezing, poor sample quality (hemolyzed or clotted), possible redraws, and/or patient injury.

(4) Position the patient in a safe chair, comfortable bed, or reclining chair.

(5) Verify dietary conditions, check for latex sensitivities if latex products are in use, and whether or not the patient has fainted before during blood collections.

(6) Exercise standard precautions and perform hand hygiene and gloving techniques.

PROCEDURE

(7) Ask about hand preference and check hand dominance; try to use the non-dominant hand.

(8) Choose a finger that is not cold, **cyanotic** (blue in color due to O_2 depletion), or swollen. Choose the tip of the third finger (or, if needed, the fourth finger) of the non-dominant hand if possible (Figure 9-5 ■).

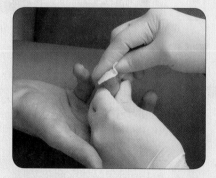

Figure ■ 9-5

(9) Warm the hand to increase the blood flow. Wrap it in a warm towel for 3 to 5 minutes or use a commercially available warming device/heat pack.

(10) Cleanse the site with an alcohol pad (70% isopropanol) and allow it to air dry. Do not blow on it.

(11) Remove the puncture device/lancet from its packaging and follow the manufacturer's instructions. Let the patient know that they will feel a prick. Hold the patient's finger (or heel, in the case of an infant) firmly with one hand, with your thumb away from the puncture site, next to the patient's fingernail (Figure 9-6 ■).

With the other hand, position the puncture device on the site. Holding it perpendicular to the finger surface activate the release mechanism. When possible, orient the cut across the fingerprints (perpendicular to the fingerprint grooves) to generate a large, round drop of blood. If the puncture is made along the lines of (i.e., parallel to) the fingerprint, a well-rounded drop will not form and the blood tends to run down the finger). Discard the puncture device in a puncture-proof biohazard container. (If a biohazard container is not within reach, discard the device immediately after completing the collections.)

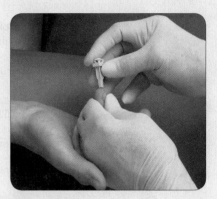

Figure ■ 9-6

(12) Wipe the first drop of blood away with clean gauze (Figure 9-7 ■) unless otherwise indicated (some point-of-care instruments do not require this step). Always follow the manufacturer's instructions.

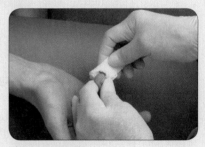

Figure ■ 9-7

(13) Collect the second drop of blood by touching it to the tip of the collection device. The blood will flow into the tube by **capillary action** whereby blood flows freely into the tube on contact, without suction. If the blood becomes jammed in the collection top, a gentle tap on a hard surface will usually dislodge it so the blood can flow freely again to the bottom of the tube (Figure 9-8 ■). Collect the blood quickly to minimize the effects of the coagulation process (microclots or platelet clumping) and to avoid prolonged exposure to air (for blood gases) and light (for bilirubin).

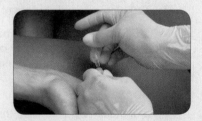

Figure ■ 9-8

(14) Gently apply pressure to the finger and hold the puncture site in a downward position to encourage the free flow of blood, thereby getting the proper amount of blood. Do not use excessive milking/massaging of the finger or forceful scraping or scooping-up of blood, because it may result in excess tissue fluid and/or hemolysis of the specimen.

(continued)

Procedure 9-1

Basic Skin Puncture for Capillary Blood Collection *(continued)*

(15) Follow the correct order of draw. Each type of microcollection laboratory test has different tube and blood volume requirements. Follow the appropriate manufacturer's instructions. Fill tubes to the correct fill volume to avoid the effects of inaccurate blood to additive ratio. Mix specimens according to the manufacturer's instructions, usually by gently inverting containers with additives to mix the blood with the additives.

Carefully and safely seal microcollection tubes with a sealant or with other commercially available devices as needed. When filling capillary tubes, do not allow air bubbles to enter the tubes, as air bubbles can cause erroneous results in many laboratory tests. Blood flow is better and air bubbles are less likely if the puncture site is held downward and gentle pressure is applied.

(16) Blood smears can also be made from subsequent drops of blood (see Procedure 9-2).

(17) Using a clean gauze pad, apply gentle pressure to the site until bleeding has stopped (Figure 9-9 ■). The hand may be slightly elevated.

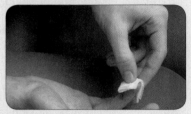

Figure ■ 9-9

(18) Label each tube correctly and in front of the patient to verify identity, and prepare the specimens for transport.

(19) Discard all other biohazardous supplies (puncture devices in puncture-resistant containers and gauze, etc., in other approved biohazard containers) before removing gloves.

AFTER THE PROCEDURE

(20) Remove and dispose of gloves in a biohazard container and perform hand hygiene.

(21) Ensure that bleeding has stopped, ask the patient to verify that the labels have his or her name, and thank the patient before allowing him or her to leave or, if in a hospital setting, before leaving with specimens and remaining supplies.

NOTES

■ In health care facilities, the puncture devices used are typically small, single-use, disposable devices. However, in home settings, a patient may have a multiuse device in which only the lancet is changed after each use with that single patient. In this case, discard the lancet and clean the multiuse device according to the manufacturer's instructions if it becomes contaminated.

■ A free flow of blood is essential to obtain accurate test results. Do not use excessive squeezing, massaging, or scraping to obtain blood.

■ If the blood drop used for the specimen is allowed to remain on the skin too long, some evaporation may occur and the drop may dry out. If this happens, wipe away this drop and use the next one; otherwise, it may result in erroneous laboratory values.

■ If the sample is not adequate and blood has stopped flowing from the puncture site, use a new sterile device to re-puncture at a *different* site. Be sure to warm the site prior to re-puncturing to improve the blood flow to the area and re-cleanse the puncture site. Avoid excessive punctures on one finger and/or hand.

If the bone is repeatedly punctured, it can lead to **osteomyelitis,** which is an inflammation of the bone caused by bacterial infection, or **osteochondritis,** inflammation of the bone and cartilage.

Manually-used blades or lancets without a retractable feature and/or depth control are *never recommended* for acquiring capillary specimens because they can cause more bruising and inflammation than automated retractable devices, they are more likely to cause accidental injuries with the exposed sharp, and they tend to be more painful.

Order of Collection

The order of filling microcollection tubes with capillary blood is different than for venipuncture. If multiple laboratory tests have been ordered, the order of collection should be as follows:[1]

- Blood gases
- EDTA specimen for hematology tests
- Other tubes with additives
- Serum tubes

Also refer to Figure 9-10 ■ which shows one manufacturer's instructions for the order of draw and mixing procedures.

There are several preexamination variables that require special attention when collecting skin puncture specimens.

- Microcollection tubes must be adequately filled and, if they contain additives, they should be gently mixed. If it takes too long to fill the tube, microclots may form. Remember that as soon as the skin is punctured, the coagulation process begins, so collect the specimen quickly to minimize the effects of platelet clumping, exposure to air (for blood gases), and light (for bilirubin).
- Excessive amounts (overfilling) can cause clot formation; inadequate amounts (underfilling) can cause cells to change morphologically because of too much anticoagulant.
- Hemolysis of the capillary blood specimen is a complication that can cause erroneous laboratory results and is usually preventable if good technique is maintained. Hemolysis is caused by:[1]

  Not removing residual alcohol or not allowing it to adequately air dry at the puncture site

  Excessive milking/massaging of the finger

  Patients having increased blood cell fragility and high packed cell volume (e.g., newborns and infants)

  Excessive shaking while mixing the specimen

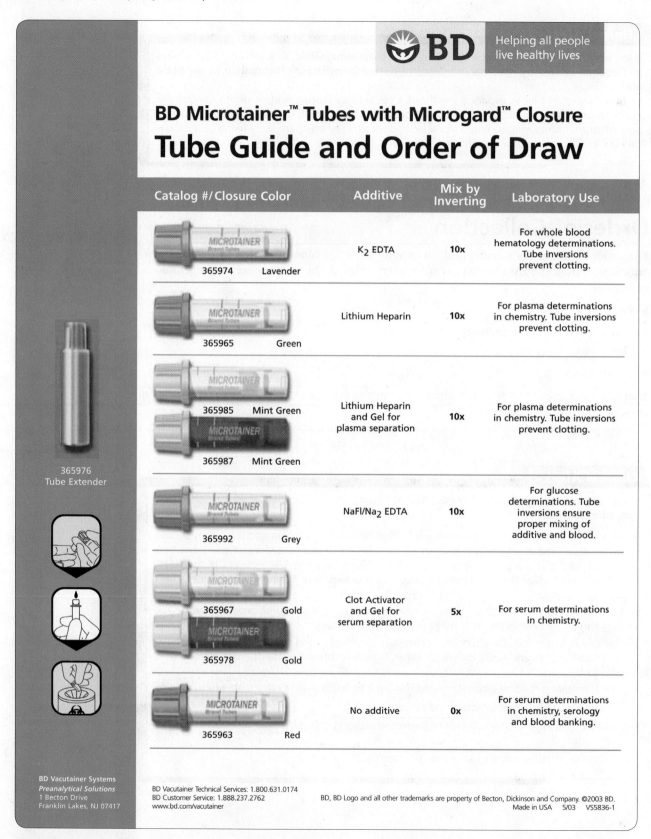

BD Microtainer™ Tubes with Microgard™ Closure
Tube Guide and Order of Draw

BD — Helping all people live healthy lives

Catalog #/Closure Color		Additive	Mix by Inverting	Laboratory Use
365974	Lavender	K_2 EDTA	10x	For whole blood hematology determinations. Tube inversions prevent clotting.
365965	Green	Lithium Heparin	10x	For plasma determinations in chemistry. Tube inversions prevent clotting.
365985	Mint Green	Lithium Heparin and Gel for plasma separation	10x	For plasma determinations in chemistry. Tube inversions prevent clotting.
365987	Mint Green			
365992	Grey	NaFl/Na_2 EDTA	10x	For glucose determinations. Tube inversions ensure proper mixing of additive and blood.
365967	Gold	Clot Activator and Gel for serum separation	5x	For serum determinations in chemistry.
365978	Gold			
365963	Red	No additive	0x	For serum determinations in chemistry, serology and blood banking.

365976
Tube Extender

BD Vacutainer Systems
Preanalytical Solutions
1 Becton Drive
Franklin Lakes, NJ 07417

BD Vacutainer Technical Services: 1.800.631.0174
BD Customer Service: 1.888.237.2762
www.bd.com/vacutainer

BD, BD Logo and all other trademarks are property of Becton, Dickinson and Company. ©2003 BD.
Made in USA   5/03   VS5836-1

FIGURE ■ 9-10 Order of Draw Using BD Microtainer Tubes
Source: Courtesy and © Becton, Dickinson and Company

Blood Films for Microscopic Slides

Blood smears are not used in all laboratories because current technologies do not require them. However, other laboratories still use this method for confirmatory purposes or as a back-up procedure. Procedure 9-2 ■ demonstrates one method for making blood smears on glass slides used for microscopic analysis for performing white blood cell **differentials** (diff), which is a hematological laboratory test to approximate percentages and determine morphology of the white blood cells. Red blood cell and platelet morphology can also be assessed. Health care facilities can vary the procedures that they use to make blood smears so appropriate procedures must be followed at each facility. It takes a significant amount of practice to learn to make slides that are acceptable for use. Health care workers must be adequately trained to make consistently good slides for microscopic analysis.

Procedure 9-2

Blood Films for Microscopic Slides

RATIONALE

Blood films on microscopic slides can be used to evaluate the morphology (form and structure) of the blood cells. The microscopic slides are prepared with a blood drop following this procedure; they are stained with special stains in the laboratory; and evaluated under a microscope. Although some facilities no longer use this manual method, it is still used in many cases for detecting cellular abnormalities, for confirmation, and/or as a back-up method.

EQUIPMENT

- Gloves
- Glass slides used for microscopic analysis
- Drying rack or other clean surface
- Same supplies used for Procedure 9-1

PREPARATION

(1) Prepare and assemble supplies.

(2) Identify the patient properly. Cleanse your hands, then don gloves.

(3) Perform the skin puncture as directed in Procedure 9-1.

PROCEDURE

(4) Make blood smears from fresh drops of blood. Perform the finger puncture in the usual way, wiping the first drop of blood away. Touch the slide to the second drop at approximately 0.5–1 in. (1.3–2.5 cm) from the end of the slide (Figure 9-11 ■). Blood smears may also be made using anticoagulated (EDTA) blood from a lavender-top tube. However, it should be done where there is minimal exposure to the blood or blood spills.

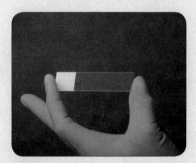

Figure ■ 9-11

(continued)

Procedure 9-2

Blood Films for Microscopic Slides *(continued)*

(5) Place the second (spreader) slide in front of the drop of blood and then pull it slowly into the drop, allowing blood to spread along the width of the slide (Figure 9-12 ■). Again, remember that procedures for making blood smears can vary so follow the methods used at your site.

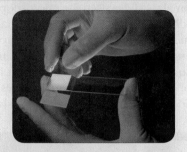

Figure ■ 9-12

(6) When the blood spreads almost to the edges, quickly and evenly push the spreader slide forward at an angle of approximately 30 degrees. Do not press downward. The only downward pressure should be the weight of the spreader slide (Figure 9-13 ■).

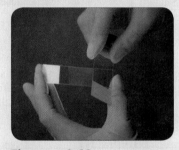

Figure ■ 9-13

(7) Allow the slide to air dry; do not blow on it (Figure 9-14 ■).

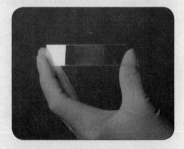

Figure ■ 9-14

(8) Blood films should have a **feathered edge,** as shown in the first slide. It has a visible curved edge that thins out smoothly and resembles the tip of a bird's feather, and it covers approximately half the surface of the glass slide. In Figure 9-15 ■, the last four slides are not acceptable for analysis.

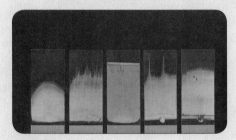

Figure ■ 9-15

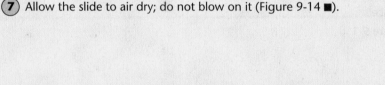

(9) No ridges, lines, or holes should be visible in the smear. Errors are often the result of too large a drop, too long a delay in making the smear, blowing on the slide, or using a chipped slide.

(10) Label the slides and prepare them for safe, secure transport to the laboratory.

AFTER THE PROCEDURE

(11) Discard any unusable or contaminated slides and all biohazardous waste in an appropriate container.

(12) Cleanse your hands. Label the slides according to the correct ID procedures at your facility, which usually includes a complete label for each slide.

(13) Thank the patient for cooperating, reconfirm identity, and allow the patient to leave (in an ambulatory setting) or depart with *all* specimens and *all* remaining supplies.

(14) Transport and/or deliver the slides to the laboratory.

Supply Disposal, Labeling the Specimen, and Completing the Interaction

Used, disposable puncture devices or lancets should always be placed into a rigid, puncture-resistant biohazard container with a lid. Contaminated supplies such as gauze, gloves, etc., should be disposed of in other designated biohazard containers. Carefully follow the disposal procedures at each health care facility. All tubes must be appropriately labeled immediately after collection and mixing and the information on the labels must be confirmed. Several tubes may be placed together in a larger labeled biohazard transport container. All supplies and equipment that were brought in should be removed or discarded appropriately. Hand hygiene must be performed again after contact with *each* patient. Before leaving the patient's side, check the puncture site to make sure that the bleeding has stopped, then thank the patient for their cooperation. An adhesive bandage may be applied; however, bandages are not recommended for infants or young children because of possible irritation and the potential of swallowing or aspirating the bandage.

Self Study

Study Questions

For the following questions, select the one best answer.

1. Which of the following is the best site for a capillary puncture on an adult?

   a. middle finger

   b. pinkie finger

   c. ankle

   d. heel

2. Controlling the depth of the skin puncture prevents:

   a. puncturing a vein

   b. sample contamination

   c. excessive bleeding

   d. osteomyelitis

3. Skin puncture is most useful in which of the following conditions?

   a. obese patient

   b. patient with a double mastectomy

   c. fragile veins

   d. healthy adults who need many laboratory tests

4. Which finger(s) are used most often for skin puncture?

   a. thumb

   b. second, or index, finger

   c. third or fourth finger

   d. fifth, or pinky, finger

5. What is the disinfectant of choice for a capillary puncture procedure?

   a. iodine preparation

   b. 100% ethyl alcohol

   c. 70% isopropyl alcohol

   d. 10% bleach solution

6. Which drop(s) of blood are most often used as the first tube is collected during a fingerstick?

   a. first

   b. second

   c. fifteenth

   d. twentieth

7. Which drop should be wiped away before beginning the capillary collection?

   a. first

   b. second

   c. fourteenth

   d. nineteenth

8. What does the *feathered edge* refer to?

   a. the point of the lancet

   b. alcohol pad

   c. edge of the blood smear on a microscope slide

   d. blood drop on a microscope slide

9. Capillary blood is composed of:

   a. venous blood only

   b. arterial blood only

   c. venous, arterial, and capillary blood, and tissue fluids

   d. venous blood and tissue fluids

10. Plastic microcollection tubes should be filled with blood in which of the following ways?

    a. using a syringe to fill the tube

    b. using capillary action to fill itself

    c. using suction to pull blood into the tube

    d. using the tube to scoop droplets off the skin carefully

Case Study

A health care worker was assigned to a collection station in the clinic where most of the patients were having fingersticks. The first patient encountered was an 18-year-old named Sarah W., who had a fear of needles. She was shaking, her hands were cold, and she was about to cry. The second patient, Henry C., had very wrinkled, dry skin and calluses on his fingers.

Question

What should the health care worker do to make the best of these two situations and collect the blood specimens?

Advocating Patient Safety Case Study

All patients hate to be re-stuck, even when it is a skin puncture on the finger. It is still painful and, depending on whether or not the patient has had multiple sticks already, the typical sites may be sore and bruised. In addition, most health care workers dread being the one to go back to a patient and inform them that another blood sample is needed, especially when one was already taken that day. It is imperative that health care workers use consistent techniques to promote "getting it done right the first time, every time" so that repeat sticks are not necessary.

Questions

1. Name two ways that the health care worker can improve blood flow to the hand area before the skin puncture is made.

2. Name two ways that the health care worker can assure an adequate blood sample is contained in the tube.

Competency Assessment

Check Yourself: Patient Preference

Think about the last time you experienced a venipuncture or a fingerstick. Discuss your preference between the two procedures. Also, explain which finger you would prefer to have stuck and why.

Competency Checklist: Capillary Blood Collection

Each step must be successfully completed. If one step is not completed successfully, the individual/student should restudy the text and seek guidance from a supervisor or educator. He or she must try again until competency has been achieved.

(1) Completed (2) Needs to improve/Repeat lesson and checklist

_____ 1. Patient identification and assessment (diet & allergy) are performed appropriately.

_____ 2. Prepares the appropriate supplies and puncture device.

_____ 3. Performs hand hygiene and gloving techniques.

_____ 4. Positions the patient appropriately.

_____ 5. Selects the most suitable finger.

_____ 6. Uses warming devices or other methods to improve blood flow to the site.

_____ 7. Cleanses the site appropriately.

_____ 8. Uses an appropriate puncture device to make an incision across the fingerprint. Discards puncture device.

_____ 9. Wipes away the first drop of blood.

_____ 10. Collects the appropriate sample tubes in the correct order, to the correct fill line, and mixes them accordingly.

_____ 11. Applies appropriate pressure to produce additional drops of blood.

_____ 12. Applies gentle pressure to stop the bleeding.

_____ 13. Handles the specimens appropriately.

_____ 14. Discards all waste in appropriate containers.

_____ 15. Labels the specimens appropriately and prepares them for transport.

_____ 16. Checks the patient status and reconfirms label identity before leaving.

_____ 17. Thanks the patient for cooperating.

Competency Checklist: Making Blood Smears for Microscopic Analysis

Many phlebotomists are no longer required to make manual blood smears or films on microscopic slides. However, it is a skill that is still required in some settings where phlebotomists are the only ones with this educational skill. Making appropriate microscopic blood smears for laboratory analysis requires repeated practice. The skill should be practiced until the phlebotomist becomes proficient.

(1) Completed (2) Needs to improve/Repeat lesson and checklist

_____ 1. Using a practice sample of blood, the phlebotomist is able to make 50 suitable blood smears.

_____ 2. Using blood from a capillary puncture on a patient, the phlebotomist wipes away the first drop of blood.

_____ 3. The glass slide is touched to the second drop on the finger about 0.5 to 1 inch from the end of the slide.

_____ 4. The second slide (the spreader) is placed in front of the drop, allowing the drop of blood to spread along the width of the slide.

_____ 5. The spreader is pushed evenly toward the other end of the slide causing the blood to evenly flow across the glass.

_____ 6. The blood smear is in the shape of a feathered edge.

_____ 7. The slide is allowed to air dry in a safe place.

_____ 8. The slide is labeled appropriately.

References

1. Clinical and Laboratory Standards Institute (CLSI): *Procedures and Devices for the Collection of Diagnostic Capillary Blood Specimens,* Approved Standard, 6th edition, document H4-A6. Wayne, PA: CLSI, 2008.

2. Niwinski, N: Becton Dickinson LabNotes, Capillary Blood Collection: Best Practices, Volume 20, No.1, 2009, www.bd.com/vacutainer/labnotes/Volume20Number1/index.asp, accessed 1/30/12.

PEARSON
myhealthprofessionskit™

Go to www.myhealthprofessionskit.com to access the Companion Website created for this textbook. Simply select "Clinical Laboratory Science" from the choice of disciplines. Find this book and log in using your username and password to access interactive learning games, assessment questions, and more.

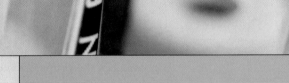

Chapter 10

Pediatric and Geriatric Procedures

KEY TERMS

Alzheimer's disease (AD)
calcaneus
capillary blood gas
    analysis
eutectic mixture of local
    anesthetics (EMLA)
geriatric
heelstick

neonatal screening
neonates
Parkinson's disease
pediatric phlebotomy
premature infant
sucrose nipple or
    pacifier

CHAPTER OBJECTIVES

Upon completion of Chapter 10, the learner should be able to do the following:

1. Describe fears or concerns that children of various ages might have regarding the blood collection process.
2. List suggestions for parents and health care workers during a venipuncture or skin puncture.
3. Identify puncture sites for a heelstick on an infant and describe the procedure.
4. Explain the special precautions and types of equipment needed to collect capillary blood gases.
5. Describe the venipuncture sites for infants and young children.
6. Discuss the types of equipment and supplies that must be used during skin puncture and venipuncture for infants and children.
7. Describe the procedure for specimen collection for neonatal screening.
8. Define five physical and/or emotional changes that are associated with the aging process.
9. Describe how a health care worker should react to physical and emotional changes associated with the elderly.

Collecting blood from **pediatric** (baby or child) and **geriatric** (elderly) patients requires much clinical knowledge about, and training for, the proper techniques. Both of these age groups require extra care in blood collection.

Pediatric Patients

Children are not just little adults, and they should not be treated as such (Figure 10-1 ■). The health care worker needs to be familiar with special types of equipment that are available, observe the various techniques as they are performed by a health care worker experienced in **pediatric phlebotomy,** and practice the techniques to develop the necessary skills. The health care worker also must learn how to talk with children of various ages to calm them for a blood collection.

Performing venipuncture or skin puncture on young patients is challenging, because children have smaller bodies and are less prepared to cope with pain and anxiety. When learning the techniques, remember to ask for help if needed and to allow adequate time to develop the necessary skills.

Preparing Child and Parent

The timing of the preparation depends on the child's age; generally, the younger the child, the closer the explanation should be to the time of the procedure.[1]

Preparing the child and the parent for the blood collection procedure involves the following steps:

1. A calm, confident approach is the first step in obtaining the cooperation of the child and parent. Introduce yourself. Be warm and friendly, establish eye contact with both the child and the parent, and show that you are concerned about the child's health and comfort. When you interact with a pediatric patient and his or her parent, provide a sense of trust and confidence.

2. Correctly identify the patient by using at least two patient identifiers.[2] The patient should have an identification bracelet with his or her name and hospital number or birth date. Verify this information. A hospitalized infant usually has the identification bracelet on his or her ankle. Newborns who have not yet been named are usually identified by their last names (e.g., Baby Boy Smith and Baby Girl Jones) and identification number. If the mother is still in the hospital after delivery, the baby may wear an identification band that is cross-referenced to the mother. Keeping identifications straight is always crucial, but especially so when specimens from twin babies must be collected and labeled.

3. Find out about the child's past experience with blood collections. Ask whether the child has ever had blood collected. The child and the parent can then tell you about their experiences with past procedures and provide you with valuable information about the approaches that worked effectively for them and those that were not as successful.

4. Develop a plan. Ask the parent how cooperative his or her child will be. Parents are excellent predictors of their child's behavior and possibility for distress. Usually, the younger child with poor venous access will have more distress. A successful plan involves not only the parent's suggestions about what will be most helpful but also the health care worker's knowledge about pediatric phlebotomy techniques. If possible, allow the child to have some control by offering a choice of which arm or finger he or she prefers for blood collection.

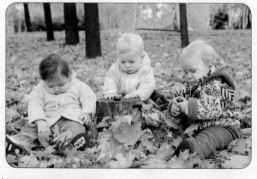

FIGURE ■ 10-1 Our Younger Generation
Source: Anatoliy Samara/Shutterstock.com

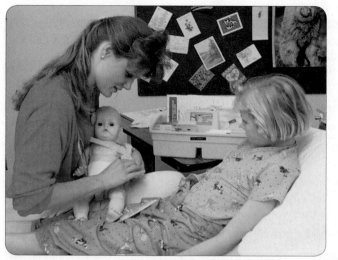

FIGURE ■ 10-2 Talking to a Child at Eye Level

5. Place yourself at the child's eye level to explain and demonstrate the procedure (Figure 10-2 ■). When explaining what you will be doing, use words appropriate for the child's age. Use of a doll, puppet, or stuffed animal in the demonstration can help you relate to the child in a nonthreatening manner. If the child has a favorite doll, blanket, or toy, he or she should be encouraged to hug it for comfort and support.

6. Establish guidelines. Tell the child and the parent that the procedure will most likely be successful on the first attempt. If not, it will be attempted only once more by another health care worker.

7. Be honest when a child asks whether the puncture will hurt. Tell the child that if the procedure hurts too much, it can be momentarily stopped, but that the more quickly the procedure is performed the less painful it will be. Instruct the child to say when he or she feels the pain or "hurt." Tell the child that saying "ouch" or making faces is acceptable but that he or she must make an effort to keep the arm absolutely still. Reassure the child that the blood will be collected as quickly as possible so that the pain will be brief.[1]

8. Encourage parent involvement.[1] Explain how the parent can assist by holding, distracting, and soothing their child during the procedure. Some parents, however, may be reluctant to participate because they do not want to be a part of a procedure that will cause their children pain. If the parent does not wish to assist but is willing to be in the room, ask him or her to maintain eye contact with the child to reduce stress. If after discussing his or her role the parent is still reluctant to be in the room, respect his or her wishes. If the parent does not wish to participate, you may ask another health care worker to assist.

PSYCHOLOGICAL RESPONSE TO NEEDLES AND PAIN

Children especially fear needles, and an emotionally upset child has difficulty separating fear from actual pain. Children 1 to 2 years old may react extremely to painless procedures, such as taking a temperature. Children 3 to 5 years old perceive pain as a punishment for bad behavior. They may react aggressively. Children 6 to 12 years old are more likely to relate pain to past experiences. Many children perceive that a "shot," or needle, hurts more than anything else that has ever happened to them. Children 13 to 17 years old are more independent and may be embarrassed to show fear. They usually need privacy and may act hostile to mask fear. With proper preparation, the child and the parent can develop coping skills to help lessen the fear and thereby diminish the "hurt."

Clinical Alert !

It is not unusual for a sick or injured child to act younger than he or she really is. If a child who is 6 behaves like a 3-year-old, use strategies appropriate for a 3-year-old.[3]

The following parental behaviors and examples will have a positive effect on relieving the child's distress.[3,4]

Behaviors	Examples
Distraction	"Look at Mommy"; "Tell us about your doll"
Emotional support	Hugging, stroking hair, patting, and talking in a soothing voice
Explanation	"We need to take a tiny bit of blood from your finger"; "You will feel a little prick"; "Mommy will help you hold your arm still so that we can finish quickly"
Positive reinforcement	"You did a great job in holding your arm still!"

DISTRACTION TECHNIQUES

Children older than 3 years respond well to distraction techniques to help them cope and lessen distress. Distraction helps the child refocus on a more pleasant experience. A parent or another health care worker can provide the distraction. Some examples of distraction are blowing bubbles, pinwheels, counting, reading a book or looking at a video, listening to music, singing, or talking in a gentle voice about something enjoyable. School-age children may respond to strategies such as picturing themselves in a pleasant setting or participating in the procedure.[3,4]

ROOM LOCATION

For psychological reasons, the best room location for a painful procedure is a treatment room away from the child's bed or play room. For a hospitalized child, the bed should be a safe, secure place to rest and sleep, not a place associated with pain. If the child shares a room with another child, performing the procedure at the bed side can be upsetting to the roommate as well. If the child cannot be moved to a treatment room, maintain privacy by drawing a curtain between the beds and speaking in a calm, quiet manner.

EQUIPMENT PREPARATION FOR A FRIENDLIER ENVIRONMENT

Just the sight of needles, syringes, and a person in a white laboratory coat can be frightening to a child. When working with children, wear bright, colorfully printed uniforms or smocks to create a child-friendly environment. Prepare the phlebotomy equipment and supplies before entering the child's room so that the child does not become even more anxious by watching the preparation. Use shorter needles if possible, and keep threatening-looking supplies (such as needles) covered and out of sight until you are ready to begin the procedure. If the hospital policy requires goggles or face shields for blood-exposure precautions, put this equipment on after greeting the child. Praise the child throughout the procedure. At the completion, reward the child with a colorful bandage, a sticker, an age-appropriate toy, or, with parental permission, a lollipop. If a parent is not present to assist in relieving the anxiety, offer a pacifier to an infant or gently stroke or talk softly to soothe a small child.

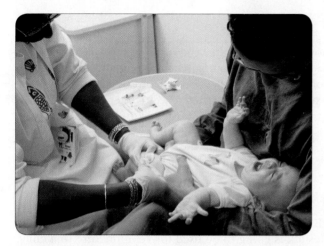

FIGURE ■ **10-3** Supine (Lying) Position for Restraining a Child to Perform Blood Collection

Positions for Restraining a Child

Holding the child may be required to ensure that the child does not move his or her limb (i.e., arm, finger, or foot) during blood collection. Restraining techniques should be compassionate, safe, and performed quickly. A supportive parent who has been properly instructed can assist with restraining while providing comfort to the child.

Two preferred comfort methods of restraining a child to immobilize the arm are the vertical position and the horizontal, or supine position (Figures 10-3 ■ and 10-4 ■).[3,4]

In both cases, the parent's face is close to the child's, thereby providing a comforting and secure feeling. The vertical technique, which works well for toddlers, requires the child to be held on the parent's lap. As the parent hugs and holds the child's body and the arm not being used, the health care worker can firmly hold the other arm to perform the procedure.

In the horizontal position, a baby can easily be held by a parent. However, more restraint may be needed for an older child. If the child lies supine, with the health care worker on one side of the bed and the parent on the opposite side, the parent can gently but firmly lean over the child, restraining the child's arm not being used while holding the opposite, extended arm securely for the health care worker.

Neonates and infants younger than 3 months usually do not require restraint and can be managed by the health care worker alone. Swaddling helps to control and comfort an upset newborn (Figure 10-5 ■).

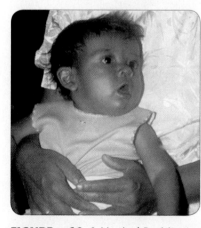

FIGURE ■ **10-4** Vertical Position for Restraining a Child to Perform Blood Collection

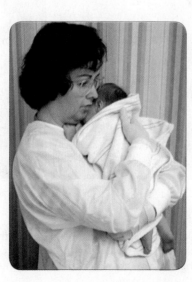

FIGURE ■ **10-5** Swaddling a Newborn

Combative Patients

At times, a child will become uncooperative even after the proper steps have been followed to gain cooperation. Children may become combative—kicking and thrashing—if force is used. Because sharps are involved in blood collection, the health care worker must be certain that the procedure can be performed safely. Using force to the point of potential physical injury is unethical and unprofessional. Therefore, if the risk of injury to the child or the health care worker is likely, discontinue the blood collection attempt and notify the nurse or the physician.

Decreasing the Needlestick Pain

A topical anesthetic (pain reliever), **EMLA (eutectic mixture of local anesthetics),** can be rubbed on the skin when a needlestick is going to be used for venipuncture to a child. This local anesthetic is ideal for use before venipuncture or starting intravenous (IV) therapy because it does not require a needle. It is applied to the skin as a patch or a cream that is then covered with a transparent adhesive dressing (see Figure 10-6 ■). Optimal anesthesia occurs after 45 to 60 minutes and may last as long as 2 to 3 hours. Drawbacks to the use of EMLA are cost, the need to apply it 60 minutes before the procedure, and having to know in advance the location of the vein to be used. Two separate locations may be anesthetized if the child has difficult veins from which to obtain blood. Do not use EMLA if the child is allergic to local anesthetics.[4,5,6]

ORAL SUCROSE

Sucrose (a sugar) is effective in reducing pain and crying time during a procedure for an infant up to 6 months old. A 25% solution of sucrose can be prepared by mixing 4 teaspoons of water with 1 teaspoon of sugar. The sucrose can be carefully administered by oral syringe, dropper, nipple, or on a pacifier. A **sucrose nipple or pacifier** is given 2 minutes before heelsticks, and its action lasts about 5 minutes. Some studies show that infants given pacifiers or sucrose have also been shown to be more alert after the procedure, to be less fussy, and to cry for a shorter duration.[5,7]

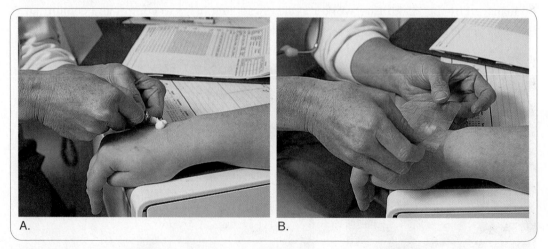

A.   B.

FIGURE ■ 10-6 Using EMLA
When a needlestick is planned, EMLA can be used to anesthetize the skin where the needlestick will occur. A. Apply a thick layer of the EMLA cream over intact skin (half of a 5g tube). B. Cover the cream with a transparent adhesive dressing for 45–60 minutes.

Precautions to Protect the Child

Premature infants, newborns, and children who are chronically ill or have extensive burns are more likely to be susceptible to infections. To protect these children from potentially harmful microorganisms, some hospitals may require protective precautions. In this instance, PPE—gowns, gloves, and masks—will be worn as indicated before entering the room. After the procedure, remove the PPE according to policy and dispose of it in the appropriately marked container. Wash your hands or sanitize them according to policy. Alcohol-based, waterless rubs, foams, or rinses are as effective as handwashing if the hands are not soiled.[8] Put on a clean gown and gloves before attending to the next infant or child.

> **Clinical Alert !**
>
> Puncturing deep veins in children may cause cardiac arrest, hemorrhage, venous thrombosis, damage to surrounding tissues, and infection.

Pediatric Phlebotomy Procedures

Two methods are used to obtain blood from infants and children: microcapillary skin puncture and venipuncture. The previously described steps for preparing the child and the parent should be taken before either procedure is performed.

MICROCAPILLARY SKIN PUNCTURE

Skin punctures are useful for pediatric phlebotomy when only small amounts of blood are needed and can be adequately tested. It is particularly important to collect only the smallest amounts of blood necessary from neonates, infants, and children so that the effects of reductions in **blood volume** are minimal. Overcollecting during phlebotomy may require packed-blood-cell transfusion in an infant. Small infants can easily become anemic if too much blood is taken. To avoid overcollection of blood by phlebotomy, the amount of blood collected from an infant and small child must be recorded and maintained.

Each hospital treating pediatric patients should determine the amounts of blood to be collected from patients on the basis of weight and the maximum cumulative amount of blood to be collected during a specified time period (see Appendix 4).

When performing skin punctures, collect the hematological specimens first to minimize platelet clumping, then collect for chemical and blood-bank specimens. Each laboratory has approved procedures for phlebotomy, including the volume of blood that is required for each test: always follow these procedures. Always record the amount of blood collected.

SKIN PUNCTURE SITES

The heel is the most desirable site for skin puncture on an infant or neonate (Procedure 10-1 ■). Use the most medial or most lateral section of the plantar, or bottom, surface of the heel (Figure 10-7 ■). DO NOT use the central area of the infant's heel for blood collection.

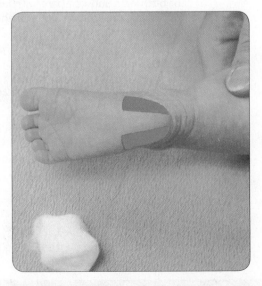

FIGURE ■ 10-7 Heel Sites for Capillary Puncture

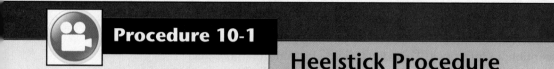

Procedure 10-1

Heelstick Procedure

RATIONALE

To perform a blood collection from the infant's heel.

EQUIPMENT

The following equipment is necessary for pediatric skin puncture:

- Sterile, automatic, disposable pediatric skin-puncture safety devices in different manufacturers' incision depths (0.65–0.85 mm for premature neonates, 1.0 mm for larger infants). (Please see Chapter 6, Blood Collection Equipment, for photo examples.)
- 70% isopropyl alcohol swabs
- Sterile 2" × 2" gauze sponges
- Plastic capillary collection tubes and sealer or caps
- Microcollection containers
- Glass slides for smears
- Puncture-resistant sharps container
- Disposable gloves (nonlatex if the child is allergic)
- Compress (towel or washcloth) to warm heel if necessary
- Marking pen
- Laboratory request slips or labels

PREPARATION

1. Prepare and assemble supplies. Remember, DO NOT place the specimen collection tray on the infant's bed or in the bassinet.

2. Introduce yourself to the parents, explain the procedure and use appropriate comfort techniques.

3. Identify the infant properly. Identify the infant by name, address, and identification number and/ or birth date and compare with laboratory test request form. If the infant is not wearing an identification bracelet the name of the person who performs this identification procedure must be documented in the medical records and charts.

PROCEDURE

4. Wash or sanitize your hands with an alcohol hand rub, then put on gloves. If required, don a gown and a mask.

5. Inspect the selected area and assess it for proper warmth. If it is cool or a blood gas specimen is to be collected, prewarm the foot ▶ with a warm, wet towel or a chemical heel-warming pack, according to policy. Wipe the heel dry after removing the warm towel.

A CLOSER LOOK

▶ **Heel Warming**

RATIONALE

The amount of blood that can be obtained from a single **heelstick** is limited; therefore, to obtain an adequate sample, prewarming the heel may be indicated. Prewarming the heel increases blood flow and arterializes the specimen. This step is essential for collecting specimens for **capillary blood gas analysis.**

PROCEDURE

(A) Prepare and assemble supplies; warm wet towel and a plastic bag or a chemical heel-warming pack.

(B) Warm the site with a commercially available warming pack or wrap a warm, wet towel at a temperature no more than 42°C around the infant's foot. If the temperature of the towel exceeds 42°C, it may burn the infant.

(C) Encase the towel in a plastic bag to help retain heat and to keep the patient's bed dry. Use caution if the towel is heated in a microwave oven, because heating is uneven and the towel may have hot spots.

(D) Prewarm the site for 3 to 5 minutes.

(E) Depending on the institution's policy, call in advance to prewarm the infant's heel.

(6) Position the baby in a supine (lying) position with the knee at the open end of the bassinet. This position allows the foot to hang lower than the torso, improving blood flow. When the baby is in an acceptable position for this procedure, clean the intended incision site on the heel with an antiseptic swab. Allow the heel to air dry. Do not touch the incision site or allow the heel to come into contact with any nonsterile item or surface (Figure 10-8 ■).

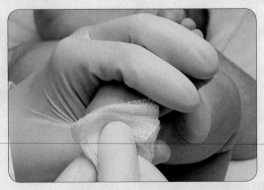

Figure ■ 10-8

Source: Courtesy of BD VACUTAINER Systems, Preanalytical Solution, Franklin Lakes, NJ

(continued)

Procedure 10-1

Heelstick Procedure *(continued)*

(7) Remove the appropriate Tenderfoot puncture device from its blister pack, taking care not to rest the blade slot end on any nonsterile surface (Figure 10-9 ■).

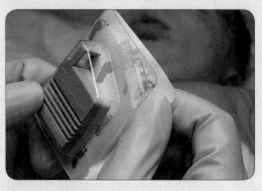

Figure ■ 10-9
Source: Courtesy of ITC

(8) Remove the safety clip. Note: The safety clip may be replaced if the test is momentarily delayed; however, prolonged exposure of any Tenderfoot device to uncontrolled environmental conditions before use may affect its sterility. Once the safety clip is removed, DO NOT push the trigger or touch the blade slot (Figure 10-10 ■).

(9) Hold the infant's foot firmly but gently to prevent sudden movement. Holding the foot too tightly may cause bruising and restrict blood flow. Also, it can lead to erroneous laboratory tests results.

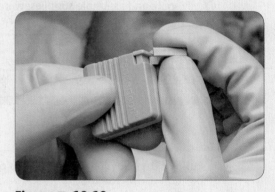

Figure ■ 10-10
Source: Courtesy of ITC

(10) Raise the foot above the baby's heart level and carefully select a safe incision site (avoid any edematous area or site within 2.0 mm of a prior wound). Place the blade-slot surface of the device flush against the heel so that its center point is vertically aligned with the desired incision site (Figure 10-11 ■).

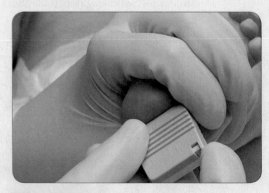

Figure ■ 10-11
Source: Courtesy of ITC

Clinical Alert !

Avoid excessive milking or squeezing, which causes hemolysis and dilutes the blood with interstitial and intracellular fluid.

11. Ensure that both ends of the device have made light contact with the skin, and depress the trigger. After triggering, immediately remove the device from the infant's heel and dispose of it in the biohazard sharps container (Figure 10-12 ■).

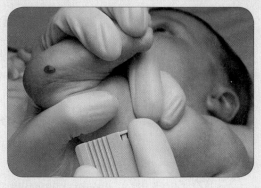

Figure ■ 10-12
Source: Courtesy of ITC

12. Using only a dry sterile gauze pad, gently wipe away the first droplet of blood that appears at the incision site (Figure 10-13 ■).

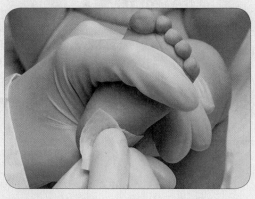

Figure ■ 10-13
Source: Courtesy of ITC

13. Taking care not to make direct wound contact with the collection container or capillary tube, fill to the desired specimen volume (Figure 10-14 ■). Take care NOT to scoop blood into the microtube as this technique can lead to hemolysis.

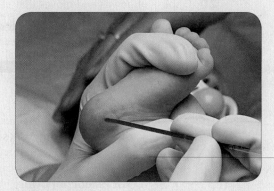

Figure ■ 10-14
Source: Courtesy of ITC

(continued)

Procedure 10-1

Heelstick Procedure *(continued)*

⑭ After blood collection, gently press a dry sterile gauze pad to the incision site until bleeding has ceased. This step will help prevent a hematoma from forming (Figure 10-15 ■).

⑮ Label the specimen container and verify identification. Record the time of collection.

AFTER THE PROCEDURE: CARE OF THE HEEL

⑯ Elevate the heel slightly above the body and ensure that bleeding has stopped.

⑰ Check the infant's heel puncture site for late bleeding or inflammation.

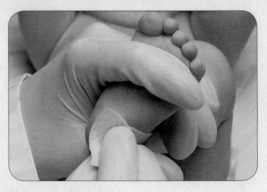

Figure ■ 10-15
Source: Courtesy of ITC

Clinical Alert !

Use of an adhesive bandage over skin-puncture sites is not recommended for children under 2 years old. Infants have delicate skin that may be irritated by the adhesive strip, and an older infant might remove it and put it in his or her mouth. Bandages can also be swallowed by older children.

CLEAN UP

⑱ Dispose of the used skin-puncture device in a sharps container with a biohazard label.

⑲ Check the infant's bed for any equipment or trash left behind.

⑳ Discard blood-soaked gauze sponges, grossly contaminated items, and gowns or gloves used in isolation rooms in biohazardous waste containers.

㉑ Dispose of gowns and gloves that are not from isolation rooms in the regular trash.

㉒ Wash or sanitize your hands after removing the gloves.

Using the proper pediatric size skin-puncture device, make an incision that is less than 2.0 mm deep (see Figure 10-16 ■). Major blood vessels lie 0.3 to 1.6 mm beneath the skin at the dermal–subcutaneous junction in newborns.[9,10] If an incision goes deeper, the **calcaneus,** or heel bone, may be hit, which may lead to osteomyelitis and/or osteochondritis.[11,12]

For children older than 1 year, the palmar surface of the distal phalanx (fingertip section) of the third (middle) or fourth (ring) finger is most frequently used, because the thumb has a pulse and the index finger may be more sensitive. The fifth finger is not used

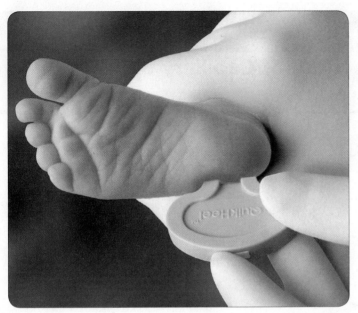

FIGURE ■ 10-16 Performing a Heelstick on an Infant
Source: Courtesy of ITC

because the skin is too thin. The plantar surface of the great toe is NOT recommended for skin puncture.

Clinical Alert !

Do not obtain blood by skin puncture from the toes or the central area of an infant's heel because this may result in injury to nerves, tendons, and cartilage; do not use fingers of infants less than 1 year old or previously punctured sites. If an infant has compromised circulation to the extremity, as in shock, or has edema, bruises, rashes, or infection at the heel, use another site (i.e., venipuncture procedure).

Capillary Blood Gases

Arterial blood is the specimen of choice for blood gas testing (i.e., pH, oxygen [O_2] content, and carbon dioxide [CO_2] content of the blood). However, capillary (skin puncture) blood can be collected from infants and small children for blood gas analysis because this procedure is safer than an arterial puncture (Procedure 10-2 ■). Skin puncture blood is less desirable as a specimen because it contains blood from capillaries, venules, and arterioles, and fluids from the surrounding tissue. In addition, common collection methods for capillary blood gas specimens use an open collection system in which the specimen is temporarily exposed to room air, which allows for a brief exchange of gases (both O_2 and CO_2) before the specimens are sealed from the air. The air exposure must be minimized to avoid falsely elevated blood oxygen levels.

Procedure 10-2

Collection for Capillary Blood Gas Testing

RATIONALE

To perform a blood collection for capillary blood gas analysis. Blood for capillary blood gas analysis is often collected from small children and babies for whom arterial punctures can be too dangerous. Samples are collected from the same areas of the body as other capillary samples, such as the lateral posterior area of the heel or the ball of the finger.

EQUIPMENT

- Sterile, automatic, disposable, pediatric skin-puncture safety devices in different manufacturers' incision depths (0.65–0.85 mm for premature neonates, 1.0 mm for larger infants)
- Heparinized safety plastic capillary tubes
- 70% isopropyl alcohol swabs
- Sterile 2" × 2" gauze sponges
- Plastic capillary collection tubes and sealer
- Microcollection containers
- Glass slides for smears
- Puncture-resistant sharps container
- Disposable gloves (nonlatex if the child is allergic)
- Warming packs or compress (towel or washcloth) to warm heel if necessary
- Marking pen
- Laboratory requisitions or labels
- Ice water
- Minute metal filing
- A magnet

PREPARATION

1. Prepare and assemble supplies.

2. Introduce yourself to the parents, explain the procedure, and use appropriate comfort techniques.

3. Identify the infant properly.

4. Warm the site according to the institution's procedures.

PROCEDURE

5. Wash or sanitize your hands with an alcohol hand rinse, then put on gloves. If required, don a gown and a mask.

6. Use a heparinized safety plastic capillary tube (Figure 10-17 ■) for the collection.

7. Perform the capillary (skin) puncture as previously mentioned and wipe away the first drop.

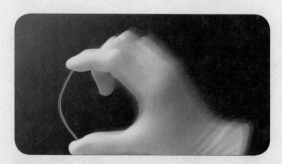

Figure ■ 10-17 SAFE-T-FILL® Capillary Blood Collection Tubes—100% Plastic for Safety

Source: Courtesy of RAM Scientific, Inc., Needham, MA

8 Fill the capillary tube with blood end-to-end to obtain the stated fill volume of the tube. Cap one end of the capillary tube, insert a small metal filing (referred to as a "flea" or "mixing wires") into the filled capillary tube, place the magnet over the tube and cap the other end of the tube (Figure 10-18 ■).

Clinical Alert !

The specimen must be collected with no air bubbles, which can cause inaccuracies in the values obtained from the specimen.

9 Use the magnet to draw the metal filing (flea) back and forth across the length of the tube to mix the specimen completely.

10 Label the tube and notify laboratory personnel of the urgent blood gas test to be performed.

11 Press the skin puncture site with a clean gauze sponge until the bleeding stops.

AFTER THE PROCEDURE: CARE OF THE HEEL

12 Elevate the heel slightly above the body and assure that bleeding has stopped.

13 Check the infant's heel puncture site for late bleeding or inflammation.

CLEAN UP

14 Dispose of the used skin-puncture device in a sharps container with a biohazard label.

15 Check the infant's bed for any equipment or trash left behind.

16 Discard blood-soaked gauze sponges, grossly contaminated items, and gowns or gloves used in isolation rooms in biohazardous waste containers.

17 Dispose of gowns and gloves that are not from isolation rooms in the regular trash.

18 Wash or sanitize your hands after removing the gloves.

19 Deliver the sample immediately to the laboratory. Delays of more than 15 minutes at room temperature will affect the results.

Capillary tube

Metal filing   Magnet   Plastic caps

Assembled:

Figure ■ 10-18 Capillary Blood Gas Tube, Metal Filing (Flea), and Plastic Caps.

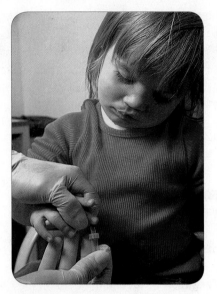

FIGURE ■ 10-19 Collecting Blood via Fingerstick from a Toddler

FINGERSTICK ON CHILDREN

A fingerstick to obtain blood for routine laboratory analysis is usually preferred for children older than 1 year (Figure 10-19 ■). Also, a fingerstick may be necessary if a child has damaged veins from repeated venipuncture or if the veins are covered with bandages or casts. Do not perform a fingerstick if the finger is swollen, edematous, cyanotic, or infected.

Use a pediatric safety skin-puncture device designed for the age and size of the child. An automatic skin-puncture device controls the puncture depth, which should not exceed 2.00 mm in small children. Automatic puncture devices are available in sizes that incise to depths of 0.85 mm for preemies, 1.25 mm for infants and 1.75 mm for toddlers. For a detailed description of collecting capillary blood specimens from the finger, refer to Chapter 9, "Capillary Blood Specimens."

NEONATAL SCREENING

In the United States, newborn babies, or neonates, are routinely screened for a variety of metabolic and genetic defects by analysis of blood collected on a special filter paper. **Neonatal screening** is important for the early detection, diagnosis, and treatment of certain genetic, metabolic, and infectious diseases. Many of these diseases can result in severe abnormalities, including mental retardation, if they are not discovered and treated early.

Blood spot testing for screening is performed before the newborn is 72 hours old (Procedure 10-3 ■). If the blood specimen is collected before the newborn is 24 hours old because of early discharge from the hospital, a second specimen for screening must be collected before 2 weeks of age.

Procedure 10-3

Collection of Capillary Blood for Neonatal Screening

RATIONALE

To perform a capillary blood collection for newborn screening specimens. The heel of the neonate is the most frequently used site for collection of blood for screening.

EQUIPMENT

The following equipment is necessary for newborn screening blood collection:

■ Sterile, automatic, disposable, pediatric, skin-puncture safety devices in different manufacturers' incision depths (0.65–0.85 mm for premature neonates, 1.0 mm for larger infants). Please see Chapter 6 (Blood Collection Equipment) for photo examples.

■ 70% isopropyl alcohol swabs

■ Sterile 2"× 2" gauze sponges

■ Newborn screening cards—appropriate collection cards are kept in the hospital laboratory or the nursery. (Do not use cards that are beyond the expiration date on the filter paper!)

■ Puncture-resistant sharps container

- Disposable gloves (nonlatex if child is allergic)
- Warming packs or compresses (towel or washcloth) to warm heel if necessary
- Marking pen
- Laboratory requisitions or labels

PREPARATION

(1) Prepare and assemble supplies (Figure 10-20 ■).

(2) Introduce yourself to the parents (if they are present), explain the procedure, and use appropriate comfort techniques.

(3) Identify the infant properly. If the infant is not wearing an identification bracelet, identify the infant by name, address, and identification number and/or birth date and compare this information with the laboratory test request form. Fill out the information on the newborn screening card shown in Figure 10-21 ■.

(4) Warm the site according to the institution's procedures.

PROCEDURE

(5) Wash or sanitize your hands with an alcohol hand rinse; then put on gloves. If required, don a gown and a mask.

(6) To prevent contamination, do not touch with hands or gloves any part of the filter paper circles before, during, or after collection. Do not allow the filter paper to come in contact with substances such as alcohol, formula, water, powder, antiseptic solutions, or lotion.

- Circles are printed on the filter paper portion of the card as shown in Figure 10-22 ■.

(7) Perform the capillary (skin) puncture as previously mentioned and wipe away the first drop of blood with a sterile gauze sponge.

(8) Allow another large blood drop to form.

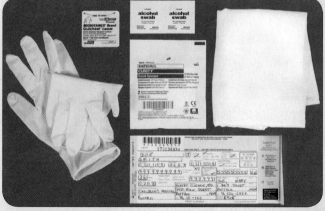

Figure ■ 10-20

Source: Courtesy of Wadsworth Center, New York State Department of Health

Figure ■ 10-21

Source: Courtesy of Wadsworth Center, New York State Department of Health

(continued)

Procedure 10-3

Collection of Capillary Blood for Neonatal Screening *(continued)*

(9) As shown in Figure 10-22, lightly touch the printed side of the filter paper with the blood drop and fill each printed circle (Figure 10-23 ■). Allow the blood to soak through and completely fill the circle with a single application of the large blood drop.

- If the circle does not fill entirely, wipe the heel and express another, larger drop to a different circle. Do not add a second drop of blood to a previously used circle.

- The filter paper must not touch the skin puncture site.

- Only use one side of the filter paper.

- Dry blood spots on a clean, dry, flat, nonabsorbent surface for a minimum of 4 hours.

- Direct application of blood from the heel to the card is the technique of choice. Most newborn screening laboratories will not accept blood spots collected by a capillary tube because the testing will not be accurate.

(10) Press the skin puncture site with a clean gauze sponge until the bleeding stops.

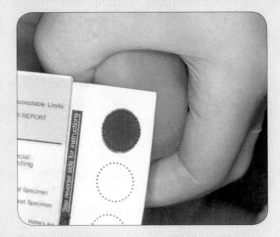

Figure ■ 10-22
Source: Courtesy of Wadsworth Center, New York State Department of Health

AFTER THE PROCEDURE: CARE OF THE HEEL

(11) Elevate the heel slightly above the body and ensure that bleeding has stopped.

(12) Check the infant's heel puncture site for late bleeding or inflammation.

CLEAN UP

(13) Dispose of the used skin-puncture device in a sharps container with a biohazard label.

(14) Check the infant's bed for any equipment or trash left behind.

(15) Discard blood-soaked gauze sponges, grossly contaminated items, and gowns or gloves used in isolation rooms into biohazardous waste containers.

(16) Dispose of gowns and gloves that are not from isolation rooms in the regular trash.

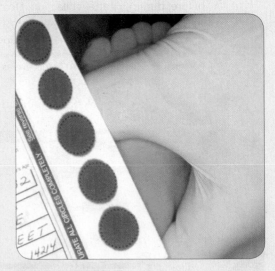

Figure ■ 10-23
Source: Courtesy of Wadsworth Center, New York State Department of Health

(17) Wash or sanitize your hands after removing the gloves.

(18) Correctly complete all the information on the screening card so that follow up can be done if the results are abnormal. Place the screening card in an appropriate envelope and send it to the laboratory within 24 hours.

INTERFERENCES IN NEWBORN SCREENING COLLECTIONS

It is important to be cautious and careful in the blood collection and transfer to the filter paper for the newborn screening.[13] Many interferences result from poor blood collection techniques. The most common include the following:

- Blood specimen not properly dried before mailing
- Filter paper circles not completely filled, not saturated with blood, or not *all* circles filled
- Contamination of filter paper circles before or after blood collection by substances such as hand lotion, powder, alcohol, antiseptic hand solution, or touching of areas with gloved or ungloved hands
- Blood applied to both sides of filter paper
- Excess blood applied (usually occurs with a capillary tube)
- Heelstick squeezed or milked, resulting in "tissue diluted" specimens
- Alcohol not wiped off heelstick site before puncture is made

VENIPUNCTURE ON CHILDREN

Venipuncture on children is used when larger quantities of blood are needed for sampling. The veins of the antecubital fossa or the forearm (Figure 10-24 ■) are the most accessible

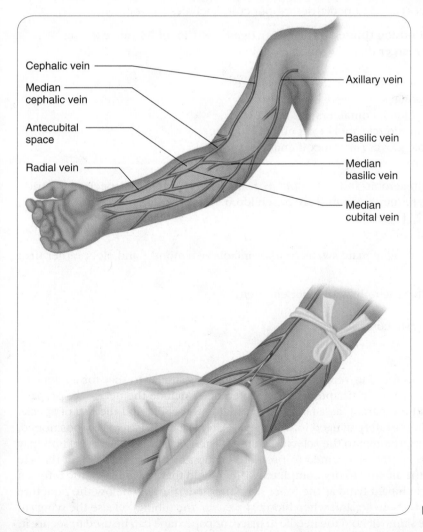

Cephalic vein

Median cephalic vein

Antecubital space

Radial vein

Axillary vein

Basilic vein

Median basilic vein

Median cubital vein

FIGURE ■ 10-24 Veins in the Arm

and are chosen for most toddlers and children. If a venipuncture is done on a child younger than age 2, the site should be limited to a superficial vein. Some studies have indicated that venipuncture, when performed by a skilled health care worker, appears to be the method of choice for blood sampling for neonates, as it is less painful and can provide adequate blood for testing.[14,15] Other sites used for venipuncture are the medial wrist, the dorsum of the foot, the scalp, and the medial ankle. Always check the policy at your facility before performing venipuncture on foot or ankle veins. If the neonate or child is receiving fluid or medication intravenously, the distal veins should be avoided for phlebotomy and preserved for IV therapy. Venipuncture is indicated for blood sampling for routine laboratory tests, erythrocyte sedimentation rate (ESR), blood cultures, cross-matching, coagulation studies, and drug and ammonia levels. Do not use veins in an extremity or area with edema or infection or if an IV line is present. Avoid deep veins in a child with hemophilia or other bleeding disorders.

Precautions

Remove the tourniquet before withdrawing the needle. Apply pressure with the gauze sponge for three minutes to prevent a hematoma. Do not use alcohol pads to apply pressure, as they will cause stinging and prevent hemostasis. Equipment of choice for venipuncture on a small child is a winged safety butterfly needle.

Equipment for Venipuncture

The equipment necessary for a pediatric venipuncture includes the following:

1. Winged safety infusion (butterfly) needle (21 gauge × 1 in. or 23 gauge × ¾ in.)
2. Syringes slightly larger than the volume of blood needed
3. Paper tape
4. 70% isopropyl alcohol swab in a sterile package
5. 2" × 2" gauze sponges
6. Appropriate specimen containers
7. Pediatric-size tourniquet (nonlatex if child is allergic)
8. Sterile disposable gloves (nonlatex if child is allergic)
9. For blood culture:
    a. Bottles, both aerobic and anaerobic. For smaller children, use a special pediatric bottle. The required volumes are for children ages 2 to 12, 2 to 4 mL; for infants under age 2, 1 mL.
    b. Iodine swabs
    c. Chlorhexidine gluconate swabs (use for infants two months and older rather than iodine)
10. Bandage strip (for use only with older children)
11. Marking pens
12. Biohazardous waste container

Procedure

The procedure for performing venipuncture on children is similar to that for adults (see Performing a Venipuncture in Chapter 8). The differences include the necessary preparation of the child and the parent, assistance in restraining the child, and the use of special pediatric-size needles or safety winged infusion sets. After the child is securely positioned, place the tourniquet proximal to the selected vein to distend it. If necessary, the limb may be lowered, rubbed gently, or warmed to promote dilation of the vein. Disinfect the site thoroughly. Allow the alcohol to dry completely. Then, hold the two wings of the infusion set together in the dominant hand as the other hand pulls taut the skin below the puncture site. After inserting the needle, and when blood appears in the tubing, release the wings of the infusion set. The skin will hold the needle in place, or paper tape can be used to secure it.

Gently aspirate the syringe until the required amount of blood is collected. Release the tourniquet and apply pressure over the puncture site with a gauze pad as the infusion set is quickly removed. Ask the parent or the nurse to hold pressure on the site until the bleeding stops. A colorful bandage strip may be used on an older child. Remove the syringe from the safety butterfly set after the needle safety guard has been engaged. Then attach the syringe to a safety syringe shielded transfer device (see Figure 6–7, page 140) for safe transfer of blood to the collecting tubes.

Geriatric Patients

The elderly, or geriatric, population is growing at an amazing rate, with 75 million United States citizens (those born between 1946 and 1964 and known as the baby boomer generation) swelling the ranks. With the life expectancy in the United States improving dramatically due to medical advances, many of these baby boomers will live into their 90s and maybe to 100. Thus, health care workers will be providing health care services for patients that have various types of chronic diseases and disorders (i.e., diabetes, cardiovascular diseases, chronic obstructive pulmonary disease [COPD], arthritis, etc.) (Figure 10-25 ■). Physical conditions, such as arthritis, **Parkinson's disease** (a disease causing tremors), **Alzheimer's disease (AD)** (a disease causing loss of intellectual abilities and mood disorders such as depression and combativeness), and other debilitating diseases in elderly persons will continue to increase point-of-care testing by skin puncture because of the difficulty of obtaining blood by venipuncture. In addition, this patient population will increasingly need point-of-care testing and other health care services in their homes, nursing homes, rehabilitation centers, and other long-term-care facilities (i.e., where the length of stay is over 30 days).

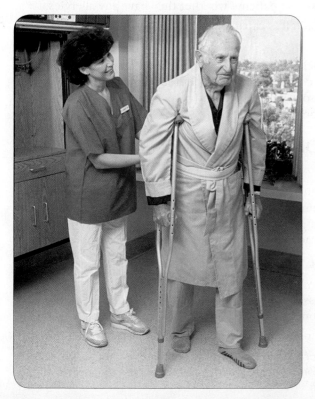

FIGURE ■ 10-25 Increasing Geriatric Population in the United States
The number of elderly citizens is rapidly increasing because of the advancing age of the baby boomer generation.

The process of aging presents physical and emotional problems that can be challenging for health care workers. Whatever the situation, treat elderly individuals with the utmost respect and dignity. Physical problems that are common in older individuals include the following:

- Hearing loss may cause embarrassment and frustration. Repeating instructions or facing the patient to speak in the "good" ear may be necessary for the patient to truly understand a procedure.

- Impaired verbal communication due to a stroke, Parkinson's disease, Alzheimer's disease, or other chronic condition.

- Failing eyesight is common, so take care to guide the elderly individual to the appropriate seat for blood collection or to the bathroom for urine collections.

- Loss of taste, smell, and feeling can accompany the aging process. Elderly people may lack an appetite, which may lead to malnourishment and dehydration. They may tend to drop things or not be able to make a fist because of muscle weakness. Make a note of these clues, particularly if the patient is homebound without a caregiver.

- Memory loss can affect the patient's ability to take medications or to remember the last time he or she ate. These factors may interfere with the interpretation of laboratory results.

- Skin tissue becomes thinner, thereby making venipuncture more difficult. Hold the skin extra taut so that the vein does not "roll." Also, do not "slap" the arm when trying to locate the vein. This causes bruising. Use of heated compresses can be helpful.

- Muscles become smaller, so the angle of penetration of a venipuncture needle may need to be more shallow.

- Increased susceptibility to accidental hypothermia (a subnormal drop in body temperature) can make the elderly patient feel cold. Thus, specimen collection may require warming of the site.

- Increased sensitivities and allergies—ask patients whether they have any allergies.

- Anxiety related to becoming older and less capable of performing everyday living activities.

Emotional problems that are associated with aging include the possible loss of career, spouse, close friends, or relatives and can be reflected by depression or anger at life in general. Remember to address elderly persons with dignity and respect by using Mr., Mrs., Miss, and so on. Also respect the patient's privacy.

CONSIDERATIONS IN HOME CARE BLOOD COLLECTIONS

Because many elderly people have limited mobility and are unable to travel to a health care clinic, it is becoming increasingly common for health care workers to travel to homes to collect blood for diagnostic and treatment purposes. If specimens are to be collected in homes, all procedures are similar to those already covered except that health care workers should:

- Take extra supplies and equipment, including biohazard containers for disposables and a temperature-regulated specimen transport container, into the home.

- Positively identify the patient if possible. If not possible, develop and follow the procedures of the health care organization.

- Place the patient in a comfortable, preferably reclining, position in case of fainting.

- Carry a hand disinfectant with other supplies and equipment and use the disinfectant on your hands before collecting blood. Locate a bathroom for access to handwashing.

- Wait for the puncture site to stop bleeding, because many elderly patients take medications that prolong bleeding (i.e., coumadin and heparin).

- Carefully inspect the area after the procedure to ensure that all trash and used supplies have been properly discarded.

- Carefully label the specimens and place them in leakproof containers with the biohazard sign on the container. Check the appropriate temperatures for transport. Locate a bathroom for access to handwashing.

- When working in high-crime areas, take security precautions, travel with a mobile phone, and carry maps or GPS to avoid getting lost on the way to or from the patient's home.

- Carefully document delays in returning specimens to the laboratory.

Chapter 8, Venipuncture Procedures, and Chapter 9, Capillary Blood Specimens, also provide procedures that apply to the elderly patient. In these blood collections, factors to consider for older patients are the types of blood collection equipment to use. For example, using a safety butterfly needle is usually more appropriate for the elderly patient's fragile veins. Consider the physiological situation of each geriatric patient in the decision to obtain a quality blood specimen for laboratory tests.

Self Study

Study Questions

For the following questions, select the one best answer.

1. Physical frailties that may affect elderly individuals include all of the following except:
   a. loss of taste, smell, and feeling
   b. memory loss about taking medications
   c. skin tissue becomes thicker
   d. susceptibility to hypothermia

2. EMLA, sometimes used for pediatric venipuncture procedure, is a:
   a. local anesthetic applied with a small needle to the child's arm before venipuncture
   b. topical anesthetic applied to the child's arm before venipuncture
   c. topical lotion applied to the child's arm before venipuncture to stop bleeding at the venipuncture site
   d. topical lotion applied to the child's arm before venipuncture to assist the phlebotomist in finding a vein

3. Which of the following is the specimen of choice for testing the pH, pO_2, and pCO_2 of the blood?
   a. venous blood
   b. skin puncture blood
   c. arterial blood
   d. heparinized plasma

4. Which of the following supplies is needed to collect blood for capillary blood gases from a newborn infant?
   a. tourniquet
   b. lidocaine
   c. metal filing
   d. syringe

5. Which of the following is a debilitating disease causing loss of intellectual abilities and mood disorders such as depression, particularly in elderly individuals?
   a. anemia
   b. Parkinson's disease
   c. Alzheimer's disease
   d. polycythemia

6. Which of the following supplies is needed to collect blood for a pediatric venipuncture?
   a. safety lancets
   b. plastic capillary tubes
   c. plastic capillary tube sealers
   d. safety winged infusion set

7. Which of the following is a complication that can result from multiple deep heelsticks on an infant?

a. hepatitis A

b. osteomyelitis

c. pneumonia

d. HIV infection

8. Blood spot testing for neonatal screening disorders should be performed before the newborn is:

a. 12 hours old

b. 24 hours old

c. 48 hours old

d. 72 hours old

9. Venipuncture in an infant and/or toddler is recommended for which of the following blood tests?

a. hematocrit

b. blood cultures

c. hemoglobin

d. fasting glucose

10. When a skin puncture is performed on an infant, which of the following specimens is collected first?

a. chemistry specimens

b. hematology specimens

c. clinical immunology specimens

d. blood bank specimens

Case Study

The phlebotomist, Maria Gibbons, must collect blood from a 3-day-old newborn baby, Baby Hernandez. This infant is to have surgery in two days. The physician has requested laboratory testing for CBC, creatinine, and ABO group and Rh typing.

Questions

In addition to the total blood collection process, including proper identification:

1. What is the proper order of collection for these laboratory tests?

2. What other record must be written down for possible future reference?

Advocating Patient Safety Case Study

Barbara Sherlock, a 6-year-old child who has had numerous blood collections due to a thyroid disorder, is known to become uncooperative (even after proper steps have been followed to gain cooperation) and will attempt to kick and thrash sometimes during blood collections.

Question

In order to avoid risk of injury to the child or phlebotomist, what would be the best approach for the blood collection attempt?

Competency Assessment

Check Yourself: Ready to Collect Blood from a 6-Month-Old Child

1. List the equipment that is needed on a blood collection tray to collect blood from a 6-month-old child.

2. After you have introduced yourself in a confident manner and then properly identified the patient (6-month-old child), describe the preparation steps for the blood collection procedure.

Competency Checklist: Pediatrics and Geriatrics

This checklist can be completed as a group or individually.

(1) Completed (2) Needs to improve/Repeat lesson and checklist

_____ 1. Lists blood collection equipment necessary for a capillary blood gas collection from a newborn infant.

_____ 2. Identifies four physical problems that are common in the elderly that can challenge blood collection efforts.

_____ 3. Lists three important considerations in blood collection from within an elderly patient's home.

References

1. London ML, Ladewig P, Ball J, Bindler R, Cowen KJ: *Maternal and Child Nursing Care.* Upper Saddle River, NJ: Prentice Hall, 2011.

2. Clinical and Laboratory Standards Institute (CLSI): Accuracy in Patient and Sample Identification: Approved Guideline GP33-A. Wayne, PA: CLSI, 2010, p.4.

3. Markenson D: *Pediatric Prehospital Care.* Upper Saddle River, NJ: Prentice Hall, 2002.

4. Schechter N, et al.: *Reducing the Anxiety and Pain of Injections: A Guide for Managing the Pediatric Patient.* Franklin Lakes, NJ: Becton Dickinson, 1998.

5. Mitchell A, Waltman PA: Oral sucrose and pain relief for preterm infants. *Pain Manag Nurs* 2003;4(2):62–9.

6. Gradin M, et al.: Pain reduction at venipuncture in newborns: oral glucose compared with local anesthetic cream. *Pediatrics* 2002;110:1053–7.

7. Lindh V, Wiklund U, Blomquiat HK, Hakansson S: EMLA cream and oral glucose for immunization pain in 3-month-old infants. *Pain* 2003; 104(1–2):381–8.

8. Centers for Disease Control and Prevention: CDC guideline for hand hygiene in health-care hygiene in health-care settings. *MMWR Recomm Rep* 2002;RR-16:51.

9. Reiner CB, Meites S, Hayes JR: Optimal depths for skin puncture of infants and children as assessed from anatomical measurements. *Clin Chem* 1990;36(3):547–9.

10. Jain A, Rutter N: Ultrasound study of heel to calcaneum depth in neonates. *Arch Dis Child Fetal Neonatal Ed* 1999;80(3):F243–5.

11. Vertanen H, Fellman V, Brommels M, Viinikka L: An automatic incision device for obtaining blood samples from the heels of preterm infants causes less damage than a conventional manual lancet. *Arch Dis Child Fetal Neonatal Ed* 2001;84:F535.

12. Meites S, Hamlin CR, Hayes JR: A study of experimental lancets for blood collection to avoid bone infection of infants. *Clin Chem* 1992;38:908–10.

13. Clinical and Laboratory Standards Institute (CLSI): *Blood Collection on Filter Paper for Newborn Screening Programs;* Approved Standard, 5th ed. Wayne, PA: CLSI Document LA4-A5, 2007.

14. Ogawa, S, Ogihara, T, Fujiwara, E, Ito, K, Nakano, M, et al.: Venipuncture is preferable to heel lance for blood sampling in term neonates. *Arch Dis Child Fetal Neonatal Ed.,* 2005; 90(5): F432–436.

15. Shah, VS, Ohlsson, A: Venepuncture versus heel lance for blood sampling in term neonates. *Cochrane Database Syst Rev.* 2007, Issue 4. Art.No.: CD001452. DOI:10.1002/14651858.CD001452.pub3

Chapter 11

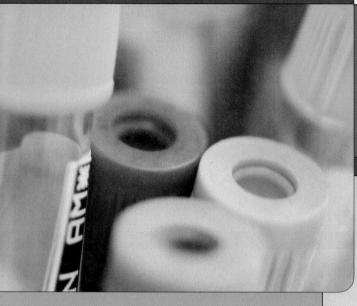

Special Collections

CHAPTER OBJECTIVES

Upon completion of Chapter 11, the learner should be able to do the following:

1. List the steps and equipment used in blood culture collections.
2. List two other terms that are synonymous with point-of-care testing.
3. Describe the most widely used applications of point-of-care testing.
4. Define quality assurance and its requirements as related to point-of-care testing.
5. Discuss the requirements for glucose testing and glucose tolerance tests.
6. Differentiate cannulas from fistulas.
7. Explain the special precautions and types of equipment needed to collect arterial blood gases.
8. List three types of urine specimen collections and differentiate the uses of the urine specimens obtained from these collections.
9. Differentiate therapeutic phlebotomy from homologous transfusion.

KEY TERMS

arterial blood gases (ABGs)
bacteremia
blood cultures
cannula
clean-catch midstream
creatinine clearance test
culture and sensitivity (C&S)
diabetes mellitus
fevers of unknown origin (FUO)
fistula
glucose tolerance test
modified Allen test
patient-focused testing
point-of-care testing
postprandial glucose test
quality control material
septicemia
sodium polyanethole sulfonate (SPS)

Depending on the specific needs of individual clinical settings, health care workers may be required to perform a variety of special tests or procedures in addition to routine skin punctures and venipunctures. This chapter presents the basic techniques and precautions for various special tests and urine collections. Extensive training is required before performing these procedures because they can harm the patient if performed incorrectly.

Blood Cultures

Blood cultures are often collected from patients who have **fevers of unknown origin (FUO).** Sometimes during the course of a bacterial infection in one location of the body, **bacteremia** (presence of bacteria in the blood) or **septicemia** (presence of pathogens in the circulating bloodstream, sometimes called *blood poisoning*) may result and become the dominant clinical feature. Septicemia is a major cause of death in the United States.[1] Blood cultures aid in identifying the specific bacterial organism causing the infections. Blood culture collections have to be performed with extreme and meticulous care and aseptic techniques. Every precaution should be taken to minimize the percentage of contaminated blood cultures that occur, usually because of poor collection technique and skills.[2]

Venipuncture is the method used for collecting blood specimens for blood cultures (see Procedures 11-1 ■, 11-2 ■, 11-3 ■, 11-4 ■, and 11-5 ■). Indwelling catheter collections for blood cultures are **not** recommended because of high contamination results. Important differences in a blood culture procedure relate to the following:

- The health care worker must explain the procedure in greater detail to the patient.
- The puncture site must be decontaminated so that it is sterile.
- The type of collection tubes used must contain culture media that enable bacteria to grow under laboratory conditions.
- The timing and number of blood cultures obtained must be clearly indicated, as well as the location of the venipuncture.

POSSIBLE INTERFERING FACTORS

- If blood culture collections are ordered along with other laboratory tests, blood culture specimens must be collected first. If an evacuated blood collection tube is used prior to the blood culture bottles or SPS evacuated tubes for blood cultures, the needle can become contaminated and cause falsely positive results.
- When the needle enters the venipuncture site, it should *not* be scraped across the skin, as this can contaminate the needle and, thus, the blood cultures.
- The anaerobic blood culture bottle must be inoculated first in all procedures except the butterfly assembly method, because injection of air into the anaerobic bottle can cause the death of some anaerobic microorganisms and result in a false-negative culture.
- Some culture bottles contain resin beads that neutralize antibiotics already in the patient's blood specimen. If these vials are not gently mixed to neutralize the antibiotics in the blood, the antibiotics can inhibit bacterial growth and cause false-negative blood culture results.
- Sometimes two sets of blood cultures are ordered, and the second set should be obtained in the same manner as the first, except that the second venipuncture should be at a different site (i.e., the other arm) and/or at a different time (i.e., 60 min. later).

■ If using a tube holder/needle assembly for evacuated tubes, there is a possibility that media from the culture bottle might flow backward into the vein (reflux action). Therefore, most manufacturers recommend that the media collection bottles not be filled directly from a tube holder/needle assembly. The blood should be collected through a butterfly attached to a tube holder or directly into a syringe.

Procedure 11-1

Site Preparation for Blood Culture Collection

RATIONALE

To obtain a sterile puncture site because bacteria normally located on the skin can contaminate a blood culture if it is not properly cleaned before the venipuncture.

EQUIPMENT

■ Personal protective equipment, gloves (recommended sterile gloves for aseptic technique), clean uniform, and laboratory coat

■ Isopropyl alcohol preps

■ 2 iodine-tincture scrub swab sticks or chlorhexidine gluconate swab sticks (2 packages)

■ 2 blood culture bottles (1 for anaerobic microorganisms and 1 for aerobic microorganisms) (2 bottles/set collected)

■ Sodium polyanethole sulfonate (SPS) evacuated tubes

■ Safety needles (21- or 23-gauge) or blood collection set

■ Safety sterile syringe or evacuated safety tube assembly and blunt-tipped cannula for syringe and direct-draw holder/adapter

■ Sterile gauze pads

■ Nonlatex bandages

■ Nonlatex tourniquet

■ Patient identification labels/requisitions

■ Pen

■ Plastic ziplock specimen bags

■ Biohazard waste container

PREPARATION

1 Identify the patient properly. Explain the test to the patient.

2 Wash or sanitize your hands with an alcohol hand rinse, don gloves (nonlatex if patient has latex allergy), and prepare and assemble equipment and supplies next to the patient. Offer to answer any questions for the patient. Place the tourniquet on the arm.

PROCEDURE

3 Locate the vein, loosen the tourniquet, scrub the site of the venipuncture with 70% isopropyl alcohol for 60 seconds to rid the site of excess dirt, and then scrub with the iodine tincture (chlorhexidine gluconate for patients sensitive to iodine or for infants older than two months)

for at least 30 seconds. The iodine swab should initially be placed at the site of needle insertion and then moved outward in concentric circles to a diameter of approximately 2.5 inches, as shown in Figure 11-1 ■. Scrub with friction.

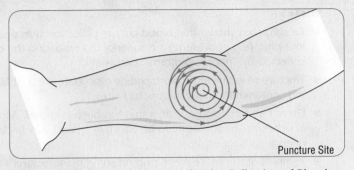

Puncture Site

Figure ■ **11-1** Arm Preparation for the Collection of Blood Culture Specimens

(4) Some health care facilities use a blood culture preparation kit that has a one-step application (e.g., Hi-Lite Orange ChloroPrep). The application has chlorhexidine gluconate/isopropyl alcohol antiseptic combined for an effective 30-second cleansing of the venipuncture site (Figure 11-2 ■).

Other blood culture preparation kits are also available commercially (Figure 11-3 ■).

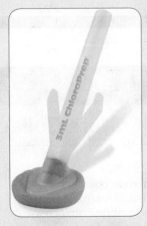

Figure ■ **11-2** One-Step 30-Second Application for Blood Culture Venipuncture Preparation
Source: Courtesy of Cardinal Health, Leawood, KS

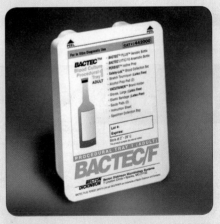

Figure ■ **11-3** BACTEC Blood Culture Procedural Tray
Source: Courtesy and © Becton, Dickinson and Company Microbiology Systems, Sparks, MD

AFTER THE PROCEDURE

(5) Collect the blood culture by vacuum tube, syringe, or safety butterfly assembly.

(continued)

Procedure 11-1

Site Preparation for Blood Culture Collection *(continued)*

NOTES

- Research has shown that blood culture collection sites prepared using iodine tincture instead of iodophor (e.g., povidone) are superior in combating the contamination of sites where cultures are collected by "nonphlebotomy" personnel.[3]

- Tincture of iodine and chlorhexidine gluconate are probably equivalent in effectiveness for combating contamination of venipuncture sites.[4]

- Do not go back over any area that has been prepped. Allow the area to dry for one to 1.5 minutes in order for the antiseptic to be effective against skin bacteria. Do not blow on the site to speed drying.

- Removal of the entire metal ring on some manufacturer's bottles introduces air into them and can cause contamination.

- Read the manufacturer's directions on blood culture bottles before using them, because they may vary as to the volume of blood specimen needed and their preparation requirements. If the fill line is not marked, place each bottle on a flat surface, and then use a marker to note a "fill-to line." Usually, the fill level is 10 mL/bottle.

- Treat the top of the blood culture bottle as a sterile area, and take care not to contaminate it.

- **Sodium polyanethole sulfonate (SPS)** in the yellow-topped evacuated tube is especially designed for blood culture collections because it inhibits phagocytosis and neutralizes biochemicals that may interfere in the blood culture recovery of microorganisms.

Procedure 11-2

Safety Syringe Blood Culture Collection

RATIONALE

For the safety *sterile* syringe collections, it is commonly recommended to do an adult collection of 20 mL and transfer the first 10 mL to the anaerobic bottle and the remaining 10 mL to the aerobic bottle. Some health care facilities collect a total of up to 30 mL from adults as it has been shown to increase the yield of pathogens.[5]

EQUIPMENT

- Personal protective equipment, gloves (recommended sterile gloves for aseptic technique), clean uniform, and laboratory coat
- Isopropyl alcohol preps
- 2 iodine-tincture scrub swab sticks or chlorhexidine gluconate swab sticks (2 packages)
- 2 blood culture bottles (1 for anaerobic microorganisms and 1 for aerobic microorganisms) (2 bottles/set collected)

- Sodium polyanethole sulfonate (SPS) evacuated tubes
- Safety needles (21- or 23-gauge)
- Safety sterile syringe, blunt-tipped cannula (connector), and direct-draw holder/adapter
- Sterile gauze pads
- Nonlatex bandages
- Nonlatex tourniquet
- Patient identification labels
- Laboratory requisition and pen
- Plastic ziplock specimen bags
- Biohazard waste container

PREPARATION

(1) Identify the patient properly. Explain the test to the patient.

(2) Wash or sanitize your hands with an alcohol hand rinse, don gloves, and prepare and assemble equipment and supplies next to the patient. Offer to answer any questions for the patient. Place the tourniquet on the arm.

PROCEDURE

(3) Locate the vein and loosen the tourniquet. Disinfect the rubber septum on the blood culture bottles with 70% isopropyl alcohol and allow it to dry (manufacturers may differ in how to disinfect culture bottles). Scrub the site of the venipuncture with 70% isopropyl alcohol for 60 seconds to rid the site of excess dirt, and then scrub with the iodine tincture (chlorhexidine gluconate for patients sensitive to iodine or for infants older than two months) for at least 30 seconds. Begin by placing the iodine swab at the site of needle insertion and then move it outward in concentric circles to a diameter of approximately 2.5 inches.

(4) Alert the patient before venipuncture. Reapply the tourniquet, anchor the vein, and smoothly insert the needle, bevel up.

(5) After the collection of the blood into the safety sterile syringe, activate the safety needle cover and aseptically dispose of the needle into the sharps container without touching the needle.

(6) Then, place a blunt-tipped cannula (connector) on the syringe tip and attach the blunt-tipped connector to the direct-draw holder/adapter (Figure 11-4 ∎).

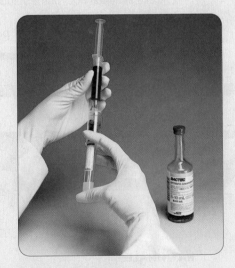

Figure ∎ 11-4

Source: Courtesy and © Becton, Dickinson and Company Microbiology Systems, Sparks, MD

(continued)

Procedure 11-2

Safety Syringe Blood Culture Collection *(continued)*

(7) Starting with the anaerobic microbiology bottle in an upright position, place the blood-transfer device on the bottle, fill to the desired amount, and remove the syringe with the blood-transfer device from the bottle.

(8) If anaerobic and aerobic microbiology bottles are to be filled with the patient's blood, fill the aerobic bottle immediately after the anaerobic bottle, and then fill the other blood collection tubes according to the "order of draw." *Never* push on the syringe plunger. Allow the vacuum in the microbiology bottles and tubes to pull the blood into the bottles and tubes.

(9) If only 3 mL or less of blood are collected, place the entire amount in the aerobic bottle.

(10) For infants and small children, only 1 to 5 mL of blood can usually be collected for bacterial culture. CLSI states that no more than 1% of the patient's total blood volume should be collected.[4] Use blood culture bottles that are designed specifically for the pediatric patient.[6]

Clinical Alert !

- For any of the blood collection procedures, the venipuncture site *must not* be repalpated after the venipuncture site is prepared for blood collection.
- Relocating the vein by repalpation after sterilization recontaminates the site.
- Make a mental note of the vein's location in relation to skin features such as a mole, crease, freckles, and so on.
- If you must repalpate, do not palpate at the actual venipuncture site.

Procedure 11-3

Safety Butterfly Assembly Blood Culture Collection

RATIONALE

To perform a blood culture collection using a safety butterfly.

EQUIPMENT

- Personal protective equipment, gloves (recommended sterile gloves for aseptic technique), clean uniform, and laboratory coat
- Isopropyl alcohol preps

- 2 iodine-tincture scrub swab sticks or chlorhexidine gluconate swab sticks (2 packages)
- 2 blood culture bottles (1 for anaerobic microorganisms and 1 for aerobic microorganisms) (2 bottles/set collected)
- Sodium polyanethole sulfonate (SPS) evacuated tubes
- Safety needles (21- or 23-gauge) or blood collection set
- Evacuated safety tube assembly
- Sterile gauze pads
- Nonlatex bandages
- Nonlatex tourniquet
- Patient identification labels
- Laboratory requisition and pen
- Plastic ziplock specimen bag
- Biohazard waste container

PREPARATION

(1) Identify the patient properly. Explain the test to the patient.

(2) Wash or sanitize your hands with an alcohol hand rinse, don gloves, and prepare and assemble equipment and supplies next to the patient.

(3) Offer to answer any questions for the patient. Place the tourniquet on the arm.

PROCEDURE

(4) Locate the vein and loosen the tourniquet. Disinfect the rubber septum on the blood culture bottles with 70% isopropyl alcohol and allow it to dry.

(5) Scrub the site of the venipuncture with 70% isopropyl alcohol for 60 seconds to rid the site of excess dirt, and then scrub with the iodine tincture (chlorhexidine gluconate for patients sensitive to iodine or for infants older than two months) for at least 30 seconds. Begin with the iodine swab at the site of needle insertion and then move it outward in concentric circles to a diameter of approximately 2.5 inches. Follow manufacturer's directions for disinfection of blood culture bottles.

(6) Alert the patient before venipuncture. Reapply the tourniquet, anchor the vein, and smoothly insert the needle, bevel up.

(7) Use a safety butterfly assembly (safety blood collection set) (see Figure 6-14) for insertion of the butterfly needle into the venipuncture site after the appropriate skin preparation.

(8) It can be helpful to place a strip of tape over the butterfly wings to keep the needle in place as the blood culture bottles are filled with the blood.

(continued)

Procedure 11-3

Safety Butterfly Assembly Blood Culture Collection *(continued)*

(9) Transfer the blood to the microbiology bottles via a direct draw adapter that fits directly over the blood culture bottle (Figure 11-5 ■). The blood culture bottles need to be in a standing position as shown in the figure and, after blood collection, the blood needs to be gently mixed with the culture media.

(10) Using this method, blood is transferred to the aerobic bottle first, because the assembly tubing contains air.

(11) If only 3 mL or less of blood are collected, place the entire amount in the aerobic bottle.

(12) For infants and small children, only 1 to 5 mL of blood can usually be collected for bacterial culture. Use blood culture bottles that are designed specifically for the pediatric patient.[6]

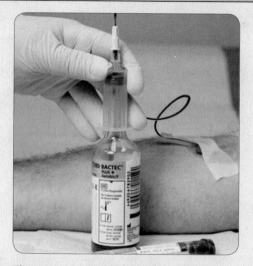

Figure ■ 11-5 Blood Culture Collection Using BACTEC Microbiology Vial with Blood Collection Safety Set
Source: Courtesy of Becton Dickinson and Company, Sparks, MD

Procedure 11-4

Evacuated Tube System for Blood Culture Collection

RATIONALE

To perform a blood culture collection using an evacuated tube system.

EQUIPMENT

- Personal protective equipment, gloves (recommended sterile gloves for aseptic technique), clean uniform, and laboratory coat
- Isopropyl alcohol preps
- 2 iodine-tincture scrub swab sticks or chlorhexidine gluconate swab sticks (2 packages)
- 2 blood culture bottles (1 for anaerobic microorganisms and 1 for aerobic microorganisms) (2 bottles/set collected)

- Sodium polyanethole sulfonate (SPS) evacuated tubes
- Safety needles
- Single-use evacuated tube holders
- Sterile gauze pads
- Nonlatex bandages
- Nonlatex tourniquet
- Patient identification labels
- Laboratory requisition and pen
- Plastic ziplock specimen bags
- Biohazard waste container

PREPARATION

(1) Identify the patient properly. Explain the test to the patient.

(2) Wash or sanitize your hands with an alcohol hand rinse, don gloves, and prepare and assemble equipment and supplies next to the patient. Offer to answer any questions for the patient. Place the tourniquet on the arm.

PROCEDURE

(3) Locate the vein, loosen the tourniquet, scrub the site of the venipuncture with 70% isopropyl alcohol for 60 seconds to rid the site of excess dirt, and then scrub with the iodine tincture (chlorhexidine gluconate for patients sensitive to iodine or for infants older than two months) for at least 30 seconds. Initially place the iodine swab at the site of needle insertion and then move it outward in concentric circles to a diameter of approximately 2.5 inches.

(4) Alert the patient before venipuncture. Reapply the tourniquet, anchor the vein, and smoothly insert the needle, bevel up.

(5) After performing a venipuncture by evacuated tube system, collect blood into the SPS tubes and then fill other tubes, as required (see Chapter 8, "Venipuncture Procedures," for additional information).

NOTE

Collecting blood directly into blood culture bottles with a needle holder designed for collecting blood into evacuated tubes is *not* recommended because of the risk of reflux of the culture media back into the vein and also because the amount of blood collected into the bottle cannot be controlled.

(6) The blood from an SPS tube can be transferred to the blood culture media.

Procedure 11-5

After Blood Culture Collection by the Previous Methods

PROCEDURE

(1) At the patient's bedside, label each culture bottle or tube with the specific site of specimen collection. Ask the patient to double check his or her name on the labels if possible.

(2) After collecting the blood, remove the iodine from the patient's skin with an alcohol prep. If chlorhexidine is used as the antiseptic, it does not have to be cleaned from the skin after the venipuncture is complete unless it is suspected that the patient may have an allergic reaction to it.[4]

(3) Document the following: (a) date and time specimen obtained, and (b) site of specimen collection.

(4) Discard the safety needle, evacuated tube holder/needle assembly, or butterfly blood collection set in the sharps biohazardous container.

(5) Discard blood-soaked gauze pads, contaminated items, and gowns or gloves used in isolation rooms in appropriate biohazardous waste containers as discussed in Chapter 4.

(6) Dispose of gowns and gloves that are not from isolation rooms in the appropriate containers.

(7) Wash or sanitize your hands.

(8) Thank the patient for cooperating and depart with all specimens and all remaining supplies. Do not leave anything at the patient's bedside.

(9) Deliver the blood specimens immediately to the laboratory.

The health care provider must initial the patient identification labels, indicate the time and date of collection on the labels, indicate the site of collection (i.e., right arm, left arm), and attach a label to each vial or tube.

Clinical Alert !

- For any of the blood collection procedures, the venipuncture site *must not* be repalpated after the venipuncture site is prepared for blood collection, even if the gloved forefinger is cleansed.
- Relocating the vein by repalpation after sterilization recontaminates the site. If palpation of the site prior to puncture is anticipated, wear *sterile* gloves.
- Make a mental note of the vein's location in relation to skin features such as a mole, crease, freckles, and so on.
- If you must repalpate, do not palpate at the actual venipuncture site.
- Microbiology culture bottles *must* be held upright during the venipuncture collection to avoid reflux of culture media into the patient.

Changing needles should *not* occur after collecting blood for culture, because it can lead to a needlestick injury to the health care worker. Careful skin cleansing has been shown to be the important factor in minimizing the specimen contamination rate.[7] Also, performing a venipuncture at a skin site that is obviously infected increases the chance of contamination of the blood culture.

Clinical Alert !

Never use the safety butterfly set without a direct draw adapter for the transfer of blood to the bottles. If the needle is not covered in this transfer of blood to the bottles, the needle poses a risk of accidental needlestick as it is pushed into the bottle.

Also, it is important to check with the manufacturers of blood collection safety-holder/needle devices before attempting blood culture collections, as some of these devices do not accommodate the blood transfer to blood culture bottles. It is important to use a blood transfer device that is compatible with the safety-holder/needle device to avoid a needlestick injury.

Glucose Tolerance Test (GTT)

The American Diabetes Association's "Standards of Medical Care in Diabetes—2011" recommends that for patients who have symptoms suggesting problems in carbohydrate (i.e., sugar) metabolism, such as **diabetes mellitus,** the **2-hour oral glucose tolerance test (OGTT or GTT)** can be an effective diagnostic tool.[8] When an OGTT is to be performed, the patient should be given complete information about the procedure so that his or her cooperation can be ensured (Box 11-1 ■).

For best results, the patient should:

1. Eat normal, balanced meals for at least 3 days before the test
2. Fast for 8–12 hours before the beginning of the test
3. Drink water
4. *Do not* drink unsweetened tea, coffee, or any other beverage during fasting or during the procedure
5. *Do not* smoke, chew tobacco, or chew gum (including sugarless gum) during the fasting time or during the procedure. (NOTE: If a patient is chewing gum before or during this procedure, note this on the requisition form, because chewing gum may interfere with the test results.)

The test is performed by first obtaining a fasting blood specimen. The fasting blood specimen should be taken to the laboratory for test results. Then the patient can be given a standard load of dextrose (glucose) (e.g., a liquid drink called Glucola), and subsequent blood and urine samples can be obtained at intervals, over a 2-hour period. If the fasting specimen is abnormal, the physician must be notified before giving the load of glucose. Each specimen is then analyzed for its glucose content. In general, glucose levels should return to normal within 2 hours after ingestion of the glucose. During the test, the patient drinks a standard dose of glucose: 75 grams for adults, approximately 1 gram per kilogram of body weight for children and small adults. A dose of 75 grams is recommended for the diagnosis of gestational diabetes.[8] Gestational diabetes occurs during pregnancy, usually during the second or third trimester (see the section on the Postprandial Glucose Test). Commercial preparations of glucose are available as flavored drinks to make the glucose more palatable. The patient must start and finish the drink within 5 minutes. Water intake is encouraged throughout the procedure. If the patient should vomit at any point in the procedure, the physician should be notified immediately to decide whether the test should be continued or stopped.

When the patient finishes drinking the solution, the time is noted, and 30-, 60-, and 120-minute blood specimens are obtained.

Examples of timed blood collections for OGTT are as follows:

■ Fasting specimen obtained and sent to the laboratory (lab result, okay to proceed with OGTT)

■ Glucose load given (i.e., Glucola) at 7:00 A.M.

| BOX 11-1 | Sample Patient Information Card |

PATIENT INFORMATION CARD: GLUCOSE TOLERANCE TEST INTRODUCTION

A glucose tolerance test (GTT) has been ordered by your physician. The purpose of a GTT is to test the efficiency of your body's insulin-releasing mechanism and glucose-disposing system.

You must prepare your body for the GTT by changing your eating and medication routines slightly for 3 days before the test. It is very important that you follow the instructions below in order for accurate results to be obtained.

Basically, you will need to follow these three guidelines to prepare for your GTT test:

1. Your carbohydrate intake must be at least 150 g per day for 3 days before the GTT.
2. Do not eat anything for 8 hours before the GTT, but do not fast for more than 12 hours before the test.
3. Do not exercise for 12 hours before the GTT.

PREPARATION: MEDICATION

Before proceeding with the GTT, you must tell your physician whether you are currently using any of the following medications, because they may interfere with test results:

- Alcohol
- Anticonvulsants (seizure medication)
- Blood-pressure medication
- Clofibrate
- Corticosteroids
- Diuretics (fluid pills)
- Estrogens (birth control pills or estrogen replacement pills)
- Salicylates (aspirin, pain killers)—only if taken in high doses, such as for rheumatoid arthritis

PREPARATION: DIET AND EXERCISE

Remember that for 3 days before your test, your diet must contain at least 150 g of carbohydrates per day. The following is a list of high-carbohydrate foods:

- **Milk and milk products**—12 g of carbohydrates per serving. One serving is equal to 8 oz. of milk (whole, skim, or buttermilk), 4 oz. of evaporated milk, or 1 cup of plain yogurt.
- **Vegetables**—5 g of carbohydrates per serving. One serving is equal to 1/2 cup of any vegetable, excluding starches (e.g., potatoes, corn, or peas).
- **Fruits and fruit juices**—10 g of carbohydrates per serving. One serving is equal to 1/2 cup of juice, 1 small piece of fresh fruit, or 1/2 cup of unsweetened canned fruit, with the following exceptions:

Apple juice	1/3 cup
Grape juice	1/4 cup
Raisins	2 Tbsp.
Watermelon	1 cup
Prunes	2 medium
Banana	1/2 small
Dates	2
Cantaloupe	1/4 6-inch melon
Honeydew melon	1/8 7-inch melon

BOX 11-1	Sample Patient Information Card *(cont.)*

- **Breads and starches**—15 g of carbohydrates per serving. One serving is equal to 1 slice of bread or 1 small roll. Other one-serving sizes are:

Bagel/English muffin	1/2
Tortilla	1
Cooked cereal	1/2 cup
Dry cereal	3/4 cup
Cooked rice, noodles, and pasta	1/2 cup
White potatoes, dried beans, and peas	1/2 cup
Yams	1/4 cup
Corn	1/3 cup
Crackers	5–6

- **Meats, cheeses, and fats**—These foods contain few or no carbohydrates.
- **Miscellaneous**

Ice cream	1/2 cup	15 g of carbohydrates
Sherbet	1/2 cup	30 g of carbohydrates
Gelatin	1/2 cup	30 g of carbohydrates
Jams and jellies	1 Tbsp.	15 g of carbohydrates
Sugar	1 tsp.	4 g of carbohydrates
Carbonated beverage	6 oz.	20 g of carbohydrates
Hard candy	2 pieces	10 g of carbohydrates
Fruit pie	1/6 pie	60 g of carbohydrates
Cream pie	1/6 pie	50 g of carbohydrates
Plain cake	1/10 cake	30 g of carbohydrates
Frosted cake	1/10 cake	38 g of carbohydrates

PREPARATION: GENERAL HEALTH

The following physical conditions should be reported to your doctor because they too may affect the results of your test:

Acute pancreatitis

Adrenal insufficiency

Diabetes mellitus

Hyperinsulinemia (excess insulin secretion, resulting in hypoglycemia)

Hyperthyroidism

Hypopituitarism (decreased function of pituitary gland)

Pregnancy

Stress

If you have any difficulty making the necessary alterations in your diet or medication schedule, please inform your doctor. For accurate test results, the instructions on this card must be followed.

Source: Courtesy of Division of Laboratory Medicine, University of Texas M. D. Anderson Cancer Center, Houston, TX.

- 1/2-hour specimen at 7:30 A.M.
- 1-hour specimen at 8:00 A.M.
- 2-hour specimen at 9:00 A.M.

The tubes should be labeled with the time as well as "30 minutes," "1st hour," and so on. Upon collection, each specimen should be sent to the laboratory for immediate testing. Venous blood is the preferred specimen for glucose tolerance tests, because normal glucose values are determined using venous blood. If serum samples are collected, the serum separator tube should be used. The grey-topped tubes have a preservative and can also be used for this procedure.

POSSIBLE INTERFERING FACTOR

The health care worker must be prepared to handle a situation when the patient becomes ill from drinking the glucose. Nausea and vomiting may occur early during the OGTT, and it is a good idea to have towels and a basin nearby. If the patient vomits within the first 30 minutes, the test should be discontinued and will probably need to be rescheduled for another day. If the patient vomits or becomes faint later in the test, have him or her lie down and complete the testing. You do not want the patient in a position (i.e., sitting in a regular chair) where he or she may faint and fall and be injured.

Postprandial Glucose Test

The 2-hour **postprandial** (after a meal) **glucose test** can be used to screen patients for diabetes, (including gestational diabetes), because glucose levels in serum specimens collected 2 hours after a meal are rarely elevated in normal patients. In contrast, diabetic patients usually have increased values 2 hours after a meal.

For this test, the patient should be placed on a high-carbohydrate diet for 2 to 3 days before the test. The day of the test, the patient should eat a breakfast of orange juice, cereal with sugar, toast, and milk to provide an approximate equivalent of 75 g of glucose. A blood specimen is taken 2 hours after the patient finishes eating breakfast. The glucose level of this specimen is then determined, and the physician can decide whether further carbohydrate metabolism tests (such as a GTT or Hemoglobin A1c) are needed.

Glucose Monitoring

With the increasing health care requirements of the growing U.S. elderly population, nurses, laboratorians, home health care specialists, and other health care providers will increasingly perform on-site laboratory testing to obtain various types of laboratory test results. The demand for **point-of-care testing** is increasing because rapid turnaround of laboratory test results is necessary for prompt medical decision making.

The other terms used for these direct laboratory services include:

- Decentralized laboratory testing
- On-site testing
- Bedside testing
- Near-patient testing
- **Patient-focused testing**

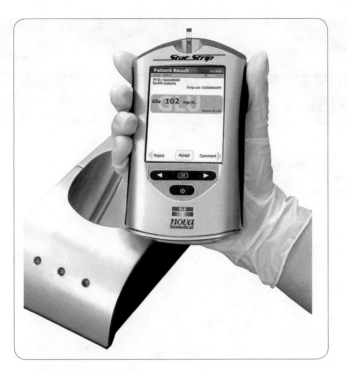

FIGURE ■ 11-6 StatStrip Glucose Analyzer
Source: Courtesy of Nova Biomedical, Waltham, MA

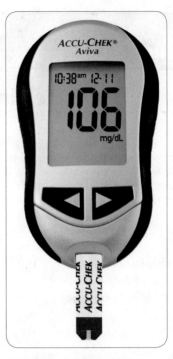

FIGURE ■ 11-7 Blood Glucose Monitor
Many types of glucose meters are available today.
Source: www.Rocheimages.com

During the past decade, small glucose testing instruments such as the one shown in Figure 11-6 ■ became commonplace in the nursing home, and at the hospital bedside. Besides glucose testing, frequently used point-of-care tests include: hemoglobin A1c, Hemoglobin, Influenza A and B, and Cholesterol among many others. These "rapid" methods (Figure 11-7 ■) require whole blood samples collected by skin puncture from the finger, heel (for infants), or a flushed heparin line. As for any blood collection procedure, appropriate safety protocols must be followed (e.g., wearing gloves), and disposal of potentially contaminated waste must be part of the quality control and safety guidelines (see Chapter 4). These bedside procedures are handy for quick screening in a hospital or outpatient setting.

To perform the blood glucose determinations, health care providers need to gather the appropriate supplies (Procedure 11-6 ■) and must be aware of the total quality assurance procedures that are required to obtain accurate and precise results.[9,10] The timing of the reaction is critical, and most of these instruments call the time to the attention of the operator by buzzing, sounding an alarm, or digitally displaying the glucose result. Also, the health care provider needs to know what type of blood—blood from a fingerstick and/or blood from venipuncture—can be used to perform glucose determinations with the point-of-care instrument, and the patient age group for whom the blood instrument can be used.

As an example, the HemoCue Glucose 201 Analyzer (Figure 11-8 ■) is an instrument that can obtain test results from capillary, venous, or arterial whole blood. It uses a microcuvette rather than a test strip and does not require blotting. Also, it can be used to monitor blood glucose in neonates as well as adults and children.

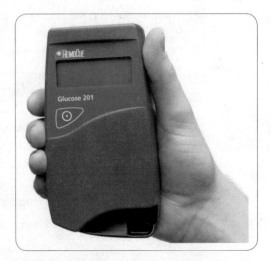

FIGURE ■ 11-8 HemoCue Glucose 201 Analyzer
Source: Courtesy of HemoCue, Inc., Cypress, CA

Procedure 11-6

Obtaining Blood Specimen for Glucose Testing (Skin Puncture)

RATIONALE

One of the most widely used applications of point-of-care testing is blood glucose monitoring, in which commercially available instruments, such as the one shown in this procedure, are used to determine blood glucose levels. Such determinations allow the physician to choose appropriate treatment regimens for patients with diabetes mellitus.

EQUIPMENT

- Gloves
- Safety automatic lancet
- Antiseptic for hand cleansing
- 3 alcohol/acetone or alcohol preps
- Sterile gauze pads
- HemoCue® blood glucose monitor

PREPARATION

(1) Gather equipment: safety automatic lancet.

(2) Identify the patient properly. Briefly explain the test to the patient.

(3) Clean your hands.

(4) Put on gloves.

PROCEDURE

(5) Select the site and cleanse it with antiseptic (especially the side of a finger) (Figure 11-9A ■).

(6) Cleanse the skin with an alcohol wipe (Figure 11-9B ■) and allow the skin to dry.

(7) Without touching the cleansed site, gently massage the finger a few times from base to tip to aid blood flow (Figure 11-9C ■).

(8) Decide on which side of the finger to make the incision (Figure 11-9D ■).

(9) Remove the safety lancet from the protective paper without touching the tip, and, as you hold the patient's finger firmly with one hand, make a swift, deep puncture with the retractable safety puncture device (Figure 11-9E ■).

(10) Wipe the first three drops of blood away with clean gauze (Figure 11-9F ■).

(11) Gently massage the finger from base to tip to obtain the needed drop of blood. Do not squeeze the fingertip, because this can cause hemolysis of the blood sample (Figure 11-9G ■).

(12) Apply the HemoCue® microcuvette to the drop of blood. The correct volume is drawn into the cuvette by capillary action (capillary, venous, or arterial blood can be used) (Figure 11-9H ■).

(13) Wipe off any excess blood from the sides of the cuvette (Figure 11-9I ■).

(14) Place the microcuvette into the cuvette holder and insert it into the photometer (Figure 11-9J ■).

(15) The laboratory test result is displayed automatically (Figure 11-9K ■).

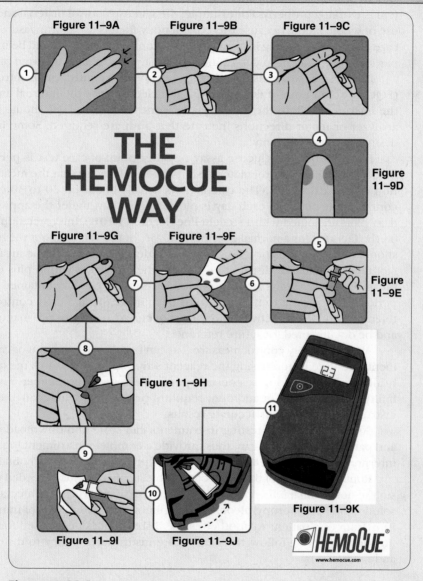

Figure ■ 11-9

Source: Courtesy of HemoCue, Inc., Cypress, CA

AFTER THE PROCEDURE

16 Discard the safety automatic lancet in the sharps container with biohazard label.

17 Discard the gauze, alcohol wipes, and gloves in biohazardous waste containers.

18 Wash or sanitize your hands.

QUALITY IN POINT-OF-CARE TESTING AND DISINFECTING POCT ANALYZERS

As described earlier, glucose-monitoring instruments and instruments that measure other analytes should be monitored daily with **quality control material**. These values must also be monitored whenever a battery is changed or the meter is cleaned. The control material should be similar to the patient's specimen in order to determine whether the analytic system is working properly. For example, the glucose control material should be based on the use of whole blood, because this type of body fluid is used for measurements with point-of-care glucose-monitoring instruments. The control material should be manufactured for that particular instrument to determine if the analytic system is working properly.

In addition, some instruments have automatic control or "electronic quality control" (EQC). The purpose of EQC is to test the electronics—the internal and analyte circuits of the instrument. Both the liquid quality control and the EQC should be performed if the analyzer or meter directions indicate that both are required. Some instruments are now designed to use EQC only.

For each day the glucose assay or other point-of-care test is performed on patients' blood specimens, control material should be analyzed so that the mean and standard deviation can be calculated. The calculations usually occur on 20 to 30 control values.[11] The control value obtained each day is plotted on a chart under the appropriate date, and the daily plots are joined with a straight line (Figure 11-10 ■). Interpretation of this chart is based on the fact that for a normal distribution, 95% of the values about the mean, or average ($\bar{x}$), should be within plus or minus 2 standard deviations (SD) of the mean (average), and the fact that for a normal distribution, 99% of the values are within plus or minus 3 SD of the mean. Tolerance limits are determined by pooling the data obtained during a 30-day test period and referring to the mean plus or minus 2 SD. If a daily control value exceeds the tolerance limits, corrective action *must* occur according to the manufacturer's directions and be documented for future reference.

Another quality control measure that can be taken when point-of-care monitoring instruments are used is purchasing the reagent strips and controls in large quantities that enable health care workers to use constant pools of the same lot number. This leads to reproducibility of the results. In addition, required preventive maintenance of each point-of-care instrument is critical for accurate results.

Some point-of-care testing instruments can store and download calibrators, controls, and patients' results and can, thus, provide a complete instrument log for quality assurance interpretation. Box 11-2 ■ provides a list of problems to avoid to obtain quality results.

Routine cleaning of the point-of-care testing instruments is needed to avoid the transmission of nosocomial infections. Using a cleaning tissue with a disinfectant such as 5% bleach solution or 70% isopropyl alcohol can minimize the possibilities of transferring microorganisms from one patient to another as the instrument is being used for testing. It is recommended to strictly follow the health care institution's policy to disinfect these analyzers and meters.

Blood Coagulation Monitoring

Similar to glucose monitoring, monitoring blood coagulation through point-of-care testing provides immediate results that can be used in monitoring bleeding or clotting disorders in patients. A blood coagulation instrument, such as the new CoaguChek XS System from Roche Diagnostics Corp., is a handheld instrument that can measure prothrombin time (PT) from an unmeasured drop of whole blood, providing results in 1 minute (Figure 11-11 ■).

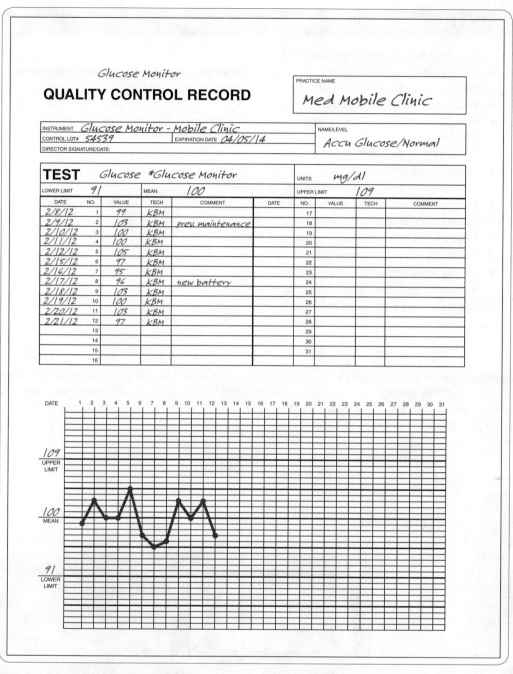

Glucose Monitor

QUALITY CONTROL RECORD

PRACTICE NAME
Med Mobile Clinic

INSTRUMENT *Glucose Monitor - Mobile Clinic*
CONTROL LOT# *54539*　　EXPIRATION DATE *04/05/14*
DIRECTOR SIGNATURE/DATE:

NAME/LEVEL
Accu Glucose/Normal

TEST *Glucose *Glucose Monitor*　　UNITS *mg/dl*

LOWER LIMIT *91*　　MEAN *100*　　UPPER LIMIT *109*

DATE	NO.	VALUE	TECH	COMMENT	DATE	NO.	VALUE	TECH	COMMENT
2/8/12	1	99	KBM			17			
2/9/12	2	103	KBM	prev. maintenance		18			
2/10/12	3	100	KBM			19			
2/11/12	4	100	KBM			20			
2/12/12	5	105	KBM			21			
2/15/12	6	97	KBM			22			
2/16/12	7	95	KBM			23			
2/17/12	8	96	KBM	new battery		24			
2/18/12	9	103	KBM			25			
2/19/12	10	100	KBM			26			
2/20/12	11	103	KBM			27			
2/21/12	12	97	KBM			28			
	13					29			
	14					30			
	15					31			
	16								

FIGURE ■ 11-10 Quality Control Record

The CoaguChek XS System can be used by home health care providers or other outpatient clinic providers to monitor long-term anticoagulation therapy in patients. The immediate test results allow rapid dose adjustments. Again, the health care provider using these instruments must be trained appropriately in the preventive maintenance and quality control parameters to obtain accurate results. Also, reading the manufacturer's directions is essential. For example, the CoaguChek XS System is calibrated to use the first drop of blood in skin puncture. Another point-of-care coagulation system is the Actalyke XL

> **BOX 11-2** | **Problems to Avoid in Point-of-Care Testing**
>
> - Specimen is inappropriately stored.
> - The blood is contaminated with alcohol. (After alcohol is used to cleanse the skin puncture site, the skin must dry completely before puncturing the site.)
> - Wrong volume of specimen is collected.
> - Instrument blotting/wiping technique is not performed according to manufacturer's directions.
> - Instrument is not clean.
> - Reagents are outdated.
> - Timing of the analytic procedure is incorrect.
> - Reagents are not stored at the proper temperature, leading to their deterioration.
> - Patient has not dieted properly for procedure.
> - Patient's result/time/date/and so on is mislabeled.
> - Recording of result is incorrect.
> - Battery for instrument is weak or dead.
> - Calibrators and/or controls are not properly used and/or recorded.
> - Results are not sent to the appropriate individuals in a timely manner.

Activated Clotting Time Test (ACT) System (Figure 11-12 ■). The Actalyke XL is designed to monitor heparin therapy during cardiac procedures and dialysis. Actalyke instruments and reagent tubes provide the sensitivity, reliability, and rapidity needed to make timely treatment decisions at the point of care.

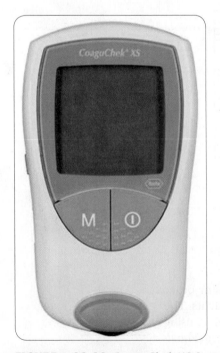

FIGURE ■ 11-11 CoaguChek XS System

Source: Courtesy of Roche Diagnostics Corp. Indianapolis, IN

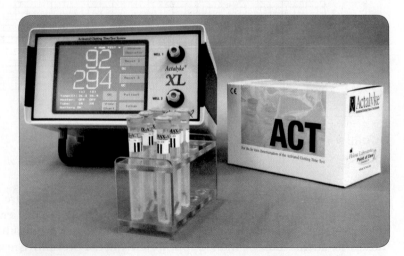

FIGURE ■ 11-12 Actalyke XL Activated Clotting Time Test (ACT) System

Source: Courtesy of Helena Laboratories Point of Care, Beaumont, TX

The INRatio2 Meter (Figure 11-13 ■) is used to measure prothrombin time (PT)INR for maintenance of proper anticoagulation therapy. These instruments are designed for use at the patient's point of care (i.e., home, intensive care unit, and physician's office) to monitor anticoagulation therapy such as heparin or warfarin sodium (Coumadin).

Hematocrit, Hemoglobin, and Other Hematology Parameters

The hematocrit (Hct, packed cell volume [PCV], or Crit) represents the volume of circulating blood that is occupied by red blood cells (RBCs). It is expressed as a percentage; thus, a hematocrit value of 38% indicates that 38 mL of each 100 mL of peripheral blood is composed of RBCs. Hematocrit values are obtained to aid in the diagnosis and evaluation of anemia, a less-than-normal number of erythrocytes. Blood collection usually occurs by skin puncture, as described in Chapter 9. For accurate test results, remember not to squeeze the tissue to obtain capillary blood because doing so will dilute the sample with tissue fluid. It is very important to follow the healthcare facility's procedures. Plastic microcapillary tubes must be used to avoid the possibility of bloodborne pathogen exposure from a broken tube.

Determining a patient's hemoglobin level is another test to aid in the diagnosis and evaluation of anemia and other blood abnormalities. The hemoglobin test has been determined by the American Medical Association (AMA) to be more accurate than the hematocrit test in diagnosis and treatment. Also, the hemoglobin procedure is a safer method for the detection of anemia. A point-of-care analyzer that can be used to measure hemoglobin is the HemoCue Hb201+ System (Figure 11-14 ■). A patient's venous, capillary, or arterial whole blood sample placed in the microcuvette and inserted into this instrument provides the patient's hemoglobin value.

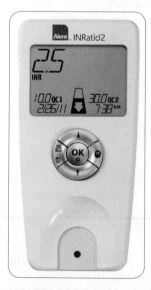

FIGURE ■ 11-13 INRatio2 Meter
Source: Courtesy of Alere: Physician Diagnostics Group

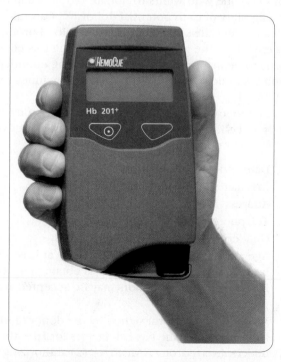

FIGURE ■ 11-14 HemoCue Hb201+ Analyzer
Source: Courtesy of HemoCue, Inc., Cypress, CA

Cannulas and Fistulas

A **cannula** is a tubular instrument that is used in patients with kidney disease to gain access to venous blood for dialysis or blood collection. Blood should be collected from the cannula of these patients only by *specially trained personnel,* because the procedure requires special techniques and experience.

A **fistula** is an artificial shunt in which the vein and artery have been fused through surgery. It is a permanent connection tube located in the arm of the patients undergoing kidney dialysis. Only *specialized personnel* can collect blood from a fistula. The health care worker should use extreme caution when collecting a blood specimen from these patients and avoid using the arm with the fistula as the site for venipuncture. If no other location can be found for the venipuncture site, the patient's arm must be cleaned thoroughly before blood collection. If the venipuncture site in this arm becomes infected, the inflammation in the blood vessels of the arm may shut down all the veins, requiring surgery to place a new shunt in the patient.

Donor Room Collections

Properly trained health care providers may be employed in a regional blood center or a hospital blood donor center to screen and collect blood from donors. Only an experienced, properly trained health care worker or technologist should be considered for this function, because a physical, emotional, or traumatic experience may keep a donor from volunteering in the future.

DONOR INTERVIEW AND SELECTION

Not everyone who wants to donate blood is eligible, so the interviewer must determine the eligibility of each potential donor.[12,13] Carefully determining donor eligibility not only helps prevent the spread of disease to blood product recipients but also prevents untoward effects on the potential donor. During this eligibility process, the health care worker needs to be in a private area for obtaining confidential donor information, and the questioning should occur in a very pleasant manner for the donor wanting to donate his or her blood.

The following confidential information on every donor should be kept on file indefinitely and is initially obtained from every prospective donor, regardless of the acceptability of his or her donation:

1. Date and time of donation
2. Last name, first name, and middle initial
3. Address
4. Telephone number
5. Gender
6. Age and birth date (Donors should be at least 17 years of age; however, minors may be accepted if written consent is obtained in accordance with applicable state law. Elderly prospective donors may be accepted at the discretion of the blood bank physician.)
7. Written consent form signed by the donor (1) allowing the donor to defer from being a donor if he or she has risk factors for HIV, the causative agent of acquired immunodeficiency syndrome (AIDS), or (2) authorizing the blood bank to take and use his or her blood

8. A record of reasons for deferrals, if any

9. Social security number or driver's license number (May be used for additional identification but is not mandatory; these data are needed for information to be retrieved in some computerized data systems.)

10. Name of patient or group to be credited, if a credit system is used

11. Race (not mandatory, but this information can be useful in screening patients for a specific phenotype [chromosomal makeup])

12. Unique characteristics about a donor's blood (Donated blood that is negative for cytomegalovirus or that is Rh-negative group-O blood is used for neonatal [infant] patients.)

To help minimize the incidence of dizziness, fainting, or other reactions to blood loss, donors are encouraged to eat within 4 to 6 hours of donating blood. Eating a light snack just before the phlebotomy may help prevent these reactions, but a donor should not be required to eat if he or she does not want to do so.

Blood bank records must link each component of a donor unit (red blood cells [RBCs], white blood cells [WBCs], platelets, etc.) to its disposition. If the donation is a "replacement for credit" for a particular patient, the donor must supply the patient's name or the group name that is to be credited.

A brief physical examination is required to determine whether the donor is in generally good condition on the day when he or she is to donate blood. The physical examination is actually a few simple procedures that are performed by the health care worker:

1. Weight. Donors must weigh at least 110 lb (50 kg); if the weight is less, the volume of blood donated must be carefully monitored and care taken that not too much blood is collected. Also, the anticoagulant in the bag must be modified for the lesser donation. Most blood banks will not routinely accept donors who weigh less than 110 lb.

2. Temperature. The donor's oral temperature must not exceed 37.5°C (99.5°F). Lower than normal temperatures are usually of no significance in healthy individuals; however, they should be repeated to verify the lower temperature.

3. Pulse. The donor's pulse should be regular and strong, between 50 and 100 beats per minute. The pulse should be taken for at least 15 seconds.

4. Blood pressure. The systolic blood pressure should measure no higher than 180 mm Hg, and the diastolic blood pressure should be no higher than 100 mm Hg. People with blood pressure outside these limits should be deferred as donors and referred to their physicians for evaluation of a possible health problem.

5. Skin lesions, piercings, and tattoos. Both arms should be examined for signs of drug abuse, such as needle marks or sclerotic veins. The presence of mild skin disorders, such as a poison ivy rash, does not necessarily prohibit an individual from donating unless the lesions are in the antecubital area or the rash is particularly extensive. The skin at the site of the venipuncture must be free of lesions. If the donor has had piercings or tattoos, he/she should wait 12 months if there is any question whether or not the instruments were sterile and free of blood contamination. This requirement is related to concerns about hepatitis.

6. General appearance. If the donor looks ill, excessively nervous, or under the influence of alcohol or drugs, he or she should be deferred.

7. Hematocrit or hemoglobin values. The hematocrit value must be no less than 38% for donors. The hemoglobin value must be no less than 12.5 g/dL. A fingerstick is commonly used to draw blood for such determinations.

8. An extensive medical history must be taken for all potential donors, regardless of the number of previous donations on record. Most blood bank donor rooms have a simple card listing all the questions to be asked and "yes" or "no" columns that are used to indicate the donor's responses. The health care provider should refer to the protocol of the donor room at the institution's blood bank or the AABB technical manual, which sets guidelines for donor screening and acceptance.

COLLECTION OF DONOR'S BLOOD

The health care worker in a donor room must operate under the supervision of a qualified, licensed physician. Blood should be collected by using aseptic technique; a sterile, closed system; and a single venipuncture. If a second venipuncture is needed, an entirely new, sterile donor set is necessary; the first is discarded according to the biohazard disposal requirements of the institution.

A donor should never be left alone either during or immediately after blood collection. The health care worker should be well versed in donor reactions, equipment safety precautions, first-aid techniques, and the location of first-aid equipment in case it is needed during the course of donation.

Sometimes a patient must have the intentional removal of blood for treatment of a disorder. When a patient is obviously ill, his or her physician or the medical director of the blood bank should be present during this therapeutic phlebotomy. Generally, the patient should be bled more slowly than a healthy donor, and the resting period should be lengthened.

The blood obtained through therapeutic bleeding may be used for homologous transfusion if the unit is deemed to be suitable by the director of the blood bank. If it is to be used, the recipient's physician must agree to use the blood from his or her patient, and a record of the agreement should be kept. The unit is then labeled and processed in the usual manner. The label must indicate that the blood is the result of a therapeutic bleed and must include the patient's diagnosis. If the unit is unsuitable for transfusion, the entire unit is disposed of in the usual manner for contaminated wastes.

Arterial Blood Gases

Arterial blood gases (ABGs) provide useful information about the respiratory status and the acid-base balance of patients with pulmonary (lung) disease or disorders.[14] In addition, critically ill patients with other diseases, such as diabetes mellitus, benefit from ABG measurement (i.e., pH, pCO_2, pO_2) which is used to help manage their electrolyte and acid-base balance. Arterial blood rather than venous blood is used because arterial blood has the same composition throughout the body tissues, whereas venous blood has various compositions relative to metabolic activities in body tissues. Capillary blood gases are used for infants, and the procedure is covered in Chapter 10, "Pediatric and Geriatric Procedures."

Arterial puncture to obtain arterial blood for blood gas evaluation requires skill and knowledge of the technique. A health care provider must undergo extensive training on arterial punctures, including demonstration of the procedure, observation, and, under the supervision of a qualified instructor, several performances on patients.

RADIAL ARTERY PUNCTURE SITE

When an ABG analysis is ordered, the experienced health care worker should palpate the areas of the forearm where the artery is typically close to the surface. The radial artery, located on the thumb side of the wrist (as shown in Figure 11-15 ■) is the artery most frequently used for blood collection for ABG analysis.

Using your index and middle fingers, palpate the pulses from the radial artery about 1 inch above the wrist (Figure 11-15). This artery has widespread collateral flow, which means that the hand area is supplied with blood from more than one artery. Arterial blood flows into the hand from both the radial and the ulnar arteries. In addition, the radial artery lies over ligaments and the bones of the wrist and can be easily compressed to lessen the chance of a hematoma during the procedure. A drawback to using the radial artery is its small size.

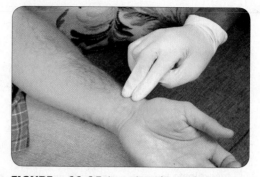

FIGURE ■ 11-15 Locating the Radial Artery

BRACHIAL AND FEMORAL ARTERY PUNCTURE SITES

The brachial artery is an alternative site for blood collection for ABG analysis. The brachial artery is in the cubital fossa of the arm, as shown in Figure 11-16 ■.

> **Clinical Alert !**
>
> The pulse of the brachial artery may be felt at the fold of the elbow on the little finger side of the arm. Puncture of a vein is a possibility because the brachial artery is close to the veins. The brachial artery lies close to the median nerve, which can be accidentally punctured.

Another choice, the femoral artery, is the largest artery used in ABG collections. It is located in the groin area of the leg, lateral to the femur bone, as shown in Figure 11-16. Even though the brachial and femoral arteries are larger than the radial artery, they are used less frequently because they lack collateral circulation. A four-year study on blood collections from the brachial artery has demonstrated that brachial artery puncture is an acceptably safe procedure and a reasonable alternative to radial artery puncture.[15] The femoral artery is sometimes used on patients with cardiovascular disorders. The possibility of releasing plaque from the inner wall of the artery in geriatric patients, however, is a definite disadvantage of using the femoral artery as a puncture site. Usually, the femoral artery is the last choice for an arterial puncture site, and the health care provider must have expertise in obtaining blood from this artery.

To use the radial artery for blood collection for ABG analysis (Procedure 11-7 ■), the health care provider must first perform the modified Allen test to make certain that the ulnar and radial arteries are providing collateral circulation (see Figure 11-17). The **modified Allen test** is performed as follows: (1) the health care provider compresses both arteries with the index and middle fingers, and the patient is asked to tightly clench his or her fist; (2) the patient is then asked to open his or her hand, and the health care provider releases the pressure on the ulnar artery; and (3) the hand should fill with blood within 5 to 10 seconds—if so, the Allen test is positive for collateral blood flow. If color does not return to the hand after 5 to 10 seconds, the Allen test is negative. A negative Allen test indicates the inability of the ulnar artery to supply blood to the hand adequately and shows a lack of collateral circulation. Thus, the radial artery should not be used in a negative Allen test, as this artery might be accidentally damaged during puncture, resulting in total lack of blood flow to the hand.

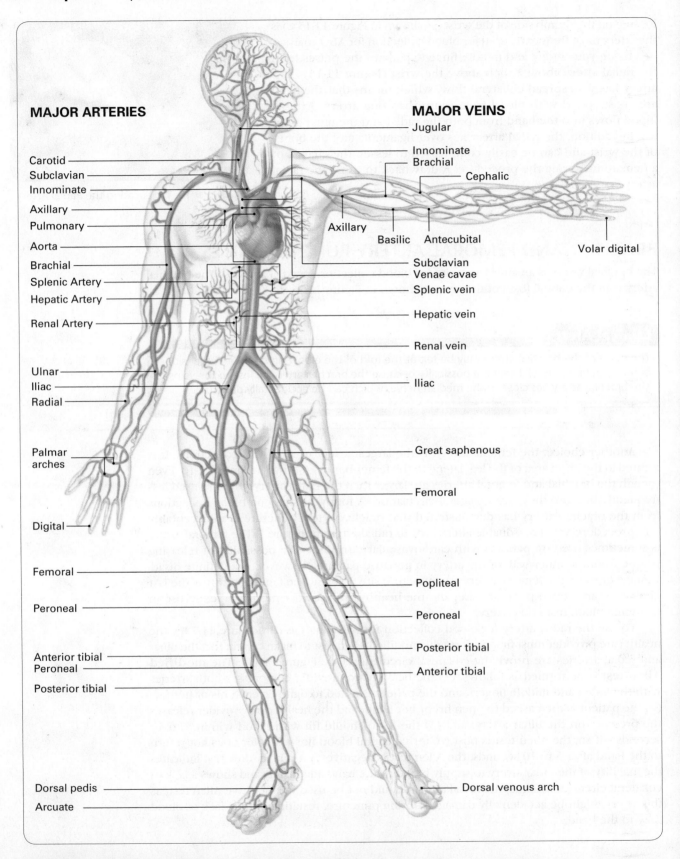

MAJOR ARTERIES

Carotid

Subclavian

Innominate

Axillary

Pulmonary

Aorta

Brachial

Splenic Artery

Hepatic Artery

Renal Artery

Ulnar

Iliac

Radial

Palmar
arches

Digital

Femoral

Peroneal

Anterior tibial

Peroneal

Posterior tibial

Dorsal pedis

Arcuate

MAJOR VEINS

Jugular

Innominate

Brachial

Cephalic

Axillary

Basilic

Antecubital

Volar digital

Subclavian

Venae cavae

Splenic vein

Hepatic vein

Renal vein

Iliac

Great saphenous

Femoral

Popliteal

Peroneal

Posterior tibial

Anterior tibial

Dorsal venous arch

FIGURE ■ 11-16 Arteries in the Arm and Leg for Puncture Sites

Procedure 11-7

Radial ABG Procedure

RATIONALE

To perform a blood collection for arterial blood gas analysis using the radial artery.

EQUIPMENT

- Tincture of iodine solution or chlorhexidine gluconate
- ½ to 1% lidocaine to numb site
- Prefilled heparinized safety syringe, 1 to 5 mL (especially designed *plastic syringe* for collections for ABG analysis)

(Collection with a plastic syringe requires the sample to be transported at room temperature and analyzed within 30 minutes. If analysis will occur after a 30-minute delay from collection, collect the blood in a *glass syringe* and transport it in a slurry of ice water.)

- Safety needles (20- to 22-gauge, for collections for ABG analysis)
- Safety needles (25- to 26-gauge, for lidocaine administration)
- Safety syringe for lidocaine administration (1- or 2-mL plastic syringe)
- Gauze squares to be held on site after puncture
- Plastic bag or cup with crushed ice and water
- Patient identification label
- Laboratory requisition
- Waterproof ink pen
- Alcohol pad
- Adhesive bandage strip
- Oxygen-measuring device to record on laboratory requisition the oxygen concentration on patient receiving oxygen
- Thermometer to record patient's temperature on laboratory requisition
- Mask
- Gloves (nonlatex if patient has latex allergy)
- Protective laboratory coat or smock
- Biohazardous waste containers for sharps

PREPARATION

1. Gather and organize the necessary equipment and supplies for a successful arterial puncture.

2. Properly identify the patient and inform him or her of the arterial puncture procedure.

3. Determine that the patient has been in a stable state for at least the previous 30 minutes (i.e., no respiratory changes).

4. Attempt to calm the patient before collecting the specimen if the patient appears anxious. The anxiety can lead to hyperventilation (i.e., rapid breathing), which will falsely alter the ABG levels.

5. Before proceeding, determine whether the patient is receiving anticoagulant therapy or is allergic to iodine or lidocaine, and record the patient's temperature, oxygen concentration from the respirator (if applicable), and respiratory rate.

(continued)

Procedure 11-7

Radial ABG Procedure (continued)

PROCEDURE

(6) Wash your hands; put on gloves, a facial mask, and a protective laboratory coat; and then palpate the radial artery in the forearm. The radial artery in the patient's nondominant hand is usually the best choice.

(7) With the forefinger or first two fingers, press at these sites to find the artery (Figure 11-15). Never use the thumb for palpating because there is a pulse in the thumb that may be confused with the patient's pulse. Avoid any site that has a hematoma or that was previously used for an arterial puncture.

(8) Position the patient's arm with the wrist slightly extended and rotated. Check for adequate collateral circulation using the **modified Allen test** ▶.

A CLOSER LOOK

▶ **Modified Allen Test**

RATIONALE

To use the radial artery for blood collection for ABG analysis, the health care worker must first perform the modified Allen test to make certain that the ulnar and radial arteries are providing collateral circulation (Figure 11-17 ■).[16]

FIGURE ■ 11-17

Modified Allen Test
A. Using the index and middle fingers, the health care worker compresses the patient's ulnar and radial arteries. The patient tightly clenches his or her fist. B. The patient opens their hand and the health care worker releases the pressure. C. If the patient's hand refills with blood (i.e., color returns) within 5 to 10 seconds, the test is positive; if not, the test is negative.

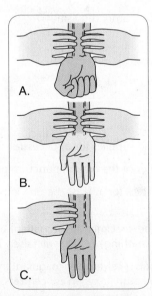

PROCEDURE

(A) Compress both arteries with your index and middle fingers, and ask the patient to tightly clench his or her fist.

(B) Ask the patient to open his or her hand, and release the pressure on the ulnar artery.

(C) The hand should fill with blood within 5 to 10 seconds; if so, the Allen test is positive. If color does not return to the hand after 5 to 10 seconds, the Allen test is negative. A negative Allen test indicates the inability of the ulnar artery to supply blood to the hand adequately and shows a lack of collateral circulation. Thus, the radial artery should *not be used* after a negative Allen test, because this artery might be accidentally damaged during puncture, resulting in a total lack of blood flow to the hand. Select an alternate artery if a negative Allen test occurs.

(9) Once the radial artery site is chosen, clean the area well with tincture of iodine or chlorhexidine. Do not touch the site after it is cleansed.

(10) If the patient desires a local anesthetic, fill a 1-mL syringe with lidocaine and inject the lidocaine with the 25- to 26-gauge needle subcutaneously around the anticipated puncture site.

(11) No tourniquet is required because the artery has its own strong blood pressure. Use a prefilled heparinized safety syringe (1 to 5 mL) with a needle to withdraw the sample.

(12) Hold the syringe or collection device in one hand as one would hold a dart, pull the skin taut with a finger of the other hand over the artery, and pierce the pulsating artery at a high angle, usually 30 to 45 degrees against the bloodstream (Figure 11-18 ■). Little or no suction is needed, because the blood pulsates and flows quickly into the syringe under its own pressure.

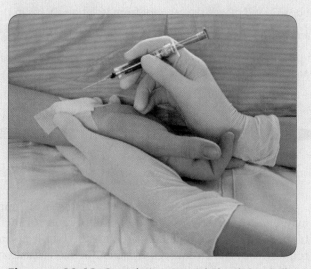

Figure ■ **11-18** Completing Arterial Blood Gas Collection
Source: Courtesy of Radiometer America, Inc.

(13) When approximately 1 mL of blood is collected, withdraw the needle carefully to avoid introducing bubbles into the syringe. Apply gauze and direct manual pressure on the site for at least five minutes.

(14) Engage the safety syringe cover to cover the needle exposure, gently mix the blood in the syringe with the heparin, and label the syringe. Mix the blood gently by inverting the syringe at least five times.

(continued)

Procedure 11-7

Radial ABG Procedure *(continued)*

(15) Before leaving the patient, clean the puncture site with an alcohol pad to remove the excess iodine or chlorhexidine solution; leave a pressure bandage on the site.

(16) If bleeding from the site persists, apply more manual pressure and ring for assistance from the patient's primary nurse. Never leave a patient who is bleeding, particularly after an arterial puncture.

AFTER THE PROCEDURE

(17) Notify the primary nurse after an arterial puncture is performed so that the area may be checked frequently for deep or superficial bleeding.

(18) Discard blood-soaked gauze pads, contaminated items, and gowns or gloves used in isolation rooms in appropriate biohazardous waste containers as discussed in Chapter 4, "Safety and Infection Control."

(19) Dispose of gowns and gloves that are not from isolation rooms in the appropriate containers.

(20) Wash or sanitize your hands.

(21) Thank the patient for cooperating and depart with all specimens and all remaining supplies. Do not leave anything at the patient's bedside.

(22) Deliver the blood specimen with the laboratory test request to the laboratory immediately.

Arterial blood results for some analytes (e.g., ammonia, glucose, lactic acid, alcohol) may differ from venous blood results because of metabolic activities. Therefore, arterial blood samples should be collected for the blood gas measurements only when specifically requested by the attending physician. In such situations, the requisition must indicate that arterial blood was collected for the analytes.

Urine Collections

In addition to collecting and transporting blood specimens, health care workers usually are involved in the collection and/or transportation of urine and other body-fluid specimens. The health care worker should be careful when transporting body fluids because they are difficult to obtain and because the quality of the clinical laboratory test result is only as good as the specimen that is collected and transported to the testing site. Also, because such specimens may be biohazardous, the health care worker must adhere to standard precautions (see Chapter 4, "Safety and Infection Control") during the collection and transportation of these specimens. Just as for blood collections, the laboratory request slip must accompany the specimen, and the specimen must be properly labeled with the patient's name, the patient's identification number, the date, the time of collection, the type of specimen, and the attending physician's name. The label should be affixed on the container, NOT the lid, as shown in Figure 11-19 ■.

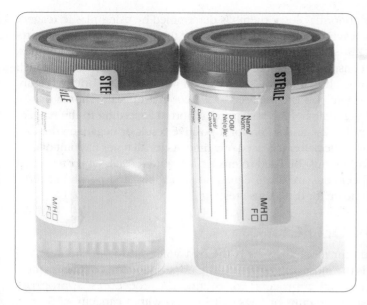

FIGURE ■ 11-19 Urine Collection Container
The label with necessary patient's information should be affixed to the container, NOT the lid
Source: Sylvie Bouchard/ Shutterstock.com

If different patients' urine specimens are in the same location for testing and the labeled lids are taken off the unlabeled containers for testing each urine specimen, it is highly likely that mismatching of the tests' results to the patients will occur.

Routine urinalysis (UA) is one of the most frequently requested laboratory procedures, because it can provide a useful indication of body health. It can be performed on a "first morning" or "random" urine specimen. Some of the more common types of urine specimen collections and their uses are provided in Table 11-1 ■. The routine UA includes a physical, chemical, and sometimes microscopic analysis of the urine sample. The physical properties include the following: color, transparency vs. cloudiness, odor, and concentration as detected through a specific gravity measurement.

Table 11-1	Types of Urine Specimen Collections and Their Uses	
Specimen Type	**Reason for Collection**	**Use**
Random	This type of specimen is most convenient to obtain.	Routine UA
		Quantitative and qualitative
First urine of the morning	This urine excretion is the most concentrated.	Protein, nitrate, microscopic analysis
		Routine urinalysis (UA)
Fasting	Metabolic abnormalities are suspected.	Glucose level determinations for diabetes mellitus testing
Clean-catch midstream	The specimen is free of contamination.	Culture for bacteria and/or microscopic analysis
Timed (e.g., 2 hour, 4 hour, or 24 hour)	The excretion rate of the analyte can be determined.	Creatinine clearance test, urobilinogen determinations, hormone studies
Tolerance test	Timed blood and urine specimens are obtained to detect metabolic abnormalities.	GTT and other tolerance tests

The chemical analysis for abnormal constituents is determined by using plastic reagent strips impregnated with color-reacting substances that test for the presence of glucose, protein, blood (red blood cells [RBCs] and hemoglobin), white blood cells (WBCs), ketones, bacteria, bilirubin, and other constituents (Figure 11-20 ■). The plastic reagent strip, which has a separate reagent pad for each chemical test, is dipped into the urine briefly (Figure 11-21 ■). The color of each reagent pad is compared to a color chart usually shown on the outer label of the reagent strip container. The results are reported according to the reagent label specifications (e.g., trace, 1+, 2+, and so on for a positive result or negative when no reaction occurs). The strip is discarded after it is used one time. As for all types of point-of-care testing, quality control monitoring must be used to ensure accurate results. Other tests that can be performed on urine specimens are the pregnancy, myoglobin, and porphyrin tests. Urine is also the specimen of choice for drug abuse testing.

SINGLE-SPECIMEN COLLECTION

The preferred urine specimen for most analyses is the first voided urine of the morning (Figure 11-22 ■), when urine is the most concentrated. The urine collection containers must be clean and dry before the collection process. For routine UA procedures, appropriate containers include plastic disposable cups or bags (for infants) with a capacity of 50 mL. The containers must be properly labeled (label on container, not the lid), free of interfering chemicals, able to be tightly capped, and leak proof (Figure 11-23 ■).

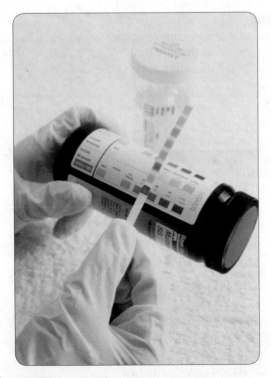

FIGURE ■ 11-20 Chemistry Urine Strip
The chemistry urine strip is used to check urine for ketone bodies. The strip is checked against the chart found on the bottle after dipping the strip into the urine
Source: Faye Norman / Photo Researchers, Inc.

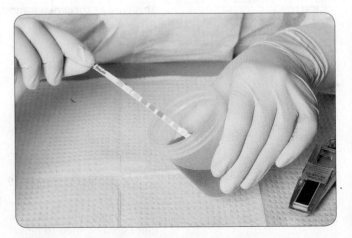

FIGURE ■ 11-21 Dipping the Plastic Urinalysis Strip into the Urine for Chemical Analysis

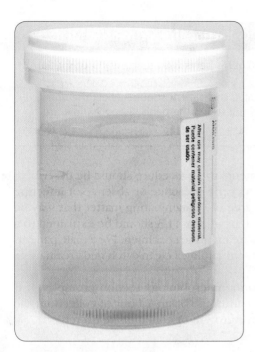

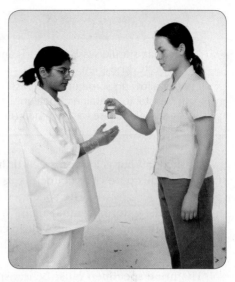

FIGURE ■ **11-23** Patient's Labeled Urine Specimen Given to Health Care Worker
Source: Dorling Kindersley Media Library

FIGURE ■ **11-22** Single Specimen Collection
Urine is most concentrated in the morning
Source: Rob Byron/Shutterstock.com

The specimen should be transported to the UA section promptly for analysis within 30 minutes after the patient voids. If transportation or analysis cannot occur within this time period, the urine should be refrigerated.

Another type of single-specimen urine test is the urine **culture and sensitivity (C&S) test**. This specimen requires a clean-catch midstream urine collection (Box 11-3 ■ and Box 11-4 ■). The patient should be instructed not to urinate for at least an hour before the test and/or to drink a glass of water about 20 minutes before sample collection. This patient preparation will help to ensure that the patient can produce enough urine for the sample. The patient is instructed to void approximately one half of the urine into the toilet, collect a portion in a readily available sterile container, and allow the rest to pass into the toilet.[17]

BOX 11-3	Clean-Catch Midstream Urine Collection Instructions for Women

1. After washing her hands, the woman should separate the skin folds around the urinary opening and clean this area with mild antiseptic soap and water or special towelettes.
2. Holding the skin folds apart with one hand and after urinating into the toilet, the patient should urinate into a sterile container. The container should not touch the genital area. It must be covered with the lid provided after urination. It is extremely important not to touch the inside or lip of the container with the hands or other parts of the body.
3. The health care worker or, sometimes, the patient will label the container with her name and the time of collection and deliver it to the requested location.
4. Health care personnel should refrigerate the urine specimen immediately.

BOX 11-4 | Clean-Catch Midstream Urine Collection Instructions for Men

1. The man should wash his hands and the end of his penis with soapy water or special towelettes and then let it dry.
2. After allowing some urine to pass into the toilet, the patient should collect the urine in the sterile container. The container should not touch the penis. Steps 3 and 4 are the same as those for a woman (Box 11-3).

If asked, "What is a clean-catch urine specimen?" the procedure should be described, stating that this type of specimen is used to detect the presence or absence of infecting (pathogenic) organisms. The specimen must be free of contaminating matter that may be present on the external genital areas. Thus, the steps in Box 11-3 should be explained to a female patient who is to obtain a clean-catch midstream urine specimen. For a male patient, the procedure in Box 11-4 should be adhered to for obtaining a clean-catch midstream urine specimen.

The urine specimen must be transported to the microbiology section promptly. If it cannot be taken to the area for microbiological culturing within 1 hour of collection, the specimen should be refrigerated to prevent an overgrowth of contaminate bacteria.

TIMED COLLECTIONS

For some laboratory assays, such as the **creatinine clearance test,** protein and hormone (e.g., cortisol) studies, 24-hour (or other timed period) urine specimens must be obtained. Incorrect collection and improper preservation of this type of specimen are two frequent errors affecting timed collections. Thus, the health care worker should be aware of the protocol for collecting a 24-hour urine specimen so that he or she can assist other health care professionals and the patient in preventing collection errors. The steps in Procedure 11-8 ■ should be followed for a 24-hour urine collection.[18]

Procedure 11-8

Collecting a 24-Hour Urine Specimen

RATIONALE

To collect a 24-hour urine specimen for a creatinine clearance test, urobilinogen determinations, or hormone studies.

EQUIPMENT

- Wide-mouthed, 3- to 4-liter container with lid and transfer cup
- Preservative, if required
- Label for specimen
- Requisition slip
- Container with ice, if required

Clinical Alert !

To obtain accurate test results, the laboratory needs the ENTIRE 24-hour urine specimen.

PREPARATION

(1) Explain the whole procedure to the patient and also provide written directions. Provide instructions in the patient's native language. Explain the importance of handwashing for the urine collection.

(2) Give the patient the transfer cup, container, and lid. Add any required preservatives to the container before giving it to the patient. Write the preservative and any precautions on the collection container label. Place the label on the container, not on the lid. Include the following information on the label:

- Patient's name
- Patient's identification number
- Starting collection date and time
- Ending collection date and time
- Name of the requested laboratory test

Other information may be required by the facility.

PROCEDURE

(3) Instruct the patient verbally and give them written instructions that the collection of the 24-hour urine specimen begins with emptying the bladder and discarding the first urine passed. This first step in the collection process should start between 6 and 8 a.m., and the exact time should be written (e.g, 7:14a) on the container label. The patient should be instructed to urinate each time in the transfer cup and then place that urine from the cup into the urine container.

(4) Except for the first urine discarded, all urine should be collected during the next 24-hour period. Remind the patient to urinate at the end of the collection period and to include this urine in the 24-hour collection. Tell the patient to urinate before having a bowel movement, because fecal material in the urine specimen will make the specimen unacceptable for collection.

(5) Instruct the patient to refrigerate the entire specimen after adding each collection during the 24-hour period.

(6) Some preservatives for 24-hour urine collection are corrosive if accidentally spilled or if the patient comes into contact with them during collection. Thus, warn the patient of any preservatives in the container.

(7) Inform the patient not to add anything except urine to the container and not to discard any urine during the collection period.

(8) A normal intake of fluids during the collection period is desirable unless otherwise indicated by the physician.

(9) Some laboratory assays require special dietary restrictions; give these instructions to the patient.

(10) If possible, discontinue medications for 48 to 72 hours preceding the urine collection as a precaution against interference in the laboratory assays.

(11) Transport the 24-hour urine specimen to the clinical laboratory as soon as possible. Place the specimen in an insulated bag or a portable cooler to maintain the cool temperature.

Self Study

Study Questions

For the following questions, select the one best answer.

1. What is a cannula?
   a. the fusion of a vein and an artery
   b. a good source of arterial blood
   c. a tubular instrument used to gain access to venous blood
   d. an artificial shunt that provides access to arterial blood

2. What is the first step in the site preparation for a blood culture collection?
   a. choose and wash patient's arm
   b. use an alcohol pad to cleanse the skin on the arm
   c. check the patient's ID according to the health care facility's protocol
   d. don gloves and locate the vein

3. Which of the following tests is measured using the CoaguChek XS system?
   a. glucose
   b. pO_2
   c. PT
   d. pH

4. Which of the following supplies is not needed to test with the HemoCue System?
   a. tourniquet
   b. safety lancet
   c. alcohol swab
   d. gloves

5. What is the reason for collecting a 24-hour urine specimen from a patient?
   a. to test for cortisol
   b. to determine whether the patient can follow the collection instructions
   c. to test for the possibility of a fistula
   d. to test for the creatine level

6. Which of the following evacuated tubes is preferred for the collection of a blood glucose during the GTT?
   a. yellow-topped evacuated tube
   b. green-topped evacuated tube
   c. light blue-topped evacuated tube
   d. gray-topped evacuated tube

7. During a glucose tolerance test, which procedure is acceptable?
   a. a fasting blood collection is performed and then a standard amount of glucose drink is given to the patient
   b. the patient should be encouraged to drink tea, water, or coffee throughout the procedure
   c. the patient is allowed to chew sugarless gum
   d. all of the patient's specimens are timed from the fasting collection

8. Of the two arteries compressed on the patient during the modified Allen Test, which one of those arteries is listed below?
   a. brachial artery
   b. femoral artery
   c. axillary artery
   d. ulnar artery

9. If blood culture collection is requested on a patient that is allergic to iodine, what alternative cleansing solution should be used?
   a. chlorophenol
   b. chlorhexidine gluconate
   c. formaldehyde
   d. 1% phenol

10. When arterial blood is collected for an ABG determination, the needle should be inserted at an angle of no less than
    a. 15 degrees
    b. 30 degrees
    c. 45 degrees
    d. 65 degrees

Case Study

As a health care worker, you provide point-of-care testing for patients in the ambulatory care center. Today, Mrs. Hoover came to the ambulatory care center and had a physician request slip for her PT to be tested. To provide the test, you collected the blood by fingerstick and applied the drop of whole blood from the patient's finger to the analyzer blood collection site for the instrument to provide the result. You waited the required number of minutes for the test result to appear on the instrument's screen, and the screen image printed out "Error in testing."

Question
Provide four possible problems that could have led to this error message.

Advocating Patient Safety Case Study

The phlebotomist, Kellie, at Jersey Clinic provides home health care visits to collect blood and perform point-of-care testing. Kellie has been performing the POC using the CoaguChek for PT on Ms. Winkler's blood every month for the past 8 months. When she tested Ms. Winkler's blood today she discovered she did not have the instrument's disposable cuvette for the blood collection. Because she was 40 miles from the clinic and in a hurry to go back to the clinic, she improvised and used a HemoCue disposable cuvette. The PT result showed an extremely increased result but she decided this was better than not turning any result in on Ms. Winkler to the clinic.

Question
Explain the consequences that could occur from this phlebotomist's actions.

Competency Assessment

Check Yourself: Providing Proper Instructions to a Patient for a 24-Hour Urine Specimen Collection

1. Write out the instructions that you would give to a patient for a proper 24-hour urine specimen collection. Also, include the types of collection containers that are used by the health care facility for this type of collection.

2. Practice giving the instruction to a friend or coworker. Practice your communication techniques by double checking that they are completely understood; ask them to give a constructive critique of your instructions.

Competency Checklist: Special Collections

This checklist can be completed as a group or individually.

(1) Completed (2) Needs to improve/Repeat lesson and checklist

_____ 1. List the dietary instructions that should be given to a patient who is going to have a GTT performed in the next few days.

_____ 2. List 12 equipment items needed for the radial ABG procedure.

References

1. Ruge, D, Sandin, R, Siegelski, S, Greene, J, Johnson, N: Reduction in blood culture contamination rates by establishment of policy for central intravenous catheters. *Lab Med* 2002;33(10):797–800.

2. Weinstein, MP: Blood culture contamination: Persisting problems and partial progress. *J Clin Microbiol* 2003; 41: 2275–2278.

3. Schifman, R, Pindur, A: The effect of skin disinfection material on reducing blood culture contamination. *Am J Clin Pathol* 1993;99: 536–8.

4. CLSI Principles and Procedures for Blood Cultures: Approved Guideline M47-A, Vol 27, No. 17, 2007, p.6)

5. Cockerill, FR III, Wilson, JW, Vetter, FA, et al.: Optimal testing parameters for blood cultures. *Clin Infect Dis.*2004;38:1724–1730.

6. Forbes, B, Sahm, D, Weissfeld, A: *Bailey & Scott's Diagnostic Microbiology.* 11th ed. St. Louis, MO: Mosby Publishers, 2002.

7. O'Hara, C, Weinstein, M, Miller, J: Manual and automated systems for detection and identification of microorganisms. In: Murray, P, Baron, E, Jorgensen, J, Pfaller, M, Yolken, R, eds: *Manual of Clinical Microbiology,* 8th ed. Washington, DC: ASM Press, 2003, 185–207.

8. American Diabetes Association. Standards of Medical Care in Diabetes—2011; December 30, 2010. Vol. 34.no. Supplement 1 S11–S61.

9. Clinical and Laboratory Standards Institute (CLSI): *Quality Management Approaches to Reducing Errors at the Point-of-Care:* Approved Guideline, POCT07-A, 2nd ed. Wayne, PA: CLSI, 2010.

10. Clinical and Laboratory Standards Institute (CLSI): *Glucose Monitoring in Settings Without Laboratory Support.* Approved Guideline, 2nd ed. Wayne, PA: CLSI, 2005.

11. Westgard, J, Klee, G: Quality management. In *Tietz Textbook of Clinical Chemistry and Molecular Diagnostics,* edited by C Burtis, E Ashwood, D Bruns. St Louis: Elsevier/Saunders Publishers, 2006.

12. Roback, JD (Chief Ed): *Technical Manual of the AABB,* 16th ed. Bethesda, MD: AABB, 2008.

13. American Red Cross Blood Donor Eligibility Requirements. http://www.redcrossblood.org/donating-blood/donation-process (Accessed website: 5/4/11)

14. Clinical and Laboratory Standards Institute (CLSI). *Blood Gas and pH Analysis and Related Measurements.* Approved Guideline, 2nd ed., Wayne, PA: CLSI, 2009.

15. Okeson, GC, Wulbrecht, PH: The safety of brachial artery puncture for arterial blood sampling. *Chest,* 1998; 114: 748–751.

16. Clinical and Laboratory Standards Institute (CLSI). *Procedures for the Collection of Arterial Blood Specimens.* Approved Standard, 4th ed. Wayne, PA: CLSI, 2004.

17. Garza, D: Urine collection and preservation. In *Textbook of Urinalysis and Body Fluids,* edited by DL Ross, AE Neely. New York: Appleton-Century-Crofts, 1983:61.

18. Sterns, R (ed): Patient information: Collection of a 24-hour urine collection. UpToDate. www.uptodate.com assessed May 11, 2011.

Appendix Contents

Finding a Job

Finding a job that is a good fit for both the applicant and the employer is a time-consuming, often challenging process. However, the time and effort spent researching and applying for a position can have a wonderful payoff in terms of job satisfaction, salary, benefits, environment, and personal gratification. The keys to finding the right job are to spend time searching, be prepared with documentation and with questions during the interview, and keep an open mind. Here are some essential factors to think about. This list can be used as a checklist for your application process.

Places to Seek Employment	Newspaper, professional journals, and Internet Health care organizations Friends and relatives School faculty and advisors Bulletin boards Employment agencies
Contacting an Employer	Check employers' Websites; research each organization Call for an appointment Send a cover letter (see example on page 300) Send a resume (see example on page 301) Complete a job application (provided by employer); online versions are usually available, if it is handwritten, print legibly
Cover Letter	Use correct spelling State where you heard about the job State the specific job for which you are applying State why you are qualified for this position List a brief summary of your education, experience, and qualifications Refer to your resume Request an interview List your name, address, and phone number
Resume	List the following: Name, address, phone number(s), and email address (Do not list personal data such as age, marital status, height, weight, religion, or national origin. Employers should consider hiring you solely on your job qualifications. Do not send a picture. Do not use abbreviations.) Career plans (provide 1 to 3 statements about your short-term and long-term career goals) Education (list most recent first, followed in reverse chronological order, only high school and beyond)

Work experience (list most recent first, followed in reverse chronological order, part-time or full-time, dates, duration of employment; if there are any gaps in employment, state the reasons for them, e.g., returned to school, left for family responsibilities, etc.)

Specific accomplishments or leadership activities at work or in community activities

Volunteer activities (community services, etc.)

Interests (sports, music, art, theater, hobbies)

Special skills and abilities (non-English language skills, experience with specific patient populations, computer skills with particular software, telephone expertise, use of special equipment, etc.)

Reference names and contact information (always ask permission of those you use as references before listing them)

Interview

Be well groomed and do not chew gum

Dress neatly and professionally

Do not use strong aftershave or perfumes

Be on time or a few minutes early

Silence or turn off your cell phone beforehand

Consider taking a briefcase or professional notebook and pen; offer your own business card if you have one and ask for business cards of those you meet; if you do not have a business card, consider printing a generic card with your contact information. Be prepared to take notes of key duties and major points made during the interview

Greet the interviewer with your name and a smile

Shake hands firmly

Stand until you are asked to sit

Answer questions truthfully and sincerely

Prepare a few questions about the job or organization

Avoid discussing personal problems

Be enthusiastic and maintain eye contact

Do not criticize former employers or teachers

Thank the interviewer for his or her time and leave promptly

After the Interview

Send a thank-you letter or email to the interviewer

If something in your application changes, make the employer aware of it immediately

---

Making a Decision

List advantages and disadvantages of your choices. Rank them based on responsibilities, salary, location, working conditions, benefits, career goals, and your "gut feeling" of the work environment

If you have an offer but are waiting to hear from another employer, it is acceptable to contact them and ask about their timeframe for a decision. If necessary, inform them that you have a firm offer from another employer

Once you have accepted a job offer, inform all those who helped you in your job search (including references) and thank them for their assistance

SAMPLE COVER LETTER FOR JOB INQUIRY

Wanda Jobs
8200 West Jersey Avenue
Lubbock, Texas 79452
511-799-9990
wjobs@nnn.com

January 20, 2012

Ms. Phoebe Thomas
Director, Laboratory Services
Muncy Hospital
P.O. Box 22333
San Antonio, Texas 78277

Dear Ms. Thomas,

I am responding to an advertisement in the *San Antonio Press* on January 5, 2012, for an entry-level phlebotomy technician. I graduated from Lamar High School in 2010. Since then, I have worked part-time and been a part-time student at Hilltop Community College. I recently completed a phlebotomy training program, and my goal is to utilize my skills while pursuing additional studies in laboratory sciences.

I have enclosed my resume, which includes a list of skills and experience. I feel that I am well qualified for this position because of my work with adults and children coupled with my organizational skills. I hope to arrange an interview as soon as is convenient for you. Please feel free to contact me at 511-799-9990 to schedule an interview or for additional information. Thank you.

Sincerely,
Wanda Jobs

SAMPLE RESUME

Wanda Jobs
8200 West Jersey Avenue
Lubbock, Texas 79452
511-799-9990
wjobs@nnn.com

Career Plans	To become an experienced phlebotomist while continuing my education in laboratory sciences
Experience	2011–present Community college phlebotomy student and part-time library assistant; responsibilities include clerical duties (filing, answering multiple telephone lines, word processing), greeting customers, and providing assistance in locating reference materials.
	2009–2010 Part-time caretaker for 3 children; responsibilities included carpooling, providing after-school snacks, assistance with homework, monitoring activities.
	2007–2009 Part-time employee at ABC Grocery; responsibilities included assisting customers in locating products, restocking groceries, checking out grocery items at cash register, assisting with inventory.
Education	2010 Graduated from Lamar High School
Skills/Strengths	Excellent verbal and written communication skills in both English and Spanish Computer skills include proficiency with both MAC and PC, word processing, Internet research, Excel, and PowerPoint
Interests	Reading, camping, art, church youth group, Girl Scouts
References	Available on request

Appendix 2

Units of Measurement and Symbols

The Joint Commission has updated the National Patient Safety Goals that includes a list of "do not use" abbreviations, acronyms, and symbols. This recommendation is to prevent confusion among caregivers when communicating test orders and results. In addition, the Institute for Safe Medication Practices (ISMP) has published a "List of Error-Prone Abbreviations, Symbols, and Dose Designations" with additional abbreviations to avoid. The aim is to eliminate misinterpretations of written information. Using both lists, selected recommendations of terms that may apply to phlebotomy practice have been incorporated into this appendix. However, this list is not exhaustive. For more comprehensive information, consult the organizations' Websites: www.jointcommission.org and www.ismp.org, respectively.

a	alpha		N	normality
Å	angstrom		n	nano- (10^{-9})
amp	ampere (unit of electric current)		ng	nanogram (1/1000 mg)
and	formerly written as symbol &, should now be spelled out		p	pico- (10^{-12})
at	formerly written as symbol @, should now be spelled out		pg	picogram (1/1000 ng)
			QNS	quantity not sufficient
c	centi- (10^{-2})		sec or s	second (unit of time)
°C	degrees centigrade or Celsius (unit of temperature)		sp g	specific gravity
			h	hecto- (10^{2})
cubic centimeter	(same as mL, ml) formerly written as cc, it should now be spelled out, *not* abbreviated		hpf	high-power field on microscope
			international unit	formerly written as IU, it should now be spelled out, *not* abbreviated
cd	candela (unit of luminous intensity)		k	kilo- (10^{3})
cm	centimeter		°K	degrees Kelvin (thermodynamic temperature)
cu mm	cubic millimeter			
d	deci- (10^{-1})		kg	kilogram (1000 g, or 2.2 lb)
discharge	formerly written as D/C, it should now be spelled out, *not* abbreviated		L, l	liter (1000 ml, unit of volume)
			less (greater) than	formerly written as symbols, should now be spelled out
discontinue	formerly written as D/C, it should now be spelled out, *not* abbreviated		lpf	low-power field on microscope
dl	deciliter (1/10 of a liter)		mcg	microgram (1/1000 mg)
°F	degrees Fahrenheit (unit of temperature)		m	meter (unit of length)
			m	milli- (10^{-3})
g or gm	gram (1/1000 of a kilogram, unit of mass)		mCi	millicurie
			mEq or meq	milliequivalent
G%	grams in 100 mL		mg	milligram (1/1000 g)
mOsm	milliosmol		mg%	milligrams in 100 ml (same as dl)

min	minutes		nanoparticles	5–200 nm
mL	milliliter (1/1000 L, same as a cubic centimeter)		TPN	total parenteral nutrition
			TPR	temperature, pulse, respirations
mm	millimeter (1/10 cm)		Unit	formerly written as U, it should now be spelled out, *not* abbreviated
mm^3	cubic millimeter			
mm Hg	millimeters of mercury		WNL	within normal limits
mmole	millimole		WNR	within normal range
mol, M	mole (unit of substance)		Wt	weight
nm	nanometer, one millionth of a millimeter		w/v	weight/volume

---

Clinical Alert !

Trailing Zeros, Decimal Points, Periods, Spacing, and Latin Abbreviations

Be particularly mindful when you are handwriting data or reading handwritten information. The following symbols are often misread and can lead to errors in patient care. If you read symbols that are unclear, you should ask for clarification before proceeding with any type of phlebotomy procedure. Here are tips for preventing errors in interpreting handwritten information.

Trailing zeros	Do not use a zero alone *after* a decimal point because the reader may not notice the decimal point (e.g., 3.0 ml might be mistaken for 30 ml; instead write 3 ml).
Decimal point	Always use a zero before a decimal point when the measurement is less than a whole unit so the reader notices the decimal point (e.g., .5 ml might be mistaken for 5 ml; instead write 0.5 ml).
Periods	Do not use a terminal period after a symbol for a unit of measurement because it may be interpreted as another symbol (e.g., 7 ml. might be mistaken for 7 ml1, which is meaningless; instead write 7 ml).
Spacing	Use adequate space between numbers and letter symbols so that they will not run together (e.g., 8ml might be mistaken as 8001 if the *m* is mistaken for zeros; instead write 8 ml).
Latin abbreviations	Use the exact meaning of words rather than Latin abbreviations (e.g., instead of the terms *q.i.d., q.o.d.,* and *t.i.d.,* write or say *once daily, every other day,* and *three times per day,* respectively).

Military Time (24-Hour Clock)

Military time uses a 24-hour time clock (Figure A3-1 ■) and eliminates the need for the A.M. and P.M. designations that are used in civilian or Greenwich time (12-hour time clock). The 24-hour clock is particularly useful in health care settings so that confusion is eliminated when documenting time for treatment procedures, specimen collections, tests, drug administration, surgical procedures, and so on. It is important that all health care workers understand and use it correctly.

Military time is expressed by four numerals; the first pair is *hours* (00 to 24), and the second pair is *minutes* (00 to 59). Each day begins at midnight, 0000, and ends at 2359.

The first 12 hours are equivalent in Greenwich and military time; that is, 3:00 A.M. is equivalent to 0300 in military time, but conversion of afternoon and evening times from a 12-hour clock to military time requires adding 12 to each hour (2:00 P.M. is 1400 in military time). The following examples illustrate:

1:00 A.M. = 0100	1:00 P.M. = 1300
5:00 A.M. = 0500	4:00 P.M. = 1600
10:00 A.M. = 1000	9:00 P.M. = 2100
11:00 A.M. = 1100	10:00 P.M. = 2200
12:00 noon = 1200	12:00 midnight = 2400/0000

Military time is usually stated in terms of hundreds (e.g., 1500 is stated as "fifteen hundred hours"; 0300 is stated as "zero three hundred").

Reference

Badasch, SA, and Chesebro, DS: *Introduction to Health Occupations, Today's Health Care Worker,* 5th ed. Upper Saddle River, NJ: Prentice Hall Health, 2000.

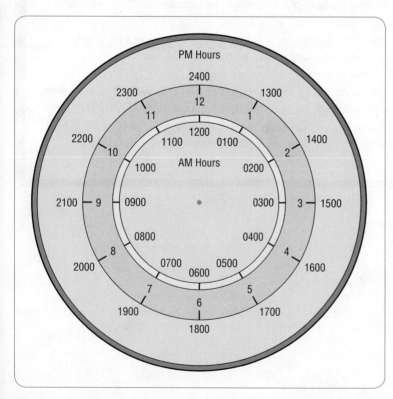

FIGURE ■ A3-1 24-Hour Clock
(Military time is indicated in the light green areas).

Appendix 4

Guide for Maximum Amounts of Blood to Be Drawn from Patients Younger than 14 Years

Patient's Weight		Maximum amount to be drawn at any one time (ml)	Maximim amount of blood (cumulative) to be drawn during a given hospital stay (1 month or less) (ml)
Pounds	Kilograms		
6–8	2.7–3.6	2.5	23
8–10	3.6–4.5	3.5	30
10–15	4.5–6.8	5	40
16–20	7.3–9.1	10	60
21–25	9.5–11.4	10	70
26–30	11.8–13.6	10	80
31–35	14.1–15.9	10	100
36–40	16.4–18.2	10	130
41–45	18.6–20.5	20	140
46–50	20.9–22.7	20	160
51–55	23.2–25.0	20	180
56–60	25.5–27.3	20	200
61–65	27.7–29.5	25	220
66–70	30.0–31.8	30	240
71–75	32.3–34.1	30	250
76–80	34.5–36.4	30	270
81–85	36.8–38.6	30	290
86–90	39.1–40.9	30	310
91–95	41.4–43.2	30	330
96–100	43.6–45.5	30	350

Appendix 5

Basic Spanish for Specimen Collection Procedures

The following translations present the health care worker with a very basic means of communicating with patients who speak Spanish. Before speaking with patients, the health care worker should practice using these phrases with someone who knows the correct pronunciation. Otherwise, the patient may become even more confused. Remember that in Spanish, the letter *h* is always silent. Also, if a word ends in *a,* it is usually feminine gender; if it ends in *o,* it is masculine. Another alternative is to have the key phrases printed on cards that the health care worker may point to or use as a reference when he or she is communicating with the patient. Also, use your hands when speaking; pantomime, point, or use facial expressions to assist in communicating your verbal or written message.

English	Spanish
one, two, three, four, five	uno, dos, tres, cuatro, cinco
six, seven, eight, nine, ten	seis, siete, ocho, nueve, diez
twenty, thirty, forty, fifty	veinte, treinta, cuarenta, cincuenta
sixty, seventy, eighty, ninety, one hundred	sesenta, setenta, ochenta, noventa, ciento/cien
Hello	Hola
Good day	Buenos dias/Buendia
Good morning	Buenos dias
Good afternoon	Buenas tardes
Good evening	Buenas noches
mother, father, sister, brother	madre/mama, padre/papa, hermana, hermano
son, daughter, husband, wife	hijo, hija, esposo/marido, esposa/marida
infant/baby	niño/niña
grandfather, grandmother	abuelo, abuela
friend	amigo/amiga
Mister, Mrs, Miss	Señor, Señora, Señorita
doctor	doctor/medico
technician	técnico
nurse	enfermera
alcohol	alcohol
fasting	enayunas
gloves	guantes
needle	aguja
sterile	estéril
syringe	jeringa

English	**Spanish**
tourniquet	torniquete
pathology	patología
procedure	procedimiento
hematology	hematología
complete blood count (CBC)	biometría hemática complete
blood bank	banco de sangre
coagulated	coagulado
reports	reportes
specimen	muestra
tubes	tubos
My name is . . .	Me llamo . . . /Mi nombre es . . .
I work in the laboratory.	Trabajo en el laboratorio.
I speak . . .	Hablo . . .
We are going to analyze	Vamos analizar
. . . your blood.	. . . su sangre.
. . . your urine.	. . . su orina.
. . . your sputum.	. . . su esputo.
Do you understand?	¿Entiende usted (ud.)?
I do not understand.	No entiendo.
Please (pls.)	Por favor (p.f.)
Thank you	Gracias.
You are welcome	De nada.
Speak slower, pls.	Hable mas despacio, p.f.
Repeat, pls.	Haga me el favor de repetir, p.f.
Can you hear me?	¿Puede oírme?
Can you speak?	¿Puede hablar?
Relax.	Relajese.
What is your name?	¿Como se llama?
What is your address?	¿Que es su domicillo?
What is your birth date?	¿En que fecha nacio?
How old are you?	¿Cuantos años tiene ud.?
Have you been here before?	¿Ha estado ud. aquí antes?
Who is your doctor?	¿Quien es su doctor?
Your doctor wrote the order.	El doctor/la doctora escribio la orden.
Here is the bathroom.	Aquí esta el baño.
Here is the call light.	Aquí esta la luz de emergencia.

English	Spanish
You may not eat/drink anything except water.	No debe de comer/beber nada solamente agua.
You may not smoke.	No puede fumar.
Have you had breakfast?	¿Ya tomo el desayuno?
We need a blood/urine/stool sample.	Necesitamos una muestra de su sangre/orina/del excremento.
Please stay in bed.	Por favor, quédese en la cama.
Do you have any allergies or are you sensitive to any substances? . . . like latex?	¿Tiene usted alergias o es sensible anormal a ciertas sustancias? . . . como el latex?
Have you fainted during blood drawing?	¿Se ha ud desmayado cuando le extrajeron sangre?
Please do not eat after midnight.	Por favor, no coma después de medianoche.
Please	Haga me el favor de
. . . make a fist.	. . . cerrar el puño.
. . . bend your arm.	. . . doblar el brazo.
. . . roll up your sleeve.	. . . levantarse la manga.
. . . open your hand.	. . . abrir la mano.
. . . sit down here.	. . . sientese aquí.
. . . change your position.	. . . cambiarse de posición.
. . . turn over.	. . . voltearse.
. . . change to the left.	. . . cambiarse a la izquierda.
. . . change to the right.	. . . cambiarse a la derecha.
I am going to lift your sleeve.	Voy levantar la manga.
I need to	Necesito
. . . take a blood sample.	. . . sacar una muestra de sangre.
. . . stick/prick your finger.	. . . picarle su dedo.
. . . two tubes of blood.	. . . sacar dos tubos de sangre.
Open your hand.	Abra la mano.
It will hurt a little.	Le va a doler un poquito.
Please do not move.	No se mueva, por favor.
This is done quickly.	Esto se hace rapido.
The needle will stay in your arm while I am collecting the blood sample.	La aguja se quedara en su brazo durante el tiempo necessario para obtener la muestra.
Could you confirm that these tubes are labeled with your name/identity?	¿Podria ud confirmar que estos tubos estan etiquetados con su nombre/identidad?
I am finished. Thank you.	Ya termine. Gracias.

English	Spanish
English	**Spanish**
Press this gauze on your arm/finger until I can make sure that the bleeding has stopped.	Comprese esta banda en su brazo/su dedo hasta que pare la sangre.
I am going to put a bandage on you.	Voy a ponerle una cinta adhesiva/un curita/un bandaid.
Are you lightheaded?	¿Esta usted mareado/mareada?
Do you feel as if you are going to faint?	¿Se siente como si se va a desmayar?
Do you feel all right?	¿Se siente bien?
You must lie down.	Necesita acostarse.
Collect the midstream portion of the urine in the container or bottle.	Coleccione la porción del medio de la orina en el vaso.
Void a little, then put urine in this cup.	Orine un poco, luego ponga la orina en esta taza.

Source: Joyce, EV, Villanueva, ME: *Say It in Spanish, A Guide for Health Care Professionals,* 2nd ed. Philadelphia: W. B. Saunders Co, 2000.

NAACLS Phlebotomy Competencies and Matrix

This table describes competencies from the National Association for Accreditation of Clinical Laboratory Sciences (NAACLS) for accredited programs in Phlebotomy. It cross-references the competencies with chapters in two textbooks where the topic or related topics are covered. It also provides a notation of the depth of coverage (beginning, intermediate, or advanced) in the context of a curriculum for phlebotomists. While some of the text discussions are not exhaustive, this matrix provides an overview of where material can be obtained and a basis on which students and instructors can seek out further information.

Depth of Coverage: B = Beginning   I = Intermediate   A = Advanced

NAACLS Competencies		*Phlebotomy Simplified, 2nd edition*	Chapter(s) where related topics are found	*Phlebotomy Handbook: Blood Specimen Collection from Basic to Advanced, 8th edition*	Chapter(s) where related topics are found
1.00	**Demonstrate knowledge of the health care delivery system and medical terminology.**	B	1	I–A	1
1.1	Identify the health care providers in hospitals and clinics and the phlebotomist's role as a member of this health care team.	B	1	I	1
1.2	Describe the various hospital departments and their major functions in which the phlebotomist may interact in his or her role.	B	1	I	1
1.3	Describe the organizational structure of the clinical laboratory department.	B	1	I	1
1.4	Discuss the roles of the clinical laboratory personnel and their qualifications for these professional positions.	B	1	B	1
1.5	List the types of laboratory procedures performed in the various sections of the clinical laboratory department.	B	3	I–A	6, 7, Appendix
1.6	Describe how laboratory testing is used to assess body functions and disease.	B	3	I–A	6, 7
1.7	Use common medical terminology.	B	3, Glossary, Key terms in all chapters	I–A	3, Glossary, Key terms in all chapters

2.00	**Demonstrate knowledge of infection control and safety.**	B	4	I–A	4
2.1	Identify policies and procedures for maintaining laboratory safety.	B	4	I–A	5
2.2	Demonstrate accepted practices for infection control, isolation techniques, aseptic techniques, and methods for disease prevention.	B	4	B	4
2.2.1	Identify and discuss the modes of transmission of infection and methods for prevention.	B	4	I–A	4, 5
2.2.2	Identify and properly label biohazardous specimens.	B	5, 8	I–A	4, 8, 10
2.2.3	Discuss in detail and perform proper infection control techniques, such as hand hygiene, gowning, gloving, masking, and double-bagging.	B	4, 8	I	4
2.2.4	Define and discuss the term *"healthcare-acquired infection."*	B	4	I	4
2.3	Comply with federal, state, and locally mandated regulations regarding safety practices.	B	4, 8	I–A	5
2.3.1	Observe the OSHA Bloodborne Pathogens Standard and Needle Safety Precaution Act.	B	4, 8	I–A	4, 5, 10
2.3.2	Use prescribed procedures to handle electrical, radiation, biological, and fire hazards.	B	4	I	5
2.3.3	Use appropriate practices, as outlined in the OSHA Hazard Communication Standard, including the correct use of the Material Safety Data Sheet as directed.	B	4	I	5
2.4	Describe measures used to insure patient safety in various patient settings, e.g., inpatient, outpatient, pediatrics, etc.	B	4, 8, 10	I–A	5, 10, 13
3.00	**Demonstrate basic understanding of the anatomy and physiology of body systems and anatomic terminology in order to relate major areas of the clinical laboratory to general pathologic conditions associated with the body systems.**	B	3	I–A	6, 7
3.1	Describe the basic functions of each of the main body systems, and demonstrate basic knowledge of the circulatory, urinary, and other body systems necessary to perform assigned specimen collection tasks.	B	3	I–A	6, 7

NAACLS Competencies		*Phlebotomy Simplified, 2nd edition*	**Chapter(s) where related topics are found**	*Phlebotomy Handbook: Blood Specimen Collection from Basic to Advanced, 8th edition*	**Chapter(s) where related topics are found**
3.2	Identify the veins of the arms and hands on which phlebotomy is performed.	B	3, 8, 10	I-A	7, 10, 11 13
3.3	Explain the functions of the major constituents of blood, and differentiate between whole blood, serum, and plasma.	B	3	A	7
3.4	Define hemostasis.	B	3	I-A	7
3.5	Describe the stages of coagulation.	B	3	I-A	7
3.6	Discuss the properties of arterial blood, venous blood, and capillary blood.	B	3	A	7, 10, 15
4.00	**Demonstrate understanding of the importance of specimen collection and specimen integrity in the delivery of patient care.**	B-I	1,5,7,8	A	10, 12, 15, 16
4.1	Describe the legal and ethical importance of proper patient/sample identification.	B-I	2, 8	I	3
4.2	Describe the types of patient specimens that are analyzed in the clinical laboratory.	B	3, 11	A	6, 7, 10, 11, 13, 14, 15, 16, 17, Appendix
4.3	Define the phlebotomist's role in collecting and/or transporting these specimens to the laboratory.	B	5, 11	A	10, 11, 12, 16
4.4	List the general criteria for suitability of a specimen for analysis and reasons for specimen rejection or recollection.	B	5, 11	A	9, 10, 12, 16
4.5	Explain the importance of timed, fasting, and STAT specimens as related to specimen integrity and patient care.	B	5, 8, 11	A	9, 10, 12, 16
5.00	**Demonstrate knowledge of collection equipment, various types of additives used, special precautions necessary, and substances that can interfere in clinical analysis of blood constituents.**	B	6, 8, 11	A	8, 9, 10, 11,13, 14, 15
5.1	Identify the various types of additives used in blood collection, and explain the reasons for their use.	B-I	6	A	8

5.2	Identify the evacuated tube color codes associated with the additives.	B	6	A	8
5.3	Describe the proper order of draw for specimen collections.	B	5, 7	I	8
5.4	Describe substances that can interfere in clinical analysis of blood constituents and ways in which the phlebotomist can help to avoid these occurrences.			A	7, 8, 9, 10, 11
5.5	List and select the types of equipment needed to collect blood by venipuncture, capillary puncture, and arterial puncture.	B	6, 8, 9	A	8, 10, 11, 13, 14
5.6	Identify special precautions necessary during blood collections by venipuncture and capillary (dermal) puncture.	B	7, 8, 9, 10, 11	I-A	8, 9, 10, 11, 13, 14
6.00	**Follow standard operating procedures to collect specimens.**	B	8	A	10, 11, 15, 16
6.1	Identify potential sites for venipuncture and capillary (dermal) puncture.	B	8, 9, 10	A	10, 11, 13
6.2	Differentiate between sterile and antiseptic techniques.	B	4, 11	A	4, 8, 10, 15
6.3	Describe and demonstrate the steps in the preparation of a puncture site.	B	8, 9, 11	A	10, 11, 15
6.4	List the effect of tourniquet, hand squeezing, and heating pads on specimens collected by venipuncture and capillary (dermal) puncture.	B	7, 8, 9, 10	A	9, 10, 11
6.5	Recognize proper needle insertion and withdrawal techniques, including direction, angle, depth, and aspiration, for venipuncture.	B	7, 8, 10, 11	A	9, 10
6.6	Describe and perform correct procedure for capillary (dermal) collection methods.	B	9, 10	A	11, 13
6.7	Describe the limitations and precautions of alternate collection sites for venipuncture and capillary (dermal) puncture.	B	8, 9, 10, 11	A	9, 10, 11
6.8	Explain the causes of phlebotomy complications.	B	7, 8	A	9, 10, 11
6.9	Describe signs and symptoms of physical problems that may occur during blood collection.	B	7, 8	A	9, 10, 11, 13
6.10	List the steps necessary to perform a venipuncture and a capillary (dermal) puncture in order.	B	8, 9	A	10, 11, 13
6.11	Demonstrate a successful venipuncture following standard operating procedures.	B	8	A	10

	NAACLS Competencies	*Phlebotomy Simplified, 2nd edition*	**Chapter(s) where related topics are found**	*Phlebotomy Handbook: Blood Specimen Collection from Basic to Advanced, 8th edition*	**Chapter(s) where related topics are found**
6.12	Demonstrate a successful capillary (dermal) puncture following standard operating procedures.	B	9, 10	A	11, 13
7.00	**Demonstrate understanding of requisitioning, specimen transport, and specimen processing.**	B	5	A	2, 12
7.1	Describe the process by which a request for a laboratory test is generated.	B	1	I-A	2
7.2	Instruct patients in the proper collection and preservation for non-blood specimens.	B	5, 11	I-A	16, 17
7.3	Explain methods for transporting and processing specimens for routine and special testing.	B	11	I-A	12, 16
7.4	Explain methods for processing and transporting specimens for testing at reference laboratories.	B	5	I-A	12
7.5	Identify and report potential preanalytical errors that may occur during specimen collection, labeling, transporting, and processing.	B	5, 7	A	7, 9, 10, 11, 12
7.6	Describe and follow the criteria for collection and processing of specimens that will be used as legal evidence, i.e., paternity testing, chain of custody, blood alcohol levels, etc.	B	2	I	3, 17
8.00	**Demonstrate understanding of quality assurance and quality control in phlebotomy.**	B	1, 11	I	1, 14
8.1	Describe quality assurance in the collection of blood specimens.	B	1	I	1
8.2	Identify policies and procedures used in the clinical laboratory to assure quality in the obtaining of blood specimens.	B	1, 8, 9	I	1, 4, 10
8.2.1	Perform quality control procedures.	B	11	I	1, 4, 10, 14

8.2.2	Record quality control results.	B	11	I	1, 4, 10, 14
8.2.3	Identify and report control results that do not meet predetermined criteria.	B	11	I	1, 3, 14
9.00	**Communicate (verbally and nonverbally) effectively and appropriately in the workplace.**	I	1	A	2
9.1	Maintain confidentiality of privileged information on individuals, according to federal regulations (e.g., HIPAA).	I	1, 2	A	2, 3
9.2	Demonstrate respect for diversity in the workplace.	B	1	I	2
9.3	Interact appropriately and professionally.	B	1, 2	I	1, 2, 3
9.4	Demonstrate an understanding of the major points of the American Hospital Association's Patient's Bill of Rights and the Patient's Bill of Rights from the workplace.	B	2	I	3
9.5	Comply with the American Hospital Association's Patient's Bill of Rights and the Patient's Bill of Rights from the workplace.	B	2	I	1, 3
9.6	Model professional appearance and appropriate behavior.	B	1	I	1, 2, 3
9.7	Follow written and verbal instructions.	B	1	I	2
9.8	Define and use medicolegal terms and discuss policies and protocol designed to avoid medicolegal problems.	B	2	I	3
9.9	List the causes of stress in the work environment and discuss the coping skills used to deal with stress in the work environment.	B	1	I	1
9.10	Demonstrate ability to use computer information systems necessary to accomplish job functions.	B	5	I	2

Competencies reprinted with permission from the National Association for Accreditation of Clinical Laboratory Sciences (NAACLS).

Answers to Study Questions, Case Studies, and Competency Checklists

Chapter 1 Phlebotomy Practice and Quality Assessment Basics

Study Questions

1. a, b, d	5. a, b	8. b
2. a, b, c	6. b	9. a
3. a, b, c	7. c	10. a
4. d		

Case Study

1. There are several tips that might help to communicate with Mrs. Gonzales:
   - Remain calm, professional, respectful, and courteous
   - Make sure she is comfortable and approach her more slowly
   - Check to see if she would prefer to speak a language other than English; if so, seek out a translator or written instructions in her language of choice
   - Ask if she has family members who might support her during the procedure
   - Double-check for understanding of your instructions

2. Factors that might contribute to her anger or anxiety are:
   - Fear of the procedure or pain
   - Inability to communicate effectively due to language barriers
   - Possible deafness or vision loss

3. Cultural issues that may affect communication with Mrs. Gonzales include the following:
   - Cultural values, such as the presence or absence of her family
   - Language preferences
   - Beliefs, such as about health care, religion, or medical staff
   - Customs and traditions

Advocating Patient Safety Case Study

Communication on the telephone should be just as professional as it is in face-to-face conversations. As discussed in this chapter, part of effective communication is active listening (concentrating on the speaker, verifying that you are listening, providing feedback, etc.). Examples of miscommunication and how these might jeopardize a patient's safety are as follows:

- Inadequate information about the time or date of the request could result in repeated venipunctures;
- Inaccurate spelling of a patient's name could result in name mix-ups and hazardous, erroneous test requests/results;
- Inaccurate recording of a patient's unique identification number could also result in patient or specimen mix-ups such that results might be reported on the wrong patient;

- Insufficient information about the case can waste valuable time in reporting results, thus increasing the time it takes for the doctor to respond to the patient's needs;
- Revealing confidential patient information to an unauthorized caller violates the patient's confidentiality;
- Hanging up too early before the caller has finished can lead to insufficient information about the patient's condition related to his or her laboratory requests or results.

Competency Checklist: Communication

Refer to pages 16–30

Competency Checklist: Quality Basics

Refer to pages 30–36

Chapter 2   Ethical, Legal, and Regulatory Issues

Study Questions

1. c
2. c
3. b
4. a

5. a
6. c
7. b

8. c
9. b
10. c

Case Study

1. Ms. Garner needs to apply pressure to the venipuncture site for additional minutes and then check to see if continuous bleeding is occurring under the skin. If the hematoma continues to enlarge, even with the pressure applied for additional minutes, the health care worker must call his or her supervisor or a nurse.

2. After the patient is provided communication to calm her, Ms. Garner and the supervisor must have the patient evaluated by the attending physician to make certain that she has not received any damage to her median nerve by the needlestick. If she is still complaining of pain, the physician can send her for diagnostic procedures to determine if there was nerve injury.

3. The health care worker must provide a written detail of everything that occurred when she attempted the blood collection from Ms. Cardo, including the patient's jumping as she entered the vein with the needle. This written statement will be the incident report that will be filed. If the patient files a malpractice lawsuit, the incident report will provide needed documentation of the venipuncture attempt. If any witnesses, such as other health care workers, or a supervisor, were in the outpatient clinic at the time of this incident and saw the event, they need to provide a written report also.

Advocating Patient Safety Case Study

The Society for Healthcare Epidemiology of America (SHEA) recommends that the health care workers who have HIV infection must have their viral loads tested routinely. Those health care workers who demonstrate HIV viral loads greater than, or equal to, 5×10^2 GE/mL must be cautiously monitored if they are working with patients. They can perform basic phlebotomies but must avoid situations such as a patient experiencing an epileptic seizure, psychiatric patients who are violent, or if a patient tries to bite a phlebotomist. Also, they must avoid resuscitation efforts on a patient.

Competency Checklist: Ethical, Legal, and Regulatory Issues

1. Refer to pages 44–45, 48
2. Refer to pages 41, 47–48

Chapter 3   Basic Medical Terminology, The Human Body, and The Cardiovascular System

Study Questions

1. b	5. a	8. c
2. c	6. a	9. c
3. c	7. b	10. d
4. d		

Case Study

The health care worker can briefly explain to the patient, "Basically, veins are thin-walled blood vessels that carry deoxygenated blood from the tissues to the heart. Venous blood is dark red, and the veins appear bluish in color. Arteries carry oxygenated blood from the heart and lungs to the tissues so arterial blood appears brighter red in color. However, if you would like a more detailed explanation, please ask your doctor. Would you like to get more information from your doctor before I continue with the blood collection procedure, or may I continue with the procedure?" It is important to provide the patient with information; however, it must be truthful and accurate. It is better not to provide any information than to make up information. Remember that the patient must agree to have the procedure done prior to the venipuncture, so it is best to assure that his or her concerns have been addressed before proceeding. If necessary, the doctor or nurse in charge of the patient can be contacted to answer further questions.

Advocating Patient Safety Case Study

1. The phlebotomist should thank the patient for the information and insight, acknowledge the patient's concern, and reassure her that a careful examination of her arms will likely result in a successful venipuncture. The phlebotomist should check the right arm first because the patient gave a hint that there was a good vein on that side.

2. The preferred area for venipunctures is in the antecubital area of the arm.

3. If the preferred area on either arm is not available for venipuncture or the phlebotomist cannot palpate a suitable vein in those locations, the back (posterior) side of the hand may be used. The anterior side of the wrist should never be used for a venipuncture because there are many superficial nerves in that area of the arm/hand. Accidental nerve damage can result from needle probing.

Competency Checklist: Prefixes

1. without, lack of	17. against	32. above, excessive	47. around
2. away from	18. ten	33. below, deficient	48. many
3. toward	19. through	34. below	49. first
4. both	20. double	35. between	50. false
5. without, lack of	21. two	36. within	51. four
6. up	22. bad, difficult	37. bad	52. five
7. before	23. within	38. large, great	53. backward
8. against	24. upon, above	39. middle	54. half
9. self	25. good, normal	40. small	55. below, under
10. two, double	26. out, away from	41. one-thousandth	56. above, beyond
11. short	27. outside, beyond	42. many, much	57. together
12. slow	28. half	43. none	58. together
13. bad	29. different	44. scanty, little	59. four
14. down	30. similar, same	45. all	60. three
15. a hundred	31. water	46. beside	61. one
16. around			

Competency Checklist: Root Words

1. vessel
2. to choke
3. artery
4. artery
5. fatty substance, porridge
6. hair-like
7. heart
8. heart
9. heart
10. elbow, forearm
11. cell
12. skin
13. electricity
14. to cast, to throw
15. work
16. red
17. blood
18. necrosis of an area
19. fat
20. study
21. thin
22. muscle
23. vein
24. vein
25. lung
26. rhythm
27. hardening
28. serum
29. pulse
30. chest
31. tension
32. clot
33. vessel
34. vein

Competency Checklist: Suffixes

1. pain
2. immature cell, germ cell
3. hernia, tumor, swelling
4. surgical puncture
5. cell
6. binding
7. pain
8. surgical excision
9. vomiting
10. a weight, mark, record
11. to write, record
12. one who specializes, agent
13. inflammation
14. study of
15. destruction, separation
16. enlargement, large
17. measure
18. resemble
19. tumor
20. to view
21. condition of
22. disease
23. deficiency
24. surgical fixation
25. to eat
26. to speak
27. attraction
28. fear
29. to obstruct
30. growth
31. formation, produce
32. surgical repair
33. paralysis, stroke
34. breathing
35. formation
36. drooping
37. spitting
38. bursting forth
39. bursting forth
40. suture
41. flow, discharge
42. rupture
43. instrument
44. to view
45. control, stopping
46. new opening
47. treatment
48. instrument to cut
49. incision
50. nourishment, development
51. urine

Competency Checklist: Identifying Medical Terms

1. coagulate
2. anticoagulant
3. hematology
4. hyperglycemia
5. leukocyte
6. erythrocyte
7. pathology
8. antecubital
9. leukopenia
10. arteriosclerosis

Competency Checklist: Spelling

1. immunology
2. phlebotomy
3. hemorrhage
4. hematocrit
5. leukemia
6. erythrocyte
7. hematology
8. embolus
9. thrombus
10. millimeter

Competency Checklist: Cardiovascular System

1. H	6. L or M	11. R	16. C
2. I	7. P	12. T	17. D
3. K	8. O	13. E	18. A
4. M or L	9. J	14. F	19. S
5. N	10. Q	15. G	20. B

Chapter 4   Safety and Infection Control

Study Questions

1. c	5. c	8. c
2. d	6. b	9. a
3. a	7. b	10. a
4. b		

Case Study

1. In this case, Ron has exposed himself to definite harm by having an open wound that could have been contaminated by the patient's blood. He must immediately cleanse the area with isopropyl alcohol and apply an adhesive bandage.

2. Even though Ron knows he made a drastic error in not taking the gloves with him for the blood collections, he must notify his supervisor, fill out the necessary incident and medical forms, and undergo the appropriate laboratory tests. In addition, Ron will need to be counseled and evaluated for HIV and hepatitis C infection at periodic intervals.

Advocating Patient Safety Case Study

Patricia should tactfully ask Danielle if she is changing gloves and washing her hands between each patient's blood collection. She might tactfully remind Danielle that hand hygiene is the number one method to control the spread of infections and that it is essential to change gloves between patients to avoid possible infectious contamination between patients and health care workers. Hopefully, Danielle will comply with the needed hand hygiene and glove changing as required. If this issue continues, then Patricia should have a discussion with the phlebotomy supervisor as Danielle is truly creating a biosafety hazard for the patients and health care professionals in that health care facility.

Check Yourself: Infection Control Procedures and Safety

1. Handwashing is essential in the performance of any phlebotomy procedure on any patient. Remember, even though you are using a different set of gloves for each patient's blood collection procedure, handwashing has to occur before another set of gloves is placed on your hands.

2. Health care workers, as well as patients, can become allergic to latex products. Many of the gloves used in health care facilities are made of latex. Also, some tourniquets, syringes, adhesive tape, and blood pressure cuffs contain latex that could lead to an allergic reaction in the patient and/or health care worker.

3. The recommendations are to:

   Wear gloves; use 1:10 bleach solution or commercially prepared solution; first clean the area with visible blood and then disinfect the entire area of possible contamination; and keep the bleach in contact with the contaminated area for at least 20 minutes to ensure complete disinfection. If it had been a "large" spill, a spill kit should have been used for the clean-up process.

Competency Checklist: Infection Control and Safety

1. Type ABC extinguishers contain a dry chemical and are used on fires of wood, cloth, paper, oil, grease, and gasoline. They are multipurpose in combating fires and are located in fire stations throughout health care facilities.

2. Always turn off and disconnect before maintenance performance on the centrifuge or any other electrical equipment.

3. Examples: gloves, facial masks, respirators, gowns, shields

4. Isopropyl alcohol   It is an antiseptic for skin.

   Iodine   It is an antiseptic for skin.

   Chloramine   It is a disinfectant for wounds.

Chapter 5   Documentation, Specimen Handling, and Transportation

Study Questions

1. a	5. c	8. b
2. b	6. b	9. c
3. b	7. a	10. c
4. a		

Case Study

1. The most likely cause of the hemolysis in so many specimens is that the phlebotomist probably shook the blood specimens too vigorously when trying to mix the anticoagulant with the specimen. Another possibility is that the specimens were not properly situated in the pneumatic tube carrier case and may have been excessively agitated during the tube transportation to the laboratory. If this had been the case, the specimen tubes may have broken or cracked and leaked, causing a serious biohazard.

2. Communication with the phlebotomist who collected the specimens should be open, and she should be asked about her technique for mixing specimens and her methods of positioning the specimen tubes for transport in the pneumatic tube. Appropriate counseling and retraining should occur. The situation should be documented for all patient specimens concerned, the physicians should be notified, and recollections should be initiated.

Advocating Patient Safety Case Study

1. Electronic medical records save time in the following ways

   ■ The time used for traditional handwritten charting is eliminated

   ■ Times and dates are automatically recorded

   ■ Electronic orders (instead of handwritten) can be generated for laboratory tests, diagnostic imaging, or other tests

   ■ Pre-established patient education materials can be retrieved and printed for a patient

   ■ Billing is automated and faster

2. Handwritten test requests and specimen labels are very prone to errors due to indecipherable handwriting and transcription errors. These are reduced or eliminated using electronic or automated laboratory requests and automatically-generated specimen labels. Technology using patient identification data on barcodes or RFID also reduces identification errors. The shift toward standardization of label format, size, and placement on the tubes themselves, are designed to reduce identification errors in the preexamination and examination phases of laboratory testing workflow.

3. In general, laboratory errors should be noted the same whether the medical record is a paper one or an electronic one. Health care workers must follow the protocol established by their facility. Essentially, the error should be mentioned to a supervisor as soon as possible. The original entry should be marked as an error and crossed out but not deleted, i.e., it should still be viewable. The correct entry should be posted with appropriate notations about the situation, and a physician should be notified.

Competency Checklist: Specimen Transportation

Refer to pages 118–128

Chapter 6   Blood Collection Equipment

Study Questions

1. b	5. d	8. c
2. b	6. b	9. b
3. d	7. b	10. b
4. d		

Case Study

1. The red-topped tube without an additive can be used if the serum is immediately taken out of the tube after the blood clots. It is preferable to use a serum separator tube that will separate the serum from the blood to avoid glycolysis. Also, the gray-topped tube can be used to collect for the glucose analysis as this tube slows the process of glycolysis.

2. No, the coagulation tests, PT and APTT, require the blood collection in a light blue–topped tube that contains sodium citrate as the additive.

Advocating Patient Safety Case Study

Ms. Halt has all of the necessary supplies EXCEPT she has only ONE tourniquet. The preferred procedure is to use a new tourniquet for each patient. This procedure will assist in reducing the spread of nosocomial infection by tourniquets and reduce the risk of cross-contamination between patients and health care workers.

Competency Assessment: Identifying the Proper Equipment for Blood Collection

1. Refer to pages 134–139
2. Refer to pages 140–147
3. Refer to pages 148–152

Chapter 7   Preexamination/Preanalytical Complications

Study Questions

1. c	5. c	8. b
2. c	6. b	9. b
3. c	7. d	10. d
4. b		

Case Study

Mary will need to assess the antecubital region of each arm to see if she can perform a venipuncture through a section of Mr. Martinez's arm that may not have tattoos to avoid any possible interference with the laboratory tests from the tattoo dyes. Also, tampering with a blood collection needle in a tattoo site could result in an infection.

In addition, the fasting time for Mr. Martinez is 14 hours and this longevity without food could result in erroneous results on his laboratory tests. The fasting time should be between 8 and 12 hours.

Advocating Patient Safety Case Study

The sight of blood before or during blood collection for some people leads to vomiting. Ms. Shilling should release the tourniquet and take the needle out of the arm immediately to avoid possible injury to the patient or phlebotomist as jerking of the patient's body may occur. Then, she should have the patient take deep breaths and use a cold compress on her head. She should follow the protocol established by the health care facility for this type of incident. The phlebotomy supervisor needs to be informed as well as the patient's physician about this complication.

Competency Checklist: Preanalytical Complications in Blood Collection

1. Refer to pages 158–160
2. Refer to page 165

Chapter 8   Venipuncture Procedures

Study Questions

1. b	5. d	8. a
2. a, b, c, d	6. d	9. c
3. b	7. b	10. b
4. d		

Case Study 1

There are several key issues that are important for the health care worker in this confusing situation: confirming the patient's identity, dealing with a comatose patient, and collecting blood from a patient with an IV.

Procedurally, the health care worker should ask the patient her name even though the patient may appear asleep or comatose. If the patient does not respond, which would be likely in this case, the health care worker should seek confirmation of the identity from an authorized nurse or family member. If the patient's armband confirms the identity on the laboratory requisitions, (e.g., Ann Beaumont), then the health care worker may proceed with the specimen collection process. However, the health care worker should notify the nurse or supervisor about the incorrect sign on the patient's bed. *Never* rely on a bed sign for identity confirmation.

Regarding the comatose condition, the health care worker should ask the nurse to assist her in positioning the patient's arm in a secure manner so that if the patient flinches during the needle puncture, it will not cause injury or disrupt the specimen collection process. And, in consideration of the IV in one arm, the health care worker should use the other arm for the venipuncture. If there are no palpable veins in the non-IV arm, the health care worker may select a dorsal hand vein on this arm or on the IV arm *below* the IV site. Remember, that venous blood is flowing from the tips of the fingers toward the heart, so IV fluid contamination into the blood specimen would be *less* likely below the IV site (on the side closest to the fingers) rather than above the IV site (on the side closest to the heart). If the specimen is collected from the dorsal side of the hand below the IV site, a notation should be made to indicate this situation. Generally speaking, the health care worker should always "go the extra mile" to confirm identity and collect an accurate specimen with the least amount of discomfort to the patient. If there is any question about identity, venipuncture site, or patient condition, seek clarification from a supervisor *before* beginning the procedure.

Case Study 2

1. Because the patient had a mastectomy on her *left* side, it would be best to draw the blood from the *right* arm in the antecubital area. If there are no suitable veins in this area, the second area to search for a good vein would be the dorsal side of the right hand.

2. The correct order of draw would be as follows:

   Blood cultures (yellow)—Keep in mind that blood cultures require sterile preparation of the site

   PT & PTT (light blue)—Coagulation tests

   electrolytes (red)—Chemistry test

   HGB & HCT, cell counts (lavender)—Hematology tests

Advocating Patient Safety Case Study

Whether a patient is ambulatory or hospitalized, there are several patient safety issues that fall under the phlebotomist's responsibilities:

- Correctly labeling the blood sample tubes—this should occur immediately after the needle has been removed, the needle safety device has been activated, and pressure has been applied to the puncture site. Labeling the sample tubes *must* be done at the patient's side (in a clinic setting) or at their bedside (in a hospital). It is not acceptable practice to label the tubes later, after leaving the patient because the risk of labeling it incorrectly increases.

- Re-confirm with the patient and/or re-check that the sample labels match the patient's identification. It is best for the patient to confirm the labels themselves if possible.

- Clean up and dispose of all contaminated supplies or equipment.

- Double-check that the patient's venipuncture site has stopped bleeding. It is important to assure that bleeding has stopped before applying a bandage. Some patients may be on blood thinners or be taking aspirin, thus causing delayed blood clotting. It will take longer for these patients to stop bleeding. It is also imperative that the phlebotomist check for hematoma formation. In all cases, applying pressure to the site usually stops the bleeding. It is the health care worker's responsibility to apply pressure, not the patient's. In cases where the patient is cooperative, it is acceptable to allow them to apply pressure to the site. However, the health care worker should apply pressure if the bleeding continues and in rare circumstances when bleeding is excessive or significantly delayed, the health care worker should call for a nurse.

- Double-check the patient to assure that they do not feel dizzy or faint. This is particularly important for patients who are ambulatory.

- Thank the patient for their cooperation. This conveys respect and leaves the patient with a more positive and cooperative attitude about the next time a venipuncture is required.

Competency Checklist: Patient Identification and Name Clarification

Refer to pages 173–176

Patient Identification

Refer to pages 173–176

Competency Checklist: Preparing for the Patient Encounter

Refer to pages 177–181

Competency Checklist: Use of a Tourniquet and Site Selection

Refer to pages 192–193

Competency Checklist: Decontamination of the Puncture Site

Refer to pages 194

Competency Checklist: Performing a Venipuncture

Refer to pages 195–199

Competency Checklist: Order of Draw

Refer to pages 203–204

Competency Checklist: Leaving the Patient

Refer to pages 207

Chapter 9   Capillary Blood Specimens

Study Questions

1. a
2. d
3. c
4. c

5. c
6. b
7. a

8. c
9. c
10. b

Case Study

In the case of Sarah W., who was obviously fearful of the specimen collection procedure and whose hands were cold, the health care worker can take several positive steps to help the situation. First, a polite, sympathetic, and professional conversation with Sarah about the procedural steps could help Sarah understand that a fingerstick is not as invasive as a venipuncture procedure. Allow Sarah to see the equipment and ask questions about it. Second, ask Sarah to hold a warming device in her hands, and/or to dangle her arm low, or to run warm water over her hand to increase the blood flow to the area. Let her know that warming her hands will facilitate the fingerstick process and help the blood flow quickly into the collection tubes. Inform her that the volume of blood needed for the procedure is very small, so it will be over quickly. Ask her if she has ever fainted during or after a blood collection procedure. If possible, place her in a reclining collection chair for comfort and safety or in a secure blood collection chair with adjustable arm rests.

As for Henry C., his skin condition may indicate that he is dehydrated. He may benefit from drinking a glass of water and coming back after a short period of time. Check the fingers of both hands, and ask him which is his dominant hand. Seek a finger site on the nondominant hand because it may be less likely to have calluses. Use of a warming device or warm water on his hand may help increase blood flow to the area. If none of these methods increases the blood flow to the hand, or the fingers appear too callused to prick, it may be best to consult a supervisor. However, if one of the fingers appears suitable, continue with the puncture procedure. Try to focus on the fleshy side, (i.e., the thick section), of the third or fourth finger tip of the nondominant hand.

Advocating Patient Safety Case Study

1. It is very easy to improve blood flow to a patient's hand and there are no excuses for not taking the time to do so. These methods significantly improve blood flow and improve the likelihood of a successful puncture and sample collection on the first try.

   - Warm the site for 3–5 minutes using warmed towels, a commercially available warming pack or heating pad, or having the patient wash/rinse his or her hands in warm water.
   - Ask the patient to lower the arm to the side so that the fingers are pointing toward the floor. This allows the blood capillaries to fill to capacity in a short time.

2. To assure that blood sample tubes are filled adequately the first time, the following tips should be utilized:
   - Wipe away the first drop of blood unless the testing instructions indicate otherwise.
   - Avoid milking, squeezing, or scooping-up the blood.
   - Collect the sample quickly to avoid clotting.
   - Fill the tubes to the correct fill volume by watching carefully.
   - Mix the sample according to the manufactures' instructions; usually this requires gentle mixing for 5–10 inversions.

Competency Checklist: Capillary Blood Collection
Refer to pages 225–229

Competency Checklist: Making Blood Smears for Microscopic Analysis
Refer to pages 221–224

Chapter 10   Pediatric and Geriatric Procedures
Study Questions

1. c	5. c	8. d
2. b	6. d	9. b
3. c	7. b	10. b
4. c		

Case Study

1. The skin puncture performed on this infant will require that the hematology specimen (i.e., CBC, hemoglobin) will be collected first, followed by the chemistry specimen (i.e., creatinine), and then the blood-bank specimen (i.e., ABO group and Rh typing).

2. The phlebotomist must *always* record the amount of blood collected from the infant. Overcollecting blood during numerous blood collections may lead to a blood transfusion in an infant. Thus, the cumulative amount of blood collected from an infant or child during a hospital stay must be continuously checked so that too much blood is not collected, leading to anemia in the infant or child.

Advocating Patient Safety Case Study

The parent should assist in having the child lie in a supine position with the phlebotomist on one side of the bed and the parent on the opposite side. The parent can gently but firmly lean over the child, restraining the child's arm not being used while holding the opposite, extended arm securely for the phlebotomist to perform the blood collection.

Check Yourself: Ready to Collect Blood from a 6-Month-Old Child

1. Refer to page 239
2. Refer to page 240–244

Competency Checklist: Pediatrics and Geriatrics

1. Refer to page 244
2. Refer to page 253
3. Refer to page 254

Chapter 11   Special Collections

Study Questions

1. c	5. a	8. d
2. c	6. d	9. b
3. c	7. a	10. b
4. a		

Case Study

Problems That Could Have Led to Point-of-Care Testing Error

Contamination of the blood with alcohol. (After alcohol is used to cleanse the skin puncture site, the skin must completely dry before puncturing the site.)

Wrong volume of specimen was collected.

Instrument blotting/wiping technique was not performed according to manufacturer's directions.

Instrument was not clean.

Reagents were outdated.

Timing of the analytic procedure was incorrect.

Reagents were not stored at the proper temperature, leading them to deterioration.

Battery for instrument was weak or dead.

In addition to this list of possible problems, the instrument will have troubleshooting guidelines to help identify the problem so that the correct result can be obtained.

Advocating Patient Safety Case Study

A health care worker should never take pieces of one POC instrument by one manufacturer to use with another POC instrument unless it states in the manufacturer's instructions that the instruments pieces are interchangeable. Kellie did not check into the interchangeability of these instruments' parts and most likely, they were not compatible. Consequently, the PT result she obtained was not accurate or reliable, especially as she did not perform any quality control checks with the other instrument's disposable cuvette to see if the quality control parameters were within the required limits to perform the patient's test. Upon receiving this elevated PT result, the physician might prescribe less blood thinning medication and that could lead to a stroke or heart attack in the patient.

Competency Checklist: Special Collections

1. Refer to page 270–271
2. Refer to page 280–282

Glossary

The terms in this glossary are defined as they would most likely be used by clinical laboratory personnel—more specifically, by phlebotomists. The definitions are not exhaustive or elaborate.

acid citrate-dextrose (ACD) an additive commonly used in specimen collection for blood donations to prevent clotting. It ensures that the RBCs maintain their oxygen-carrying capacity.

active listening a set of skills that enables an individual to become a more effective listener. The skills include concentrating on the speaker, getting ready to listen by clearing one's mind of distracting thoughts, use of silent pauses when appropriate, providing reassuring feedback, verifying the conversation that took place, keeping personal judgments to oneself, paying attention to the body language of the person speaking, and maintaining eye contact.

additives substances (gels, clotting activators, or anticoagulants) that are added in small amounts to specimen collection tubes to alter the specimen so as to make it appropriate for laboratory analysis or handling.

age-specific care considerations providing services that are age-appropriate and considerate (e.g., special considerations are needed for different ages of children (toddler versus teen) and also for geriatric patients). Factors typically relate to age-related fears/concerns, communication styles, procedures for comforting the patient, and safety.

alcohol colorless liquid that can be used as an antiseptic.

aliquot a portion of a blood specimen that has been removed/separated from the original primary specimen tube after initial processing (centrifugation) and is considered to be identical to all other portions of the original sample of serum, plasma, urine, and cerebrospinal fluid. Each aliquot should be labeled with a unique identifier that can be linked to the primary collection container.

Allen test a procedure used prior to drawing specimens (for ABGs) from the radial artery. It assures that the ulnar and radial arteries are providing collateral circulation to the hand area. Basically, it entails compressing the arteries to the hand and emptying the hand of arterial blood, then releasing the compression to see if the circulation is immediately restored. A negative test would indicate that collateral circulation is not sufficient and an alternative artery (brachial or femoral) should be used for ABG collections.

Alzheimer's disease (AD) a disease that causes loss of intellectual abilities and mood disorders such as depression and combativeness. It is more prevalent in the elderly.

ambulatory care health care services that are delivered in an outpatient or nonhospital setting. It implies that the patients are able to ambulate, or walk, to the clinic to receive their services.

American Society for Clinical Laboratory Scientists (ASCLS) professional organization for laboratory personnel that provides continuing education and conference activities for laboratory professionals.

American Society for Clinical Pathology (ASCP) professional organization offering clinical and research conferences, many types of continuing education activities, and ongoing certification programs. Certification is through the Board of Certification (BOC) for many types of laboratory professionals and specialties.

analyte a substance being analyzed, i.e., a chemical analysis.

analytic phase refers to the phase in laboratory testing whereby the specimen is actually assessed or evaluated, and results are confirmed and reported.

anatomic pathology major area of laboratory services whereby autopsies are performed and surgical biopsy tissues are analyzed.

anemia medical condition in which there is a reduction in hemoglobin thus lowering the O_2 carrying capacity of blood cells.

antecubital area of the forearm (around the crease of the elbow) most commonly used for selecting veins prior to venipuncture.

anterior surface region of the body characterized by the front (or ventral) area and including the thoracic, abdominal, and pelvic cavities.

anticoagulant substance introduced into the blood or a blood specimen to keep it from clotting.

antiglycolytic agent an additive used in blood collection tubes that prevents glycolysis.

antimicrobial chemical or therapeutic agent that destroys microorganisms such as bacteria, viruses, and fungi.

antiseptic hand rub applying/rubbing a waterless antiseptic product onto all surfaces of the hands to reduce the number of microorganisms present; the hands are rubbed until the product has dried.

antiseptic hand wash washing hands with soap and water or other detergents containing an antiseptic agent.

antiseptics chemicals (e.g., 70 percent isopropyl alcohol, chlorhexidine, chlorine, hexachlorophene, chloroxylenol, quarternary ammonium compounds, iodine, and triclosan) used to clean human skin by inhibiting the growth of microorganisms.

aorta the largest artery in the body.

arterial blood gases (ABGs) analytical test that measures oxygen and carbon dioxide in the blood. Provides useful information about respiratory status and the acid–base balance of patients with pulmonary disorders.

arterioles smaller branches of arteries.

artery highly oxygenated blood vessel that carries blood away from the heart.

aseptic a degree of cleanliness that prevents infection and the growth of microorganisms. The technique to achieve this condition includes frequent use of hand hygiene procedures, use of barrier garments and personal protective equipment (PPE), waste management of contaminated materials, use of proper cleaning solutions, following standard precautions, and using sterile procedures when necessary.

assault a legal term referring to the unjustifiable attempt to touch another person or the threat to do so in circumstances that cause the other person to believe that it will be carried out, or to cause fear. An assault may be permissible if proper consent has been given (e.g., consent to obtain a blood specimen).

assessments a measurement term referring to factors that affect both the analytic (quantitative) and nonanalytic (qualitative) components of health care. Competency assessments are used to measure an individual's ability to perform specified job tasks.

atria plural of atrium; a chamber of the heart that receives blood from the veins and forces it into a ventricle or ventricles.

automated skin-puncture safety device a single-use apparatus that pierces the skin with a lancet that automatically retracts into a protective casing.

bacteremia presence of bacteria in the blood; an infection of the blood.

bar codes series of light and dark bands of varying widths that relate to alphanumeric symbols. They can be one or two-dimensional symbologies and may correspond to the patient's name and/or identification number, and/or patient specimen numbers. The codes are read by optical devices referred to as scanners.

basal state for phlebotomy procedures, this refers to the patient's condition in the early morning, approximately 12 hours after the last ingestion of food. In hospitals, most laboratory tests are analyzed on basal state specimens.

basilic vein vessel of the forearm that is acceptable for venipuncture; however other veins in the antecubital area are preferred because the basilic vein lies in close proximity to the median nerve and brachial artery.

battery a complex legal term referring to the intentional touching of another person without consent, and/or beating or

carrying out threatened physical harm. Battery always includes an assault and is therefore commonly used with the term in *assault and battery*.

beta-carotene a photosensitive analyte.

bevel slanted surface at the end point of a needle.

bilirubin a photosensitive analyte.

blood circulating fluid and cells in the cardiovascular system.

bloodborne pathogens (BBPs) pathogenic microorganisms, including hepatitis B virus and human immunodeficiency virus, that are present in human blood and can cause disease in humans.

blood cells components of blood, the three main types of circulating blood cells are erythrocytes, leukocytes, and thrombocytes.

blood cultures tests that aid in identifying the specific bacterial organism causing infections in the blood. In the case of a patient that is experiencing fever spikes, it is recommended that the blood culture specimens be collected before and after the fever spike, when bacteria are most likely present in the peripheral circulation. Care must be taken by the phlebotomist not to contaminate the specimen, so special sterile preparation of the collection site is required.

blood-drawing chair a chair specifically designed to hold a patient comfortably and safely in a proper position during and after a blood collection procedure. The design typically includes a moveable armrest on both sides of the chair.

blood gas analysis see *arterial blood gases*.

blood sample a portion of blood removed that is small enough so as not to cause harm.

blood specimens discrete portions of blood taken for laboratory analysis of one or more characteristics to determine the character of the whole body.

blood urea nitrogen (BUN) analytic testing procedure to determine the amount of urea in the blood.

blood vessels key components of the circulatory system, these vessels transport blood throughout the body.

blood volume the total amount of blood in an individual's body. This is particularly important in pediatric phlebotomies because withdrawing blood can cause a significant decrease in the total blood volume of a small infant, thus resulting in anemia. Blood volume is based on weight and can be calculated for any size person.

body planes imaginary dividing lines of the body that serve as reference points for describing distance from or proximity to different portions of the body. Body planes include the sagittal, frontal, transverse, and medial planes.

brachial artery an artery located in the cubital fossa of the arm and used as an alternative site for ABG collections. Phlebotomists must be specially trained to perform collections from this site.

breach of duty a legal term referring to an infraction, violation, or failure to perform.

buffy coat in blood specimens that contain anticoagulants, the WBCs and platelets form a thin white layer above the RBCs called the *buffy coat.*

butterfly needle also referred to as a blood collection set or winged infusion set, it is the most commonly used intravenous device. It is a stainless steel beveled needle and tube with attached plastic wings on one end and a Luer fitting attached to the other. Most butterfly needles come with safety sheaths for needlestick protection after use.

butterfly system also called a winged infusion system or scalp needle set, the system can be used for difficult venipunctures due to small or fragile veins. The needle is typically smaller, and has a thin tubing with a Luer adapter at the end so that it can be used on a syringe or an evacuated tube system during venipuncture. Most models have needle safety devices such as retractable needles and/or needle coverings/sheaths.

calcaneus heel bone.

cannula a tube that can be inserted into a cavity or blood vessel and used as a channel for transporting fluids. The term is most commonly used in dialysis for patients with kidney disease. The cannula is used to gain access to venous blood for dialysis or for blood collections. Specialized training and experience are required to draw blood from a cannula.

capillary microscopic blood vessel that carries blood and links arterioles to venules.

capillary action a term used when referring to microcollection procedures that indicates the free flowing movement of blood into the capillary tube without the use of suction.

capillary blood a specimen from a skin puncture that contains a blend of blood from venules, arterioles, and tissue fluid.

capillary blood gas analysis using microcollection methods on infants (usually the heel site) to collect specimens for blood gas analyses; these analytical tests measure oxygen and carbon dioxide in the blood. Provides useful information about respiratory status and the acid–base balance of patients with pulmonary disorders.

capillary tubes disposable narrow-bore pipettes that are used for pediatric blood collections and/or microhematocrit measures. The tubes may be coated with anticoagulant such as heparin, and for safety reasons are usually made of plastic.

cardiopulmonary resuscitation (CPR) the method used to revive the heart breathing of a patient whose heart or respiration has stopped. It is advisable for health care workers to be appropriately trained in the use of CPR.

cardiovascular system body system that provides for rapid transport of water, nutrients, electrolytes, hormones, enzymes, antibodies, cells, and gases to all cells of the body. It includes the heart, the vascular system, and the blood.

cause-and-effect diagrams (Ishikawa) a quality improvement tool that uses diagrams to identify interactions between equipment, methods, people, supplies, and reagents.

Centers for Disease Control and Prevention (CDC) federal agency responsible for monitoring morbidity (disease) and mortality (death) throughout the country.

centrifugation the process of separating cellular elements from the liquid portion of a blood specimen. It is done by spinning the specimen in a specially designed centrifuge.

centrifugation phase period of time when a blood specimen is inside the centrifuge.

cephalic vein a vein of the forearm that is acceptable for venipuncture.

cerebrospinal fluid (CSF) fluid that surrounds the brain and meninges within the spinal column.

chain of infection the process by which infections are transmitted; components include the source of the infection (nonsterile items, contaminated equipment or supplies, etc.), the mode of transmission (direct contact, airborne, medical instruments, etc.), and the susceptible host (patient).

Chlorhexidine an antibacterial chemical used to cleanse the skin for venipuncture. Should not be used on infants younger than 2 months old.

circulatory system also called the cardiovascular system, the body system referring to the heart, blood vessels, and blood; responsible for transporting oxygen and nutrients to cells and transporting carbon dioxide and wastes until they are eliminated; transports hormones, regulates body temperature, and helps defend against diseases.

citrate type of anticoagulant additive for blood collection tubes; prevents the blood clotting sequence by removing calcium and forming calcium salts.

citrate-phosphate-dextrose (CPD) anticoagulant additive typically used for specimens collected for blood donations.

civil law different from criminal law; in civil law, the plaintiff sues for monetary damages.

clean-catch midstream a urine specimen that is used for detecting bacteria and/or for microscopic analysis. Normally, the specimen should be free of contamination because the patient should be instructed to clean and decontaminate themselves prior to urination. The urine specimen should be collected into a sterile container. Urine should be voided and the specimen should be collected mid-urination.

clinical laboratory a workplace where analytic procedures are performed on blood and body fluids for the detection, monitoring, and treatment of disease.

Clinical Laboratory Improvement Amendments (CLIA) federal guidelines that regulate all clinical laboratories across the United States. Regulations apply to any site that tests human specimens, including small POLs, or screening tests done at the patient's bedside.

Clinical and Laboratory Standards Institute (CLSI) a non-profit organization that recommends quality standards and guidelines for clinical laboratory procedures.

clinical pathology major area of laboratory services where blood and other types of body fluids and tissues are analyzed.

clinical (or medical) record see *medical records*.

coagulation a phase in the blood-clotting sequence in which many factors are released and interact to form a fibrin mesh-work, or blood clot.

competency statements performance expectations that include entry-level skills, tasks, and job roles.

confidentiality the protected right of the patient and duty of health care workers not to disclose any information acquired about a patient to those who are not directly involved with the care of the patient.

constituents chemical or cellular elements that make up blood.

contaminated sharps used objects that can penetrate the skin, including needles, scalpels, broken glass, broken capillary tubes, and exposed wires.

contamination presence of blood or potentially infectious substances on an item or surface.

continuous quality improvement (CQI) a theoretical framework and management strategy to improve health care structures, processes, outcomes, and customer satisfaction. It is ongoing and involves all levels of the administrative structure of an organization.

creatinine clearance test analytic procedure to determine whether or not the kidneys are able to remove creatinine from the blood.

criminal actions acts against the public welfare; these actions can lead to imprisonment of the offender.

critical test result a term that should be defined by each health care organization and typically includes test results that are abnormal, STAT test results, or other results that require an immediate response.

critical value a laboratory result that indicates a pathophysiologic state at such variance with normal as to be life threatening; these values should be defined and reported to the patient's physician as soon as possible.

culture a system of values, beliefs (spiritual, family bonding), and practices (food, music, traditions) that stem from an individual's concept of reality. Culture influences decisions and behaviors in many aspects of life.

culture and sensitivity (C&S) microbiologic test to determine the growth of infectious microorganisms in bodily specimens (e.g., urine), and to determine which antibiotics are most therapeutic and effective in killing the microorganism.

cyanotic skin bluish in color due to oxygen deficiency.

date of birth (DOB) personal information, i.e., birthday, included in a patient's medical record and on laboratory test requests.

decontaminate use physical or chemical means to remove or destroy bloodborne pathogens on a surface (including skin) or item so that pathogens are no longer able to transmit disease. Prior to venipuncture, decontamination involves cleaning with a sterile swab or sponge to prevent microbiological contamination of either the patient or the specimen. This is usually accomplished with a sterile swab containing 70 percent isopropyl alcohol (or isopropanol).

defendant individual (e.g., a health care worker), against whom a legal action (civil or criminal) or lawsuit is filed.

dehydration loss of water from the body (due to conditions such as excessive sweating, reduced fluid intake, vomiting, blood loss, etc.).

diabetes mellitus metabolic disease in which carbohydrate utilization is reduced due to a deficiency in insulin and characterized by hyperglycemia, glycosuria, water and electrolyte loss, ketoacidosis, and in serious conditions, coma. In milder forms of noninsulin-dependent diabetes mellitus, dietary regulation may keep the disorder under control.

diagnostic test results the results from all tests performed on the patient: laboratory, radiology, and so on.

diastolic pressure the second measure reported in a blood pressure measurement.

differentials a laboratory test that categorizes blood cells and any abnormalities present.

digestive system body system referring to organs in the gastrointestinal (GI) tract that break down food chemically and physically into nutrients that can be absorbed by the body's cells and allow the elimination of waste products of digestion.

disinfectants chemical compounds used to remove or kill pathogenic microorganisms; typically used on medical instruments or countertops.

disposable sterile puncture device (disposable sterile lancet) sterile sharp device, preferably retractable, and designed for a single use in skin puncture collections. It should penetrate the skin at specified depths (e.g., no more than 2.0 mm for infant heelsticks) that are safe enough for withdrawing blood samples without causing complications or injuries.

distal distant or away from point of attachment (e.g., the birthmark was *distal* to the wrist).

diurnal rhythms opposite of nocturnal (nighttime) rhythms, "diurnal" rhythms are variations in the body's functions or fluids that occur during daylight hours or every 24 hours (e.g., some hormone levels decrease in the afternoon). Also referred to as circadian rhythms.

dizziness lightheadedness, unsteadiness, loss of balance.

dorsal surface region of the body characterized by the back (or posterior) area and including the cranial and spinal cavities.

double bagging practice of using two trash bags for disposing of waste from patient's rooms, particularly those in isolation.

edema swelling

edematous condition in which tissues contain excessive fluid; it often results in localized swelling.

electronic medical record (EMR) or electronic health (or health care) record (EHR) computerized, legal record for each patient that describes the patient's visits, tests and procedures, and clinical progress.

email electronic mail often used in health care facilities. Guidelines for using email, including a patient's consent to use email, are now required of health care facilities.

engineering controls refer to devices that isolate or remove bloodborne pathogen hazards from the workplace (e.g., needleless devices, shielded needle devices, plastic capillary tubes). "Work practice" controls are activities that reduce the risk of exposure (e.g., "no-hands" procedures for discarding sharps).

Environmental Protection Agency (EPA) federal agency that, among its other responsibilities, regulates the disposal of hazardous substances and monitors and regulates disinfectant products.

ethics a branch of philosophy that deals with distinguishing right from wrong and with moral consequences of human actions.

ethylenediaminetetraacetic acid (EDTA) anticoagulant additive used to prevent the blood-clotting sequence by removing calcium and forming calcium salts. EDTA prevents platelet aggregation and is useful for platelet counts and platelet function tests. Fresh EDTA samples are also useful for making blood films or microscopic slides, because there is minimal distortion of platelets and WBCs.

eutectic mixture of local anesthetics (EMLA) a topical anesthetic (pain reliever) that is an emulsion of lidocaine and prilocaine and can be applied to intact skin.

evacuated (vacuum) tube system method of blood collection using double-sided needles whereby the needle is attached to a holder/adapter and allows for multiple specimen tube fills and changes without blood leakage.

expiration date the date after which products or supplies should not be used.

exposure control plan a document required in health facilities that details the process for medical treatment, prophylaxis, and/or follow-up after an employee has been exposed to

potentially harmful or infectious substances (e.g., in the case of a percutaneous needlestick injury).

extrinsic factors substances involved in the clotting process that are stimulated when tissue damage occurs.

fainting see *syncope*.

fasting refers to no food or drinks (except water).

fasting blood tests tests performed on blood taken from a patient who has abstained from eating and drinking (except water) for a particular period of time.

feathered edge a term used to describe blood smears on microscopic slides; it is a visible curved edge that thins out smoothly and resembles the tip of a bird's feather.

femoral artery located in the groin area of the leg and lateral to the femur bone, it is the largest artery used as an alternative site for ABG collections. Phlebotomists must be specially trained to perform collections from this site.

fevers of unknown origin (FUO) indicates the patient has an undiagnosed infection, which usually results in ordering blood cultures.

fibrin substance that forms a blood clot.

fibrinolysis the final phase of the hemostatic process whereby repair and regeneration of the injured blood vessel occurs and the clot slowly begins to dissolve or break up (lyse).

fistula an artificial shunt or passage, commonly used in the arm of a patient undergoing kidney dialysis; the vein and artery are fused through a surgical procedure. Only specially trained personnel can collect blood from a fistula.

fomites inanimate objects that can harbor infectious agents and transmit infections (e.g., toilets, sinks, linens, door knobs, glasses, phlebotomy supplies).

frontal plane imaginary line running lengthwise on the body from side to side, dividing the body into anterior and posterior sections.

gauge number refers to the size (diameter) of the internal bore of a needle. The larger the number, the smaller the bore size, and vice versa.

gauze loosely woven material used for bandages that are sterile or chemically clean.

geriatric refers to an elderly patient.

gestational diabetes diabetes that begins during pregnancy (often the second or third trimester). It occurs in 1–4% of pregnancies and usually subsides after delivery.

glucose tolerance test (GTT) diagnostic test for detecting diabetes. The test is performed by obtaining blood and urine specimens at timed intervals after fasting, then after ingesting glucose. Each specimen is analyzed for its glucose content to determine if the glucose level returns to normal within 2 hours after ingestion.

glycolytic inhibitor an additive used in blood collection tubes that prevents glycolysis.

granulocytes (basophils, neutrophils, eosinophils) mature leukocytes (WBCs) in the circulating blood; when stained and viewed microscopically, granules are present.

hand hygiene term that applies to handwashing (with non-antimicrobial soap and water), antiseptic handwashing, antiseptic hand rub (with waterless antiseptic), or surgical hand antisepsis.

health care–acquired (HIAs) or health care associated (nosocomial) infection infections acquired after admission into a health facility.

Health Insurance Portability and Accountability Act (HIPAA) federal law (1996) expanded in 2000 to protect security, privacy, and confidentiality of personal health information.

heart a key component of the cardiovascular system, it is the pump that forces blood throughout the body.

heelstick pediatric phlebotomy procedure that requires puncturing the skin of specified areas of an infant's heel with a device that controls for the depth of the puncture. The designated areas should be used to reduce the risk of bone injuries or complications such as infections.

hematocrit a commonly ordered laboratory test to assess the circulatory system; it describes the concentration of RBCs and therefore provides an indirect measure of the oxygen-carrying capacity of the blood.

hematology the study of blood.

hematoma a localized leakage of blood into the tissues or into an organ. In phlebotomy, it can occur as a result of blood leakage during the vein puncture, thereby causing a bruise.

hematopoiesis the process of blood cell formation that occurs in the bone marrow.

hemoconcentration increased localized blood concentration of large molecules such as proteins, cells, and coagulation factors. This can be caused by excessive application of a tourniquet.

hemoglobin the molecules that carry oxygen and carbon dioxide in the RBCs.

hemolysis rupture or lysis of the blood cells.

hemostasis maintenance of circulating blood in the liquid state and retention of blood in the vascular system by prevention of blood loss.

heparin an anticoagulant that prevents blood clotting by inactivating thrombin and thromboplastin, the blood-clotting chemicals in the body.

histograms bar graphs often used as quality improvement tools.

holder (adapter) plastic apparatus needed in specimen collecting using the evacuated tube method. The adapter/holder secures the double-pointed needle: one end of the needle goes into the patient's vein, and on the other end of the needle is placed an evacuated tube.

home health care services provision of health care services in a patient's home under the direction of a physician.

homeostasis means literally "remaining the same"; also referred to as a steady-state condition, it is a normal state that allows the body to stay in a healthy balance by continually compensating with necessary changes.

human immunodeficiency virus (HIV) a virus spread by sexual contact or exposure to infected blood.

hypoxia a condition in which body tissues are not receiving enough oxygen.

iatrogenic anemia a type of induced blood-loss resulting in anemia when too much blood is withdrawn in a short period of time; a patient who has this may require a blood transfusion.

immunology the study of diseases of the immune system.

incision a cut into the skin. The term is used to describe the puncture made by an automatic skin puncture device.

infection control programs guidelines designed to address surveillance, reporting, isolation procedures, education, and management of community-acquired and health-care-associated infections.

informed consent a complex legal term; basically, it refers to voluntary permission by a patient to allow touching, examination, and/or treatment by health care workers after the patient has been given information about the procedures and potential risks and consequences. It allows patients to decide what may be performed on or done to their bodies.

inpatients hospitalized patients.

insulin a chemical produced by the pancreas that is released into the bloodstream to facilitate glucose absorption from the blood into the tissues where it is used for energy. When insulin is not produced (as in diabetes mellitus), blood glucose levels increase because the glucose cannot be absorbed into the tissues.

integumentary system body system referring to skin, hair, sweat and oil glands, teeth, and fingernails; involved in protective and regulatory functions.

interstitial space between tissues and/or organs.

interstitial (tissue) fluid minute amounts of liquid forming between gaps/layers of tissue; a natural component of capillary blood.

intravenous (IV) catheter vascular access device inserted into a blood vessel for administration of medications and nutrients and for blood collection.

intrinsic system part of the coagulation process that involves the clotting factors contained in the blood.

invasion of privacy a legal term referring to objectionable or personal intrusion upon an individual such that it is offensive (e.g., the publishing of confidential information).

invasive description for medical procedures whereby a medical instrument is inserted directly into a body cavity or organ, e.g., withdrawing spinal fluid requires an invasive procedure.

iodine used to make tincture of iodine (2% solution) which is used as a skin disinfectant. Some patients are allergic to iodine.

isolation procedures methods used to protect individuals (health care workers) from patients with infectious diseases. Formerly divided into two types (category-specific and disease-specific), newer guidelines combine isolation practices for moist and potentially infectious body substances, to be used for all patients. The new categories of isolation are based on the mode of transmission and include airborne, droplet, and contact precautions.

The Joint Commission independent, nonprofit organization that sets quality standards for health care.

judicial law legal processes designed to resolve disputes.

lancet/lancing device a sharp apparatus or blade used to puncture or cut through skin for the purpose of acquiring a capillary blood specimen. The preferred device is a single-use, retractable, safety mechanism that performs a puncture of predetermined depth.

lateral directional term meaning toward the sides of the body.

latex allergic having a reaction to certain proteins in latex rubber, a natural ingredient in some varieties of gloves. Allergic reactions range from skin redness, rash, hives, or itching to respiratory symptoms and, in rare instances, shock.

law societal rules or regulations designed to protect society and resolve conflicts; laws are rules that must be observed.

liable a legal term that refers to a legal obligation when damage occurs.

light sensitive refers to laboratory specimens; some chemical constituents (bilirubin, vitamin B_{12}, carotene, folate, urine porphyrins) decompose if exposed to light and therefore should be protected/covered during transportation and handling.

lipemic when referring to serum, it is a cloudy or milky appearance, usually due to a temporarily elevated lipid level after the ingestion of fatty foods.

lithium iodoacetate antiglycolytic agent and anticoagulant; not to be used for hematology testing or enzymatic determinations.

litigation process a legal action to determine a decision in court. Many malpractice cases are negotiated and settled out of court.

lymphatic system body system responsible for maintaining fluid balance, providing a defense against disease, and absorption of fats and other substances from the blood stream.

lymphocytes type of white blood cell that is nongranular in appearance; plays a role in immunity and in the production of antibodies.

lymphostasis obstruction and/or lack of flow of the lymph fluid.

malice a legal term referring to a reckless disregard for the truth (e.g., knowing that a statement is false).

malpractice a legal term referring to improper or unskillful care of a patient by a member of the health care team, or any professional misconduct, unreasonable lack of skill, or infidelity in professional or judiciary duties; often described as "professional negligence."

mastectomy removal of a breast; a double mastectomy refers to the surgical removal of both breasts.

medial directional term meaning toward the midline of the body.

median cubital vein forearm vein that is most commonly used for venipuncture.

Medicaid a shared federal- and state-funded program designed to provide health insurance for individuals with low incomes.

medical records definitive documents, paper or electronic medical records (EMR), that contain a chronological log of a patient's care. It must include any information that is clinically significant or relevant to the patient's care.

Medicare federal program designed to provide health insurance for the elderly and members of special groups.

melanin pigment in the skin that provides color and protects underlying tissues from absorbing ultraviolet rays.

metabolism an important bodily function that allows the formation or breakdown of substances (e.g., proteins) for the purpose of using energy.

microbiology the study of microbes.

microcollection process by which small amounts of blood are collected in small containers or tubes using specially designed devices.

microcontainers specialized collection devices designed for small quantities of blood; some containing anticoagulants. These devices are typically used for pediatric or geriatric patients with fragile or inaccessible veins, and/or for fingersticks.

microorganisms living organisms that are too small to see with the naked eye such as bacteria, viruses, and fungi.

misdemeanor a legal term referring to many types of criminal offenses that are not serious enough to be classified as felonies.

mode of transmission refers to the method by which pathogenic agents are transmitted (e.g., direct contact, air, medical instruments, other objects, and other vectors).

monocytes type of white blood cell that is nongranular and also plays a role in defense.

multiple-sample needles used with the evacuated tube method of blood collection, these needles are attached to a holder/adapter and allow for multiple specimen tube fills and changes without blood leakage.

muscular system body system referring to all muscles of the body.

National Fire Protection Association (NFPA) developed the labeling system for hazardous chemicals that is used in health-care facilities.

National Phlebotomy Association (NPA) professional organization for phlebotomists that offers continuing educational activities and a certification examination for phlebotomists.

needleless system a device that does not use needles for procedures that are normally associated with needle use. This includes collection of bodily fluids or withdrawal of body fluids after initial venous or arterial access is performed. It refers to procedures that have a risk for occupational exposure to blood-borne pathogens from contaminated sharp objects.

needlestick skin puncture using a needle.

negligence a legal term referring to the failure to act or perform duties according to the standards of the profession.

neonatal screening typically refers to mandatory (required by law) laboratory testing of infants for specified disorders such as PKU and hypothyroidism. There is wide variability in what tests are required by each state.

neonate a newborn infant; term used during the first 28 days after birth.

nervous system body system that includes organs that provide communication in the body, sensations, thoughts, emotions, and memories.

obesity an unhealthy abundance of body fat.

occluded veins closed or constricted veins.

occult blood analysis that detects hidden (occult) blood in the stool.

occupational exposure contact via skin, eye, mucous membranes, or parenteral with potentially infectious materials as a result of an individual's work duties.

Occupational Safety and Health Administration (OSHA) an agency of the U.S. Department of Labor requiring employers to provide a safe work environment including measures to protect workers exposed to biological and occupational hazards.

osteochondritis inflammation of the bone and its cartilage.

osteomyelitis inflammation of the bone due to bacterial infection.

osteoporosis a condition of the bone whereby the mineral density is reduced, making the bone more fragile.

outcomes used as a quality improvement term to refer to what is accomplished for the patient (e.g., healing, return to wellness, or return to normal functions). Poor patient outcomes have been described as the "5 Ds": death, disease, disability, discomfort, and dissatisfaction.

oxalates anticoagulants that prevent blood-clotting sequence by removing calcium and forming calcium salts.

panic value see *critical value*.

parental involvement during pediatric phlebotomy procedures, a parent's support and presence is often helpful in reducing stress/anxiety for the patient. On the other hand, some parents are reluctant to be involved, so the phlebotomist must assess each situation to determine the level of parental involvement that would optimize the phlebotomy encounter.

Parkinson's disease a neurological disease characterized by muscular tremors and rigidity of movement.

pathogenesis the origin of a disease.

pathogenic agents disease-causing bacteria, fungi, viruses, or parasites that are transmitted by direct contact, air, medical instruments, other objects, and other vectors.

pathology the study of all aspects of disease and abnormal conditions of the body.

patient confidentiality see *confidentiality*.

patient-focused testing laboratory services usually designed around a team concept and focused on convenience to the patient.

patient–physician relationship the professional communication linkage that a patient has with his or her doctor.

Patient's Bill of Rights a statement developed to affirm the rights of patients. Key elements involve the right to respectful and considerate care; accurate information about diagnoses, treatment, and prognoses; informed consent; refusal of treatment; privacy; confidentiality; advance directives; reviewing records about own treatment; knowing identity and role of personnel involved in care; information about research procedures; billing information; and knowing business relationships of those providing care.

peak a term used for therapeutic drug monitoring to describe the blood sample that is taken when the drug is at its highest concentration in the patient's serum (e.g., "the *peak* level").

pediatric phlebotomy procedures performed on infants and children and which require specialized training and management. Often done by skin puncture, pediatric phlebotomies also entail matching the procedure with the specimen requirements for testing, the patient's age and emotional condition, and possible parental involvement.

percutaneous through the skin.

peripheral circulation near the surface of the body.

personal protective equipment (PPE) equipment designed to protect the health care worker from hazards in the workplace (e.g., goggles, gloves, gowns).

petechiae minute, pinpoint hemorrhagic spots in the skin that may be indicative of a coagulation abnormality. For phlebotomists, it should be a warning sign that the patient may bleed excessively.

phenylketonuria (PKU) a congenital disorder, usually diagnosed at birth, that can cause brain damage resulting in severe retardation, often with seizures and other neurologic abnormalities.

phlebotomist individual who practices phlebotomy (i.e., a blood collector); *phlebo* is related to "vein," and *tomy* relates to "cutting."

phlebotomy a cut or incision into the vein.

photosensitive sensitive to light.

physician–patient relationship the association between the patient and the physician providing clinical and consultative services; the communication between them is private and confidential.

physician's office laboratories (POLs) nonhospital laboratories usually based in a physician's office/clinic at the private practice.

plasma liquid portion (unclotted or anticoagulated) of the blood in which blood cells are suspended.

platelets (thrombocytes) blood cells that aid in blood clot formation.

pleural fluid fluid from the lung cavity.

pneumatic tube systems transportation system used in many health care facilities for specimens and paper-based documentation. Considerations for use of these systems involves evaluation of speed, distance, control mechanisms, shock absorbency, sizes of carriers, and breakage/spillage rates.

point-of-care (POC) testing refers to tests and procedures that are actually performed at the patient's bedside or at the "point of care." The tests are not sent to a laboratory in a remote location; rather, they are rapid methods designed to produce quick results.

porphyrins a type of photosensitive analyte.

postcentrifugation phase period of time after a specimen has been centrifuged but before serum or plasma has been removed for testing.

posterior surface region of the body characterized by the back (or dorsal) area and including the cranial and spinal cavities.

postprandial glucose test a glucose test performed after ingestion of a meal; useful for screening patients for diabetes, because glucose levels in serum specimens drawn 2 hours after a meal are rarely elevated in normal patients. In contrast, diabetic patients have elevated glucose values 2 hours after a meal.

precentrifugation phase period of time after a blood sample has been collected but before centrifugation.

preexamination (preanalytical) phase laboratory testing phase in which tests are ordered and specimens are collected and prepared for testing. Preanalytical variables include patient variables (fasting versus nonfasting, stress, availability, etc.), transportation variables (specimen leakage, tube breakage, excessive shaking, etc.), specimen processing variables (centrifugation, delays, contamination of the specimen, exposure to heat or light), and specimen variables (hemolysis, inadequate volume, inadequate mixing of the tube, etc.). Preexamination procedures include steps from the clinician's test request, to specimen collection, to transporting and processing within the laboratory, and up until the analysis begins.

premature infant an infant born before 37 weeks of gestation (normal gestation is 40 weeks).

primary care health care services that are provided to maintain and monitor normal health and provide preventive services.

primary tube tube containing the patient's blood sample.

privacy the patient's right to respectful consideration of the confidential nature of his or her health information.

proficiency testing (PT) testing that is part of the quality management of laboratory services and involves subscribing to an outside source to provide "unknown" or "blind" specimens to see how one laboratory's results compare with other laboratories' results. Performance reviews on proficiency tests are part of the accrediting process for most laboratories.

protective (reverse) isolation precautionary measures and procedures designed to protect patients who are particularly susceptible or at increased risk of acquiring infections (e.g., patients with low WBC counts (neutropenic or leukopenic), patients with burns, and/or immunosuppressed patients).

proximal near the point of attachment (e.g., the leg broke on the *proximal* side of the knee).

pulmonary arteries the lungs receive deoxygenated (without oxygen) blood from the right side of the heart via the *pulmonary arteries*.

pulmonary circuit the circulatory pathway where blood leaves the heart and enters the right and left pulmonary arteries.

pulmonary veins 2 veins from each lung that return blood with oxygen to the heart.

puncture proof a surface that can withstand punctures from sharp objects such as needles, e.g., puncture proof biohazard disposal container.

qualitative test pertains to the presence or absence (positive or negative) of a substance in the specimen.

quality refers to a specimen that is correctly identified, collected, and transported.

quality control material daily controls that are used in analytic testing to determine acceptable ranges of test results (i.e., tolerance limits).

quantitative test pertains to the exact measurement or quantity of substance in the specimen.

radial artery located on the thumb side of the wrist, this artery is most commonly used to collect blood specimens for arterial blood gases. Phlebotomists must be specially trained to perform collections from this site.

radio frequency identification (RFID) a form of identification/labeling with the following characteristics: labels or tags contain tiny silicon chips that transmit data to a wireless receiver, does not require line-of-sight reading with a scanner, can be detected at various distances, identifies and/or tracks many items simultaneously, and can be used in combination with a bar code for multiple purposes.

random urine sample urine sample taken at random time(s).

red blood cells (RBCs or erythrocytes) blood cells that function to transport oxygen and carbon dioxide in the body.

reference ranges when referring to laboratory values, these are laboratory test value ranges that are considered within "normal" limits.

reproductive system body system referring to organs involved in sperm production, secretion of hormones (e.g., testosterone, estrogens, and progesterone), ovulation, fertilization, menstruation, pregnancy, labor, and lactation.

requisition form paper-based method for requesting laboratory tests. Electronic requisitioning involves similar procedures but without the paper trail.

respiratory system body system referring to parts that assist in respiration or breathing (e.g., nose, pharynx, larynx, trachea, bronchi, and lungs).

sagittal plane imaginary line running lengthwise on the body from front to back, dividing the body into right and left halves.

sample one or more parts (e.g., blood or tissues) taken from a system (the patient's body), and intended to provide information on the system.

sample integrity quality or completeness of a blood sample.

sclerosed veins veins that have become hardened.

secondary tube or specimen tube or specimen containing removed plasma/serum (an aliquot) *after* specimen centrifugation of a primary tube containing the patient's blood sample.

separated plasma/serum serum or plasma that has been removed or separated from contact with blood cells. It is referred to as an *aliquot*. It can be removed from the primary tube after centrifugation using a pipette, or separated from cellular contact with a chemical or physical barrier.

septicemia formerly called "blood poisoning," the term now means the presence of toxins or multiplying bacteria in the blood.

serum when blood is allowed to clot, sera (fluid portion) separates from the blood cells that form a fibrin clot. Serum contains the same constituents as plasma except that the clotting factors are contained within the blood clot.

sharps any devices or tools that can potentially cut, puncture, or cause injury.

single-sample needle used for collecting a blood sample from a syringe.

skeletal system body system referring to all bones and joints.

skin (dermal) puncture a cut into the skin or dermis (e.g., of the finger or heel) preferably with a single-use retractable puncture device.

sodium fluoride an additive (antiglycolytic agent) present in specific blood collection tubes that is used for glycolytic inhibition tests.

sodium polyanethole sulfonate (SPS) an additive typically used in blood culture bottles to prevent clotting.

source the origin of an infection (e.g., human hands, lab coats or other clothing, contaminated medical instruments).

specimen the discrete portion of a body fluid (e.g., blood or urine) or tissue taken for examination, study, or analysis of one or more characteristics (analytes), to determine the character of the whole.

specimen collection manual electronic or paper-based document required by accrediting agencies that includes instructions for patient preparation, type of collection containers, amounts of specimen required for specified tests, timing requirements, preservatives or anticoagulants needed, special handling instructions, proper labeling requirements, and other test-specific or situation-specific requirements for specimens.

specimen integrity high quality blood sample that can be adversely affected or compromised by the method of transport, timing delays, temperature, agitation, exposure to light, and centrifugation methods.

specimen rejection relates to the suitability of a specimen for testing or when it may *not* be used for laboratory analyses.

stakeholders individuals, groups, organizations, and/or communities that have an interest in or are influenced by health care services. Stakeholders can be internal to the organization or external (i.e., outside the organization).

standard of care the practices or guidelines that a reasonably prudent person would follow in any particular circumstance. Many agencies, licensing boards, certifying boards, and accrediting organizations write standards of care or standards of practice to guide health care workers in their duties.

standard operating procedures (SOP) instructions to achieve uniform or consistent performance of a function.

Standard Precautions a set of safeguards designed to reduce the risk of transmission of microorganisms; guidelines apply to *all patients and all body fluids, nonintact skin, and mucous* *membranes and include the use of barrier protection (protective equipment such as gloves, gowns, etc.), hand hygiene, and proper use and disposal of needles and other sharps.* Policies must comply with OSHA. Standards are available from the U.S. Centers for Disease Control and Prevention.

STAT an emergency situation that requires immediate action; in the case of blood collection and analysis, tests that are ordered "STAT" should be given the highest priority for collection, delivery to the laboratory, analysis, and reporting.

steady state also referred to as homeostasis, it is a condition that allows the normal body to stay in balance by continually compensating with necessary changes, thereby remaining in a healthy condition.

sterile gauze pads typically used in blood collection procedures either during the decontamination process and/or after blood collection to aid in stopping the bleeding; it is a sterile cotton mesh pad that is packaged in individual units.

sterile technique use of procedures that produce an aseptic condition (i.e., free from all living microorganisms and their spores).

sucrose nipple or pacifier a sucking device for infants and toddlers that is used to pacify or comfort the child.

superficial near the surface of the body (e.g., *superficial* veins show up easily on the skin).

superior vena cava one of the two large veins that brings oxygen-poor blood to the heart from the head, neck, arms, and chest region.

supine reclining position.

susceptible host a component in the chain of infection; the degree to which an individual is at risk for acquiring an infection. Factors affecting susceptibility are age, drug use, degree and nature of the patient's illness, and status of the patient's immune system.

syncope the transient (and frequently sudden) loss of consciousness due to a lack of oxygen to the brain (i.e., fainting) and resulting in an inability to stay in an upright position. Patients usually recover their orientation quickly, but injuries (e.g., abrasions, lacerations) often result from falling to the ground.

synovial fluid joint fluid.

syringe method method whereby a syringe is used to collect blood, which is then placed in a transfer device for safely moving the blood from the syringe into collection tubes.

systemic circuit part of the cardiovascular system that carries blood to the tissues of the body.

therapeutic drug monitoring (TDM) testing procedures to evaluate drug levels in a patient's blood. This is valuable for drug dosage and to monitor the patient for a variety of other factors (clinical effectiveness, toxicity, etc.).

therapeutic phlebotomy removal of blood for therapeutic reasons (i.e., in conditions where there is an excessive production of blood cells).

thermolabile constituents that degrade if exposed to warm temperatures.

thrombi blood clots formed somewhere within the cardiovascular system; they may occlude a vessel or attach to the wall of a vessel.

timed specimen a test is ordered to be drawn at a particular time.

tissue (interstitial) fluid fluids (that are not blood) found in between and around tissues.

tourniquet a soft flexible strip, preferably latex free, typically about 1 inch wide and 15 to 18 inches long that is used temporarily on the arm to help find a site for venipuncture. The ends are stretched around a patient's arm about 3 inches above the venipuncture area. The tightening of the tourniquet causes venous filling in the veins and enables better feel and/or visualization of the prominent veins in the area. Leaving the tourniquet on the patient's arm for more than 1 minute at a time may cause hemoconcentration and have adverse effects on laboratory test results. Single-use tourniquets are preferred to reduce the spread of infections.

transmission-based precautions categories of precautionary measures based on the route of transmission of disease. Three types of transmission-based precautions are airborne, droplet, and contact precautions.

transverse plane imaginary line running crosswise, or horizontally, on the body, dividing the body into upper and lower sections.

trough a term used for therapeutic drug monitoring to describe the blood sample that is taken just prior to the next dose, or when the drug is theoretically at the lowest concentration in the patient's serum (i.e., the "trough" level).

turbid cloudy or milky in appearance.

Turn-around time (TAT) the time it takes for a blood specimen to be ordered, collected, transported, processed, analyzed, and a result reported.

Ulna thin long bone in the forearm, located opposite the thumb side.

Universal Precautions (also called "Standard Precautions" or "Standard Universal Precautions"). Refers to an infection control concept of bloodborne disease control, requiring that all human blood and other potentially infectious materials be treated as if known to be infectious for HIV, HBV, HCV, or other bloodborne pathogens, regardless of the perceived risk. Other concepts in infection control are referred to as "Body Substance Isolation" (BSI) and Standard Precautions, meaning that all body fluids and substances are potentially infectious.

urinary system body system referring to processes enabling the production and elimination of urine. Consists of kidneys, ureters, bladder, and urethra.

vacuum (evacuated) tube color-coded specimen collection tube that contains a vacuum so as to aspirate blood when a needle enters a patient's vein. The tubes are part of a blood collection method that also requires a double-pointed needle and a special plastic holder (adapter). One end of the double-pointed needle enters the vein, the other pierces the top of the tube, and the vacuum aspirates the blood into the tube. Tubes may contain anticoagulants.

vascular a network of blood vessels that includes veins, arteries, and capillaries.

vasoconstriction rapid constriction of the blood vessels to decrease blood flow to the area.

veins blood vessels that carry blood toward the heart after oxygen has been delivered to the tissues.

vena cavae largest veins of the body.

venipuncture withdrawing a venous (from a vein, not an artery) blood sample using a needle attached to an evacuated tube system or other collection devices.

ventral surface region of the body characterized by the front (or anterior) area and including the thoracic, abdominal, and pelvic cavities.

ventricles two lower chambers (of the four chambers) of the heart; they are referred to as the right and left ventricles, depending on which side of the heart they are located.

venules minute veins that flow into larger veins.

virology study of viruses.

visceral (nonstriated, smooth, involuntary) muscles muscles that line the walls of internal structures (e.g., veins and arteries).

volume space occupied by a liquid and usually measured in liters or milliliters.

whistle blowing disclosure of a legal wrongdoing by an employee of the same organization (e.g., an illegal action is reported by an employee to appropriate authorities such as a governmental agency or accreditation agency). Employees who speak out to reveal illegal actions may fear reprisals that could jeopardize their safety or their job. Thus, numerous laws are in place to protect employees who report legitimate wrongdoings.

white blood cells (WBCs or leukocytes) blood cells that provide for defense against infectious agents.

winged infusion system (set) also called a butterfly set or scalp needle set, the system can be used for difficult venipunctures due to small or fragile veins. The needle is typically smaller, and it has a thin tubing with a Luer adapter at the end so that it can be used on a syringe or an evacuated tube system during venipuncture.

work practice controls practices that diminish the likelihood of exposure to hazards by altering the manner in which the work is performed (e.g., prohibiting the recapping of needles with a two-handed approach).

zone of comfort area of space surrounding a person/patient that is considered "private or personal"; if a stranger (or phlebotomist) gets too close to the individual (i.e., beyond the zone of comfort), the person/patient may begin to feel uncomfortable.

Index

Note: page numbers with *b* indicate boxes, page numbers with *f* indicate figures, and those with *t* indicate tables.